Connective Tissues
in Arterial and Pulmonary Disease

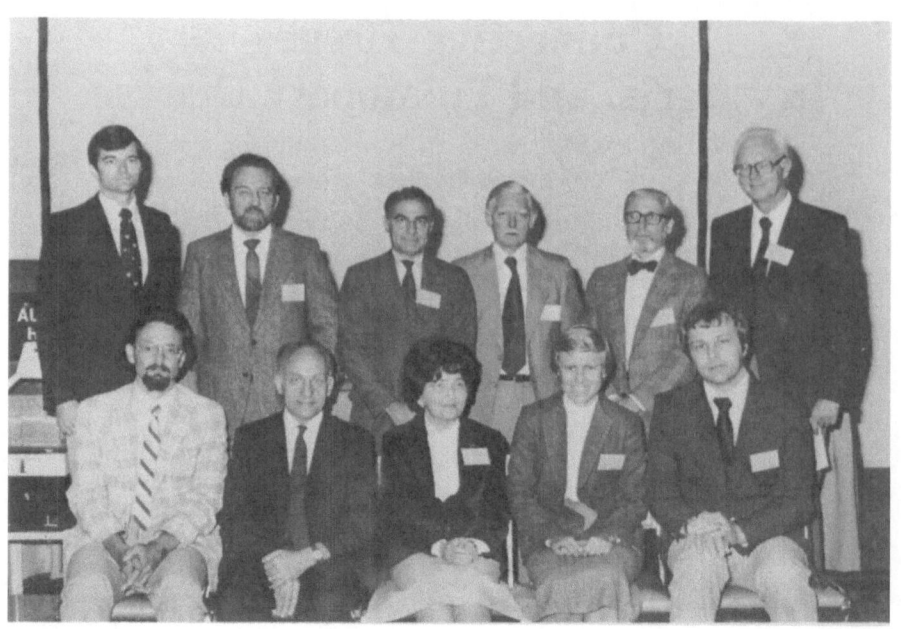

Participants: Seated, left to right: Drs. Rosenquist, Glagov, Puchtler, Foster, Oegema; standing, left to right: Drs. Rhodes, Kramsch, Turino, Caulfield, Snider, Schiebler

Connective Tissues
in Arterial and Pulmonary Disease

Edited by

Thomas F. McDonald, Ph.D.
Professor of Anatomy
Associate Dean for Basic Sciences
Medical College of Georgia

A. Bleakley Chandler, M.D.
Professor of Pathology
Chairman, Department of Pathology
Medical College of Georgia

With 66 Figures

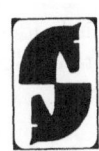

Springer-Verlag
New York   Heidelberg   Berlin

Thomas F. McDonald, Ph.D.
Associate Dean for Basic Sciences
School of Medicine
Medical College of Georgia
Augusta, Georgia 30912, U.S.A.

A. Bleakley Chandler, M.D.
Chairman, Department of Pathology
School of Medicine
Medical College of Georgia
Augusta, Georgia 30912, U.S.A.

Sponsoring Editor: Larry W. Carter
Production: William J. Gabello

Library of Congress Cataloging in Publication Data
Connective tissues in arterial and pulmonary disease.
    "Proceedings of a symposium held in honor of
Holde Puchtler, M.D., on October 15, 1980 in Augusta,
Georgia"—Copyright page.
    Includes bibliographical references and index.
    1. Connective tissues—Congresses. 2. Connective
tissues—Diseases—Congresses. 3. Atherosclerosis—
Congresses. 4. Lungs—Diseases—Congresses. 5. Pucht-
ler, Holde. I. McDonald, Thomas F. (Thomas Francis),
1927– . II. Chandler, A. Bleakley (Arthur
Bleakley), 1926– . III. Puchtler, Holde.
[DNLM: 1. Connective tissue—Physiopathology—Con-
gresses. 2. Vascular diseases—Physiopathology—
Congresses. 3. Arteries—Physiopathology—Congresses.
4. Lung diseases—Physiopathology—Congresses.
QS 532.5.C7 C751 1980]
QP88.23.C68   616.1'307   81-13595
                                       AACR2

9 8 7 6 5 4 3 2 1

ISBN-13: 978-1-4612-5969-5   e-ISBN-13: 978-1-4612-5967-1
DOI: 10.1007/978-1-4612-5967-1

Contents

Part I
Connective Tissues in Arterial Disease
James B. Caulfield, Chairman

Part II
Connective Tissues in Pulmonary Disease
Thomas H. Rosenquist, Chairman

Part III
Holde Puchtler: An Appreciation

Preface

The processes of distention and recoil have an essential role in the functions of arteries and lungs. In both organ systems, these processes involve to a great extent the connective tissues, in particular the manner in which the extracellular materials are arranged to afford such movements. This book concerns the microenvironment of the connective tissues in the walls of arteries and the stroma of lungs.

Proteoglycans, collagen, and elastic fibers and their interrelationships are discussed by eight scientists who are established researchers in this area. Their reports include important findings on how this microenvironment is altered in diseases such as atherosclerosis, emphysema, and pulmonary fibrosis. The concepts developed result from studies at the biochemical, macromolecular, ultrastructural, and light microscopic levels. Taken collectively, the reports focus attention upon the role of the connective tissues in arterial and lung distensibility and how alterations in the connective tissues result in the loss of this function.

Medical researchers and physicians interested in arterial or lung functions or diseases will find the scientific approaches and findings of the authors innovative and provocative. Students of stereologic morphometry will be particularly interested in the quantitative studies of cells and fibers in arterial walls; histologists and pathologists will find the chapter on histochemical staining interesting from both a scientific and historic viewpoint.

The papers were presented at the Symposium on Connective Tissues in Arterial and Pulmonary Disease conducted in honor of Dr. Holde Puchtler, October 15, 1980, in Augusta, Georgia. Since the discussions following presentation of the papers were informative and often illuminating, they have been edited and included here.

Thomas F. McDonald
A. Bleakley Chandler

Acknowledgments

This Symposium was held in Augusta, Georgia, in conjunction with the 20th annual meeting of the Southern Society of Anatomists and was sponsored by the Department of Pathology, Medical College of Georgia.

The Organizing Committee consisted of Thomas F. McDonald, Chairman; Dale E. Bockman, President, Southern Society of Anatomists; A. Bleakley Chandler, Faye Sweat Waldrop, Linda L. Vacca, David A. Welter, J. Robert Teabeaut II, and Benjamin O. Spurlock. The endorsement and support of the officers and members of the Southern Society of Anatomists are especially appreciated. Many others contributed to the success of this Symposium, including Eric Weiss, D. Greer Falls, Mark B. Barrett, Louise M. Markwalter, Marie F. Hiller, W. Thomas Broome, J. Michael Barrett, Fannie M. Mitchell, Heidi L. Valenzuela, Frank H. Gearhart, W. Clay Adamson, Susan N. Meloan, Octavia Garlington, Julie G. Guillebeau, Stanley R. Leida, Deborah I. Pomeroy, Delmar R. Staecker, Alex H. Vaughn, Dale W. Sickles, Gurkirpal S. Sohal, and Patricia O'Meara, all on the staff and faculty of the Medical College of Georgia.

The generous contributions of all those participants who made this Symposium so successful through their formal presentations and lively, productive discussions are gratefully acknowledged.

It is a special pleasure to acknowledge the excellent and thoughtful editorial direction in the preparation of this volume from the medical editor and staff of Springer-Verlag New York, Inc.

The Symposium was made possible by the generous financial support of the following contributors: Brenda W. Branch, A. Bleakley Chandler, Harold M. Conner, Nancy O. Doss, John G. Etheridge, A Friend, Geneva S. Gray, Sophie Gropp, Alexander S. Haraszti, Rosalie B. Haraszti, John T. Harper, Sr., Albert S. Hollingsworth, James B. Hurst, James G. Jackson, James G. Kuhns, Susan N. Meloan, James W. Mitchener, Lynn L. Ogden, James L. O'Quinn, Walter G. Rice, Ashburn P. Searcy, Walter R. Stern, J. Robert Teabeaut II, The Upjohn Company, Faye Sweat Waldrop, Pauline Woo Saito, American Hoechst Corporation.

Authors and Discussants

Sergio E. Bustos-Valdes, Ph.D., Department of Dental Biochemistry, Medical College of Georgia, Augusta, Georgia 30912, U.S.A.

James B. Caulfield, M.D., Department of Pathology, University of South Carolina, School of Medicine, Columbia, South Carolina 29208, U.S.A.

A. Bleakley Chandler, M.D., Department of Pathology, Medical College of Georgia, Augusta, Georgia 30912, U.S.A.

Ronald R. Cowden, Ph.D., Department of Basic Sciences, East Tennessee State University College of Medicine, Johnson City, Tennessee 37601, U.S.A.

Tukaram V. Darnule, Ph.D., Department of Medicine, Columbia University College of Physicians and Surgeons, New York, New York 10032, U.S.A.

Judith A. Foster, Ph.D., Department of Biochemistry, University of Georgia, Athens, Georgia 30602, U.S.A.

Rogers M. Fred III, B.S., Department of Zoology, University of Georgia, Athens, Georgia 30602, U.S.A.

Seymour Glagov, M.D., Department of Pathology, University of Chicago, Chicago, Illinois 60637, U.S.A.

Joseph Grande, Ph.D., Department of Pathology, University of Chicago, Chicago, Illinois 60637, U.S.A.

Stephen Keller, Ph.D., Department of Pathology, Columbia University College of Physicians and Surgeons, New York, New York 10032, U.S.A.

Dieter M. Kramsch, M.D., Department of Medicine and Biochemistry, Boston University Medical Center, Boston, Massachusetts 02118, U.S.A.

Ines Mandl, Ph.D., Department of Obstetrics and Gynecology, Columbia University College of Physicians and Surgeons, New York, New York 10032, U.S.A.

Thomas F. McDonald, Ph.D., Department of Anatomy, Medical College of Georgia, Augusta, Georgia 30912, U.S.A.

Susan N. Meloan, Department of Pathology, Medical College of Georgia, Augusta, Georgia 30912, U.S.A.

William H. Moretz, M.D., President, Medical College of Georgia, Augusta, Georgia 30912, U.S.A.

Theodore R. Oegema, Jr., Ph.D., Department of Orthopedic Surgery, University of Minnesota, Minneapolis, Minnesota 55455, U.S.A.

Harry B. O'Rear, M.D., Vice Chancellor for Health Affairs, University System of Georgia, Atlanta, Georgia 30334, U.S.A., and former President, Medical College of Georgia, Augusta, Georgia, U.S.A.

Mohamed M. Osman, D.V.M., Department of Medicine, Columbia University College of Physicians and Surgeons, New York, New York 10032, U.S.A.

Holde Puchtler, M.D., Department of Pathology, Medical College of Georgia, Augusta, Georgia 30912, U.S.A.

R. Kent Rhodes, Ph.D., Department of Biochemistry and Institute of Dental Research, University of Alabama, Birmingham, Alabama 35294, U.S.A.

Celeste B. Rich, M.S., Department of Biochemistry, University of Georgia, Athens, Georgia 30602, U.S.A.

Thomas H. Rosenquist, Ph.D., Department of Anatomy, Medical College of Georgia, Augusta, Georgia 30912, U.S.A.

Theodore H. Schiebler, M.D., The Anatomical Institute, University of Würzburg, Würzburg, Federal Republic of Germany

Gordon L. Snider, M.D., Department of Medicine, Boston University School of Medicine, Boston, Massachusetts 02118, U.S.A.

Gerard M. Turino, M.D., Department of Medicine, Columbia University College of Physicians and Surgeons, New York, New York 10032, U.S.A.

Draga Vesselinovitch, D.V.M., Department of Pathology, University of Chicago, Chicago, Illinois 60637, U.S.A.

Faye Sweat Waldrop, Department of Pathology, Medical College of Georgia, Augusta, Georgia 30912, U.S.A.

Shiu Yeh Yu, Ph.D., Department of Pathology, St. Louis University School of Medicine, St. Louis, Missouri 63125, U.S.A.

Christopher K. Zarins, M.D., Department of Surgery, University of Chicago, Chicago, Illinois 60637, U.S.A.

Part I
Connective Tissues in Arterial Disease

JAMES B. CAULFIELD, *Chairman*

Introduction

JAMES B. CAULFIELD

The presence of connective tissue throughout many phyla has been well demonstrated for many years (Homgren E [1907] Ueber die Trophospongien der quersteiften Muskelfasern nebst Bemerkungen über den allgemeinen Bau dieser Fasern. Arch Mikr Anat 71: 165–247). Early workers tended to use heavy metal impregnation techniques which outline in exquisite detail some of the fibrillar components of connective tissue. This reaction seemed to be more dependent upon the size of the fibrils than upon their chemical composition. The heavy metal approach was supplemented by tinctorial dyes, with the color variations empirically determined rather than being predetermined by specific chemical reactions defined by the investigator. These procedures, when augmented by polarizing optics and reasonably specific enzyme digestion techniques, allowed further identification and definition of the function of some of the extracellular components (Bairati A, [1937] Struttura e proprietà fisiche del sarcolemma della fibra muscolare striata. Z Zellforsch 27: 100–124; Banus PJ, Chur BM, Wayland H [1969] On the mechanical behavior of elastic animal tissue. Trans Soc Rheology 13: 83–102).

A more complete understanding of the disposition of connective tissue requires careful identification of the components and development of specific techniques for localizing and quantitating these materials in tissue. The results can then be related to the physical properties of the various materials present, and an idea of the relationship of connective tissue to specific organ function can be synthesized.

The first session of this symposium approaches a number of these problems with respect to the arterial wall. Clearly, connective tissue is a complex of fibrillar and nonfibrillar components. The chemistry and structure of two of these components, proteoglycans and collagen, are covered in the first and fourth papers. The new information does not yet tend to simplify the problems of understanding the form and function of vascular connective tissue; rather it clearly indicates the complexity built into vessel walls. Utilizing morphometric techniques, the second paper points the way to identifying and quantitating the components, both cellular and matrical, of the aortic wall. The third paper, utilizing many of the techniques derived from basic chemistry and morphometry, approaches a major problem in the Western world, atherosclerosis.

The contributions of Dr. Holde Puchtler to the basic question of identifying and localizing the connective tissue components are presented in the final paper of this symposium. Morphometry requires precise identification, which Dr. Puchtler's histochemical techniques provide on a scale that permits sampling of large amounts of tissue. This is important in examining normal tissue and crucial to investigating the abnormal. The symposium emphasized the need to combine various techniques in order to work with and eventually understand the role of connective tissue.

Structure and Function
of Aorta Proteoglycan

THEODORE R. OEGEMA, JR.

Ever since the extracellular matrix was first viewed through early microscopes, the matrix has been the subject of much speculation and its components the bearers of such fanciful names as amorphous ground substance. In recent years, major strides have been made in the development of methods to study the matrix. They include new techniques for exploring the biochemistry of two major components of the matrix, collagen and proteoglycan; advances in methods for culturing cells from these tissues; and new staining and other microscopic procedures for viewing the tissue and localizing the components. This multidiscipline approach is now in the process of revolutionizing the understanding of connective tissue structure and metabolism. This discussion outlines the current status of a study of proteoglycan structure and speculates on possible relationships to function in aorta.

PROTEOGLYCAN STRUCTURES

Proteoglycans are covalent complexes of protein and glycosaminoglycans. Although Morner isolated glycosaminoglycans from aorta as early as 1895, the major structural features of the molecules were not worked out until the 1950's by Meyer and others (Rodén and Horowitz 1978). The subtle features such as the

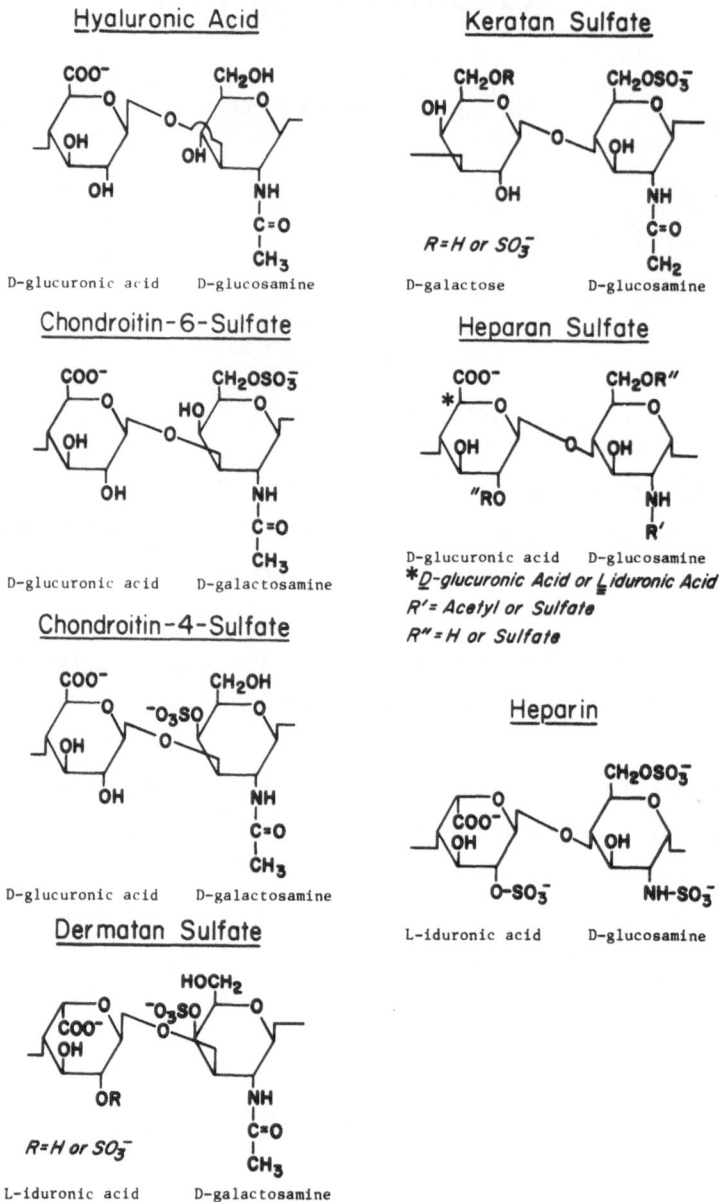

FIG. 1.   Structure of repeating units of glycosaminoglycans.

antithrombin active sequence of heparin are still under investigation (Laurent et al. 1978; Danielsson and Bjole 1978).   Figure 1
shows the generalized repeating structure for the glycosamino-

glycan. The carbohydrate linkage region to the protein core is the same for chondroitin sulfate, dermatan sulfate, heparin, and heparan sulfate. This linkage region is O-β-D-glucopyranurono-syl (1→3)O-β-D-galactopyranosyl(1→3)O-β-D-galactopyranosyl-(1→4)O-β-D-xylopyranosyl-L-serine (Rodén et al. 1972). Chon-droitin-4- and 6-sulfate and dermatan sulfate residues occur as hybrid structures on the same carbohydrate chain (Rodén and Horowitz 1978). Keratan sulfate doesn't follow the pattern in that it doesn't have a hexuronic acid in the repeating sequence. Keratan sulfate is attached to the protein backbone via galactos-amine to a serine or threonine hydroxyl. On the 3 position, approximately 70% of the chains contain a sialic acid - galactose disaccharide (Kieras 1974; Choi and Meyer 1975). The repeating disaccharide chain is believed to initiate from the 6 position of the galactosamine. In corneal keratan sulfate, the chain is at-tached to the protein via N-glycosidic bonds through aspargine residues, i.e., 2-acetamido-1-(L-β-aspartamido)-1,2, dideoxy-β-D-glucose (Baker et al. 1975). The linkage region for hyal-uronic acid is unknown. Even carefully purified preparations of hyaluronic acid that are isolated under nondegrading conditions contain a small amount of protein (0.1% - 0.2%) (see review, Rodén and Horowitz 1978). Purification is difficult due to the tremendous molecular weight ($1 - 4 \times 10^6$) of the hyaluronic acid molecule.

GLYCOSAMINOGLYCAN BIOSYNTHESIS

Glycosaminoglycans are built up stepwise by the addition of a single sugar from an activated sugar nucleotide intermediate (Rodén et al. 1972). At present, there is no evidence for the participation of lipid intermediates with the possible exception of the synthesis of the linkage region of corneal keratan sulfate (Hart and Lennartz 1978). The availability of the protein core seems to be the rate-limiting step in chain synthesis, although the possibility that it is the availability of xylosyltransferase has not been completely ruled out. After chain initiation, there is a rapid chain elongation and then sulfation with the active sulfate donor adenosine-3'-phospho-5'-sulfophosphate (PAPS) (Rodén and Horowitz 1978). The process seems to be all or none with little chondroitin sulfate of intermediate chain size being detected (Richmond et al. 1973).

Xylosyltransferase is the only soluble enzyme involved in chain elongation of chondroitin sulfate; the other enzymes are membrane bound (Rodén et al. 1972). An association between xylosyltransferase and the first galactosyltransferase has been suggested (see review, Rodén and Horowitz 1978). Although it has not been specifically demonstrated, available information is consistent with the presence of a "factory" that takes the core protein and spews out completed glycosaminoglycan chains, but whether the mitiation process is ordered or random along the protein core is not known. Also, little is known about the relative contribution of enzyme levels, enzyme affinity, and precursor pool size on the final overall length of the chondroitin sulfate chains.

If chains synthesis in chondrocyte cultures is uncoupled with β-xylopyranosides, the chondroitin sulfate chains are initiated on this sugar rather than the protein cores (Lohmander et al. 1979). Under these conditions, the rate of synthesis of chondroitin sulfate in the chondrocyte cultures are stimulated two- to threefold with only a 25% decrease in chain size. These observations suggest that, within limits, the chain length may be determined by such factors as enzyme affinity for the growing chain and the progression of the protein core through the Golgi apparatus of the cells rather than enzyme or precursor pools.

The chondroitin-4- and 6-sulfotransferases compete for substrate, with sulfation generally taking place in blocks of residues (Roden and Horowitz 1978). Generally, 10% - 20% of the chondroitin residues remain unsulfated, usually near the protein core. The chondroitin sulfate chains terminate almost equally with a galactosamine or glucuronic acid; heparin with a hexuronic acid

or glucosamine. Dermatan sulfate arises by the C-5 epimeriza-
tion of the carboxyl group with an exchange of the C-5 hydrogen with water in the medium (Fig. 1). This is a freely reversible reaction that appears to stabilize in the L-ido form by subsequent 0-sulfation (Rodén and Horowitz 1978).

Heparin and heparan sulfate synthesis is currently under intense investigation. Information available suggests that a sequential modification takes place, involving the synthesis of a
β-linked glucuronic acid α- N-acetylglucosamine polymer. This
serves as a substrate for an N-deacetylase and the free amino
group is subsequently N-sulfated. This is a substrate for the
epimerase which is then followed by 6-sulfation on the glucosamine, 2-sulfation of the iduronic acid, and possibly some 3-sulfa-
tion on the glucosamine residue (Rodén and Horowitz 1978; Malmström et al. 1980). At present, there is no information as to
the signal that determines whether the xylose-initiated chain will
become a chondroitin sulfate or heparan sulfate or if the synthesis process involves separate complexes within the Golgi apparatus.

PROTEOGLYCAN PURIFICATION AND STRUCTURE

At the end of the 1960s, Vincent Hascall and the late Stanley
Sajdera published a series of papers that introduced a technique
of dissociative extraction for purifying proteoglycans from cartilage (Fig. 2). The technique involves the use of high concentrations of certain salts such as 4M guanidine hydrochloride to
dissociate the proteoglycans in the tissue, prevent interaction of
the components, and allow the proteoglycans and other molecules
to diffuse out. If cesium chloride is added to the extract and
the solution is centrifuged at 40,000 rpm for 40 hours, a linear
isopynic cesium chloride density gradient forms and the proteoglycans migrate to the equilibrium density position in the gradient. This position is at very high density because of the contributions of the sulfate to the overall density of the molecule

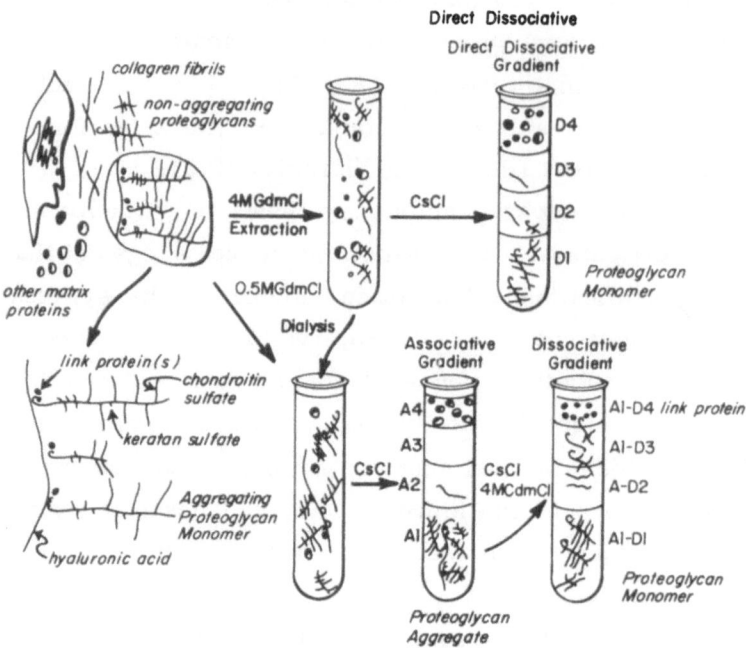

FIG. 2.   Scheme for the isolation of tissue proteoglycans.

(generally greater than 1.7 g/ml for cartilage proteoglycans into protein contents of less than 8%) and the molecules will be separated from the most common contaminates (protein, glycogen, etc.). Proteoglycan monomers are prepared from the bottom fractions of such gradients. If, however, the solution is dialyzed to lower salt concentrations, i.e., 0.5M guanidine hydrochloride, other components that can interact with proteo molecules assemble. If cesium chloride is added subsequently and a gradient is formed as described for the monomer, proteoglycan aggregates are isolated in the bottom fractions of the density gradients where nonproteoglycan components interact with proteoglycan molecules.

Detailed structural analysis of proteoglycans aggregates

Over the past decade as the result of work from several laboratories, the detailed structural analysis of aggregates isolated

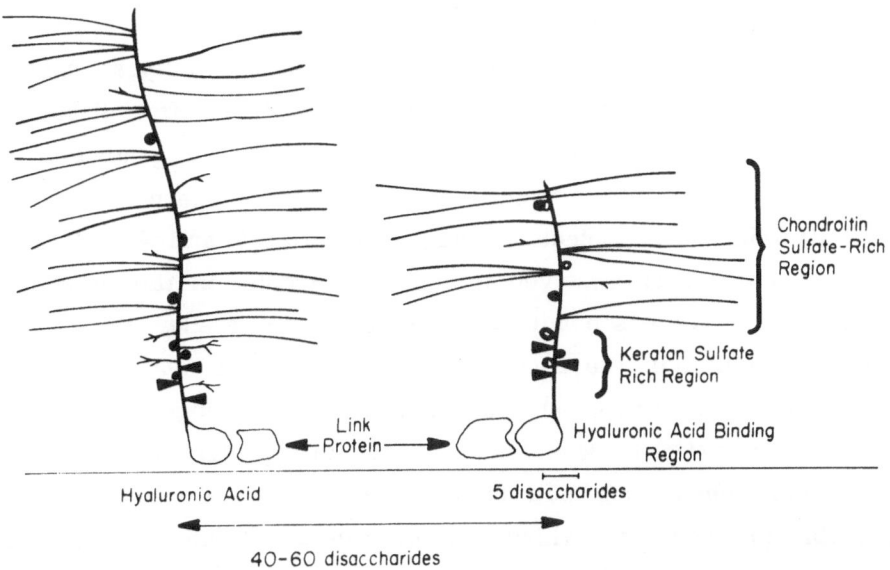

FIG. 3. Generalized structure of the cartilage progeoglycan aggregate. ◄ , aspargine link mannose oligosaccharide; ○ galactosamine linked oligosaccharides.

in the above manner has been reported (Hascall 1977; Rodén and Horowitz 1978). This has resulted in the generalized structure shown in Fig. 3. For proteoglycan from both bovine nasal septa and Swarm rat chondrosarcoma, the core protein molecular weight has been reported to be about 2×10^5 (Hascall and Riolo 1972; Oegema et al. 1975). The core protein molecule is organized into various domains that have been described respectively as the hyaluronic acid-binding region, the keratan sulfate-rich region, and the chondroitin sulfate-rich region. The hyaluronic acid-binding region comprises about 30% of the molecule. It is a globular region that specifically interacts with hyaluronic acid. This interaction, involving the five repeating disaccharides or ten monosaccharides, has been specifically characterized as requiring the glucuronic acid carboxyl group and as having an absolute requirement for the orientation of the C-4 hydroxyl of the glucosamine residue since unsulfated chondroitin will not bind

(Hascall 1977). The distance occupied on the hyaluronic acid by the hyaluronic acid binding region would be about 5 nm.

The interaction with hyaluronic acid and proteoglycan monomers is further stabilized by a link protein that, after dissociation from the aggregate fraction in a dissociative gradient, is found in the top 1/5 or A1-D4 fraction. In bovine nasal septa, link proteins have molecular weights of 51,000 and 47,000 and have recently been resolved by chromatography in the presence of detergent (Caterson and Baker 1978). The smaller link is the only link found in the Swarm rat chondrosarcoma (Oegema et al. 1975), the rat (Pita et al. 1979), and rabbits (Oegema, unpublished observation), whereas a large link protein is found in developing chick limb bud systems (Hascall et al. 1976). The possible presence of a third link protein in bovine cartilage has been reported recently by Baker and Caterson (1977). In the bovine system, at least a portion of the large 51,000 component can be converted to the 47,000 molecular weight component by reduction. This may be due to the partial cleavage of peptide bonds located in such a position that the fragments are still held together by a system of disulfide bridges (Baker and Caterson 1979).

The exact role of link protein is still being investigated. Based on the stoichiometry of isolation (Oegema et al. 1977) and biosynthetic studies (Kimura et al. 1979) link protein and proteoglycan occur as a one-to-one complex. There is also evidence that hyaluronic acid can interact with proteoglycan alone (Hascall 1977) or with the link protein alone (Heinegård and Hascall 1974a; Oegema et al. 1977). In addition, binding between only proteoglycan and link protein has been detected (Caterson and Baker 1978). Recent work using proteolytic enzyme digestion has demonstrated that the link protein and proteoglycan protect each other from digestion by trypsin (Hascall 1977) and that in aggregate, specific regions of the molecules are protected from chemical modification (Heinegård and Hascall 1979b), showing specific interaction between the two molecules. Also, proteoglycan monomers are capable of self interaction through the protein core (Sheehan et al. 1978).

From the Swarm rat chondrosarcoma, it has been possible to isolate aggregates that have not been dissociated by using 0.5M guanidine hydrochloride as the extractant (Faltz et al. 1979). Results of these studies suggest that as initially isolated there was one link protein per hyaluronic acid binding region and that this complex contained an average of 97 monosaccharide units of hyaluronic acid for each complex. After exhaustive treatment with chondroitinase ABC, one hyaluronic acid binding region and one link protein complex was bound to about 41 monosaccharides of hyaluronic acid. A value of approximately 50 monosaccharides was found after the complex was digested with hyaluronidase from Streptomyces. If the core protein was treated with chondroitinase ABC to remove the chondroitin sulfate chains, leaving only the keratan sulfate and oligosaccharides, and this core protein was added in amounts sufficient to saturate a limited amount of hyaluronic acid, the spacing of the core proteins along the core was approximately 20 hyaluronic acid monosaccharides (Heinegård and Hascall 1974).

The proteoglycan monomer spacing from reconstituted aggregates, as opposed to that isolated under associative conditions where the aggregate is not reassembled, has been compared by electronmicroscopy. The spacing for 4M guanidine hydrochloride extracted and reassembled aggregates from 8-day chick limb bud cartilage cultures is 48 nm, whereas 0.5M guanidine hydrochloride extracted aggregates from the same type of tissue has an average spacing of only 32 nm, suggesting that there is a closer packing between nondissociated native aggregates as opposed to reassembled aggregates (Kimura et al. 1978).

In the proteoglycan immediately adjacent to the hyaluronic acid binding region is the keratan sulfate-rich region, which contains about 60% of all keratan sulfate present in bovine nasal septa proteoglycan (Heinegård and Axelsson 1977). This region contains approximately three keratan sulfate chains for each chondroitin sulfate chain and is relatively resistant to trypsin and chymotrypsin digestion. The region occupies about 10% of the protein core ($M_r = 2 \times 10^4$).

The remainder of the molecule is the chondroitin sulfate-rich region and contains about 40% of the keratan sulfate chains and a majority of the chondroitin sulfate chains. These chains tend to occur in clusters of two to eight chains (average five chains) between trypsin or chymotrypsin sensitive regions (Heinegård and Hascall 1974b). This would mean that an average proteoglycan molecule weight of 2.5×10^6 would contain 80 - 100 chondroitin sulfate chains and 30 - 50 keratan sulfate chains.

Recent studies by Hascall and co-workers have identified two new moities in proteoglycan structures (Lohmander et al. 1980; DeLuca et al. 1980). They are a mannose-rich aspargine linked glycopeptide and a class of oligosaccharides that are released by sodium hydroxide - sodium borohydride treatment consisting of 0-linked glycosidic oligosaccharides linked through galactosamine to the hydroxyl group of serine or threonine. The structures of these molecules are shown in Fig. 4. There are approximately 15 of the N-glycosidic-linked mannose glycopeptides per core protein, and they are located primarily in or near the hyaluronic acid binding region. In the Swarm rat chondrosarcoma proteoglycan there are approximately 1.3 of these oligosaccharides for every chondroitin sulfate chain. The distribution along the protein core of these oligosaccharides suggests that they are related to the keratan sulfate, being enriched in the regions near the hyaluronic acid binding region. In the developing chick limb bud system, 0.25 keratan sulfate chains are present for every chondroitin sulfate chain and one 0-linked oligosaccharide is present per chondroitin sulfate chain, giving a ratio for the total keratan plus oligosaccharides of about 1.25 per chondroitin sulfate chain, a value in agreement with the chondrosarcoma study. This additionally suggests that there is a reciprocal relationship between the keratan sulfate and the oligosaccharide, with oligosaccharides being prematurely terminated keratan sulfate chains, a suggestion

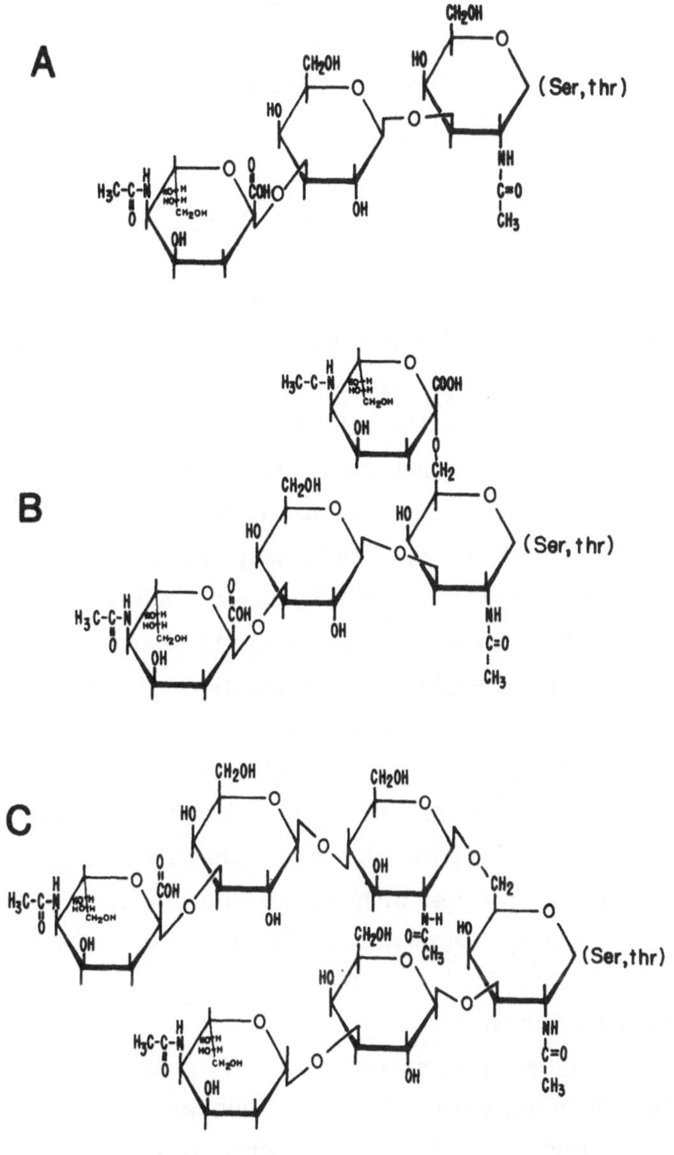

FIG. 4. Structure of oligosaccharides isolated from Swarm rat chondrosarcoma.

that was made previously for the chondrosarcoma system (Oegema et al. 1975). In view of the structure of these oligosaccharides a controlling point for the synthesis of keratan sulfate chains could be the glucosamine transferase that would transfer the glucosamine to the terminal galactose and glucosamine which would be the first sugar of the repeating disaccharide of keratan sulfate (DeLuca et al. 1980).

PROTEOGLYCAN SYNTHESIS

Studies on the biosynthesis of cartilage proteoglycans have yielded some equally interesting observations. Upholt et al. (1979) using antibodies to proteoglycan core and a cell free poly-ribosome system, found that the initially synthesized proteogly-can protein core had a molecular weight of 340,000 prior to pro-cessing. The work of Kimura et al. (1978) indicated that proteo-glycans, when initially secreted, may be complexed with link proteins but not associated with hyaluronic acid, and that assem-bly into a stable aggregate may take in excess of 30 minutes. Recently, Oegema (unpublished observation) has detected a tran-sient appearance in some human disease states, such as osteo-arthritis and steroid-induced avascular necrosis, of a nonaggre-gating intermediate in cartilage that, either with increased chase time or by treatment with the rat chondrosarcoma, can be in-duced to form complexes with hyaluronic acid. These observa-tions taken together suggest that there may be processing of the core protein before final secretion and assembly into extracellular aggregate structures.

All proteoglycan preparations contain a small amount of non-aggregating proteoglycan. Recently Heinegård and Hascall (1979) isolated the nonaggregating fraction from bovine nasal septa pro-teoglycan and found that the nonaggregating molecules contained extra peptides not present in the aggregated molecules. In studies on proteoglycan separated by chromatography and stud-ied with electron microscopy, a large polydispersity in the length of the protein core has been noted (Kimura et al. 1978). At the present time, it is not known whether this arises from a syn-thetic or catabolic process. To further complicate the picture, a

low buoyant density proteoglycan comprising about 3% of the proteoglycan present in developing chick epiphyseal cartilage has
been identified as small dermatan sulfate proteoglycan (Kimata et
al. 1978). This suggests that within the cartilage system there
may be at least three different types of proteoglycan: a large
nonaggregating monomer similar to the aggregating monomer but
with extra peptide; the aggregating monomer; and a small low
buoyant density proteoglycan containing dermatan sulfate.

PROTEOGLYCAN DEGRADATION

Studies on the degradation of cartilage proteoglycans by cartilage cells are rather limited. Sandy et al. (1978) have presented evidence that in rabbit articular cartilage, the initial step
in degradation is a cleavage near the hyaluronic acid binding
region, releasing a large fragment without the hyaluronic acid
binding region. Chick chondrocytes have been shown to have
the system of enzymes necessary to completely degrade chondroitin sulfate (Glaser and Conrad 1979). Although little is
known about the mechanism by which the fragments are transported into the chondrocyte, in fibroblast systems it apparently
involves recognition of polyanionic compounds at the cell surface
and then pinocytosis (Truppe and Kresse 1978).

PROTEOGLYCANS FROM OTHER TISSUES

The 4M guanidine hydrochloride extraction procedure coupled
with cesium chloride density gradients for purification have been
used to characterize proteoglycans from several other tissues.
Proteoglycans from the anulus fibrosis and nucleus pulposis of
intervertebral disc have been characterized from several species
(Stevens et al. 1979; Adams and Muir 1976; Emes and Pearce
1975). In anulus fibrosis, proteoglycans tend to be aggregated
(40% - 50%) and have K_{av}s on Sepharose CL-2B of the monomer
similar to corresponding hyaline cartilage proteoglycans, whereas

the nucleus pulposis has a lower percent aggregate (generally in the range of 10% - 30%) and a smaller proteoglycan as measured by K_{av}s on Speharose CL-2B.   Stevens et al. (1979) have recently proposed that the nucleus pulposis proteoglycan has a relatively shortened chondroitin sulfate-rich region as opposed to the corresponding articular cartilage.   Oegema et al. (1979) in a recent study have suggested that human nucleus pulposis displays an interesting biosynthetic pathway.   The initially synthesized proteoglycan may in fact have the same properties as the hyaline cartilage proteoglycan in that it has a long chondroitin sulfate-rich region and is synthesized primarily as aggregate. In a series of pulse-chase experiments they found that all of the initially synthesized proteoglycan in human nucleus pulposis was synthesized as large aggregating proteoglycan and that about 10% of the total proteoglycan persisted as this species. Because of the large avascular nature of the nucleus pulposis, the authors felt that the majority of the proteoglycan present in the disc, which gives the biomechanical properties to the disc, are retained as a result of the impermeability of the surrounding tissues to the breakdown products.

Using hot urea, a dermatan sulfate proteoglycan was isolated by Öbrink (1972) from porcine skin.   It had an average molecular weight estimated by light scattering at 2.9 x 10^6, although the presence of noncovalent aggregates could not be excluded. The protein content was 58% and the molecule contained dermatan sulfate chains with molecular weights of about 15,000.   Damle et al. (1979) isolated a low molecular weight dermatan sulfate proteoglycan from pig skin by 4M guanidine hydrochloride extraction in the presence of protease inhibitors.   After purification by precipitation in ethanol KSCN to separate them from collagen, the proteoglycans were fractionated into two components on cesium chloride density gradients under associative conditions.   Dermatan sulfate proteoglycan containing 50% - 60% protein was found in the top of the gradient and a small chondroitin sulfate-rich proteoglycan containing about 4% - 5% protein, 85% chondroitin-4, and 15% chondroitin-6-sulfate chains with a molecular weight of about 20,000 was found in the bottom fraction. The latter proteoglycan contained 8% of the hexosamine as glucosamine that was probably either heparan sulfate or keratan sulfate. Having a molecular weight of about 1×10^6, the molecule would contain about 50 chondroitin sulfate chains. It did not interact with added hyaluronic acid. The dermatan sulfate proteoglycan with a protein content of 50% - 60% had a $M_r = 1.3 \times 10^5$, which is considerably smaller than that reported by Öbrink (1972).

In the same vein, a recent report by Coster et al. (1979) suggested that at least a fraction of the proteoglycans synthesized by human embryonic fibroblasts contain large molecular weight dermatan sulfate proteoglycans that show reversible association-disassociation when chromatographed on Sepharose CL-2B columns in the presence of phosphate buffered saline or 4M guanidine hydrochloride, respectively. The association was markedly increased by the addition of hyaluronic acid.

Hassell et al. (1979) have identified the presence of two proteoglycans in the Rhesus monkey corneal stroma. They were characterized as a chondroitin dermatan proteoglycans consisting of approximately 70% protein, having a M_r equal to approximately 1.0×10^5 to 1.5×10^5 and, containing one dermatan sulfate chain, $M_r = 5.5 \times 10^4$ per molecule, and a keratan sulfate proteoglycan consisting of 74% protein with a M_r of 4.0×10^4 to 4.7 $\times 10^4$ and containing only one or two keratan sulfates with $M_r = 7.0 \times 10^3$ per molecule. This work is essentially in agreement with that of Axelsson and Heinegård (1978), who partially fractionated a keratan sulfate and dermatan sulfate proteoglycan and found they aggregate in the absence of hyaluronic acid.

Margolis et al. (1976) have isolated from brain a soluble chondroitin sulfate proteoglycan that had a sedimentation coefficient of 6.5, eluted as a single peak on Sepharose CL-4B in the presence of 4M guanidine hydrochloride, and contained 56% protein, 24% glycosaminoglycans (the majority of which was chondroitin sulfate), and 20% glycopeptide. This molecule contains an unusual oligosaccharide that is linked through mannose to a threonine (Finne et al. 1979).

Hascall and co-workers (Yanagashita et al. 1979; Yanagishita and Hascall 1979) have recently isolated the proteoglycans from porcine ovarian follicular fluid and looked at early aspects of biosynthesis. The molecule contained about 20% protein, 50% dermatan sulfate, and 20% oligosaccharides (rich in sialic acid, galactose mannose, glucosamine, and galactosamine) linked through galactosamine to threonine or serine. The dermatan sulfate chains had a M_r equal to 5.6×10^4. The molecular weight of the proteoglycan was about 2×10^6 to 2.5×10^6 with a core protein of about 4×10^5. It contained an average of 20 dermatan sulfate chains and 350 sialic acid-linked oligosaccharides. The molecule did not interact with hyaluronic acid.

In cultured glial cells using $[^{35}S]$sulfate as a precursor for proteoglycans, Norling et al. (1978) described a small percentage of the proteoglycans present as large molecular weight chondroitin sulfate proteoglycans that were capable of interacting with hyaluronic acid.

Nakamura and Nagai (1979) have isolated from bovine blood a small proteoglycan containing undersulfated chondroitin-4-sulfate. It has a molecular weight of approximately 4.4×10^4 and is composed of 77% protein and 23% glycosaminoglycan, with only one glycosaminoglycan chain per molecule. The amino acid composition suggests that it is not derived from other tissue proteoglycans.

A chondroitin-4-sulfate proteoglycan has been isolated from platelets and characterized as the carrier for heparin neutralizing activity (platelet 4 factor) (Barber et al. 1972). This molecule has a molecular weight of 5.9×10^4 and contains four chondroitin-4-sulfate chains with $M_r = 1.2 \times 10^4$. In a fully saturated state, the complex has a molecular weight of 3.5×10^5, so each proteoglycan is the carrier of four molecules of platelet 4 factor and 2 moles of proteoglycan are in the complex.

Several heparan sulfate proteoglycans of low molecular weight have been isolated from various sources, including human dentin (Bradford-White 1978), mouse mastocytoma (Chandrasekaran et al. 1975), plasma membranes of an ascites hepatoma (Mutoh et al. 1978), and a cell surface heparan sulfate from rat liver membranes (Oldberg et al. 1979). The latter proteoglycan was characterized as having a total molecular weight of about 7.5×10^4 and a core molecular weight estimated at 1.7×10^4 to 4.4×10^4 after removal of the heparan sulfate oligosaccharides by different enzymatic and chemical methods. A molecular weight of 1.4×10^4 was estimated for the chains released by alkaline treatment. This would be consistent with a proteoglycan containing four polysaccharide chains attached to a protein core and would be similar to the general findings on heparan sulfate proteoglycans that have been purified.

Horner, Lindahl, and co-workers in collaboration (Robinson et al. 1978) have partially characterized a heparan proteoglycan from rat skin presumably synthesized by mast cells and stored in mast cell granules. They have a molecular weight greater than 9×10^5, the protein core has a molecular weight of 2.0×10^4 and consists of almost equal molar amounts of glycine and serine with only traces of other amino acids. The heparan chains have a M_r of 6.0×10^4 to 10.0×10^4 and can be degraded to active heparin fragments, M_r equal to 7×10^3 to 2.5×10^3. This molecule would contain 15 chains of heparan with 2 out of 3 serines being substituted.

PHYSIOLOGIC FUNCTION IN CONNECTIVE TISSUES

Glycosaminoglycans and sulfated proteoglycans have a series of physical properties that are important in the organization of the respective tissues (for review, see Comper and Laurent 1978). One of these properties is hydrodynamic volumes that are extremely large relative to the dry volumes. For example, those of hyaluronate and cartilage proteoglycan are 1000 and 100 times larger, respectively, than the volume of dry molecules.

The solution domains are extremely large, so that for concentra-tions on the order of 1 mg/cm^3 and 10 mg/cm^3 for hyaluronate and cartilage proteoglycans, respectively, molecule domains will begin to overlap (Comper and Laurent 1978). At higher concen-trations they form continuous networks in which individual mole-cules cannot be distinguished. The exact nature of the interac-tion of this entanglement is not understood but it means that solutions are viscoelastic, where at low strain frequency the solutions exhibit predominantly viscous behavior and at high strain frequency they exhibit elasticity, the elasticity increasing with increasing concentrations.

A second important concept is that the proteoglycan molecules can be immobilized in the tissues. This means that they can be viewed as similar to an ion exchange resin and the properties interpreted in a similar manner. The negatively charged domain of the glycosaminoglycan chain can be seen as a continuous domain with the counter ions appearing to condense along the proteoglycan molecules at a fixed distance such that only 40% of the sulfated proteoglycan counter ions are active at low ionic strength (Comper and Laurent 1978). A Donnan distribution between polyionic-containing compartments and a nonpolyionic-containing compartment will occur. The counter ion concentra-tion will be higher in the polysaccharide compartment and the co-ion concentration, lower. The condensation in a micro-ion environment will be dependent on the nature of the ions, with divalent ions being more strongly affected than monovalent ions (Comper and Laurent 1978). This appears to be a property of the glycosaminoglycan chain since no marked differences were noted, for example, with the interaction of calcium ions with pro-teoglycan aggregate, monomer, or free glycosaminoglycan chains (Cuervo et al. 1973). However, there is a pronounced differ-ence on the affects of aggregate versus monomer and the ability to inhibit mineral growth in vitro (Cuervo et al. 1973). Some evidence favors a relatively high affinity of calcium for proteo-glycan fractions associated with collagen (MacGregor and Bowness

1971). Mathews (1970) found that calcium and sodium ion binding to proteoglycan appears to be freely exchangeable. However, with large polycations, such as lysozyme, apparently specific salt linkages are formed (Greenwald and Schwartz 1974).

A common feature of glycosaminoglycan is that the osmotic
behavior is extremely nonideal in that the osmotic pressure is
not proportional to concentrations but rises rapidly with increased concentrations and it is considerably higher than serum
albumin, which has the molecular weight of approximately 50 -
100 times lower (Comper and Laurent 1978). This behavior tends
to amplify osmotic forces in homostasis in vitro. Fluid loss from
a proteoglycan containing tissue under compression will cause a
large increment in the osmotic restoring force, whereas dilution
will cause relatively small diminution in the osmotic pressure.

Proteoglycans will affect micro-ion transport only in tissues
where they contribute an extremely large amount of negative
charge such as in the intervertebral disc and nasal septum
where fixed charge densities are as high as 0.6 mmoles/cm^3
(Comper and Laurent 1978). Because of the interaction with the
negative charge, for example, the sodium permeability across the
tissue would be increased 2 - 3 times. However, the chloride
ion would be retarded $0.1 - 0.3$ fold of that in free solution and
sodium chloride migration would be reduced to approximately 0.8
times of the value in water. However, on the basis of a direct
obstruction affect, articular cartilage and nucleus pulposis retard
the movement of water and small molecules to the rate of 50% -
60% of the migration rate in water. This suggests that even in
these highly dense tissues, the charge on the proteoglycan molecule has little affect on ion or small molecule transport.

Glycosaminoglycan - Glycosaminoglycan Interaction

In addition to the specific interactions mentioned for the aggregation of hyaluronic acid in proteoglycan molecules, it has
also been demonstrated that copolymeric dermatan - chondroitin-
4-sulfates will interact specifically with each other (Fransson

1976). This was demonstrated by attaching chondroitin-4 and dermatan sulfate hybrids to an agarose gel and looking at the interaction of glycosaminoglycans chromatographed over this material. The nature of the aggregates have not been sufficiently investigated to provide a detailed structure.

Proteoglycan - Collagen Interactions

Glycosaminoglycans and proteoglycan interactions with collagen have been shown by a number of techniques such as electrophoresis, precipitation, chromatography, light scattering, circular dichromism, and equilibrium binding. Sulfated glycosaminoglycans, with the exception of keratan sulfate, bind to collagen at physiologic pH and with ionic strength and this has the characteristics of an ionic interaction (see review, Comper and Laurent 1978). Proteoglycans interact more strongly than individual chains. For example, using monomeric lathyritic collagen, Öbrink (1973) was able to use quantitative light scattering to show an interaction between collagen and glycosaminoglycans and proteoglycans. He showed binding to chondroitin-4- and 6-sulfate, dermatan sulfate, heparan sulfate, and heparin, but not to keratan sulfate and hyaluronic acid, although hyaluronic acid showed a larger steric exclusion affect for collagen. The presence of iduronic acid instead of glucuronic acid resulted in more pronounced binding. This goes along with the observation that dermatan sulfate is more difficult to extract from collagen-rich tissues than chondroitin sulfate (Toole and Lowther 1968). The number of glycosaminoglycan chains bound to each collagen molecule is limited to the range of 2 - 4 (Öbrink and Sundelöf 1973), values that have been confirmed by other studies (Öbrink et al. 1975). Gelman and Blackwell (1974) found that tissue glycosaminoglycans were able to stabilize the collagen triple helix such that the melting point was raised from 38° to 46°.

In studies where soluble collagen was allowed to form fibrils at physiologic salt concentrations and pH at 37°, the presence of proteoglycan inhibited fibril formation and the proteoglycan was specifically bound to the newly formed fibers (Oegema et al. 1975), with about one proteoglycan being bound per 20 - 25 collagen molecules. Aggregate was as effective as monomer in this system. The nature of the interaction or at what stage of fibril formation it occurred has not been defined.

Proteoglycan Glycosaminoglycan - Lipoprotein Interaction

Sulfated high molecular weight polymers precipitated β-lipoproteins at low ionic strength. Iverius (1972) investigated the binding of various lipoprotein fractions to connective tissue glycosaminoglycans using glycosaminoglycans covalently attached to agarose gels. He found that at physiologic ionic strength, heparin, and dermatan sulfate to a lesser degree, bound low-density lipoprotein and very low-density lipoprotein. The other glycosaminoglycans interacted only at much lower salt concentrations. He did not find an interaction of the glycosaminoglycans with high-density lipoprotein. The reaction did not require divalent ions, but the stability of the complex was enhanced by the presence of Ca^{+2}, Mg^{+2}, or Mn^{+2}.

Steric Exclusion

Two particles cannot occupy the same space at the same time. They therefore will exclude a certain space from each other. For example, a spherical particle excludes the center of another sphere for the volume eight times greater than the volume of the particle itself. The steric exclusion phenomenon will affect enzyme reactions, depending on the molecular size of the enzymes and substrate or inhibitor and on the relative volumes that the molecules have access to in the tissues. Steric exclusion will affect large molecules that can take up different orientation in solutions if the conformations occupy different volumes by affecting the equilibrium between different conformational states and favoring the more compact conformation. This suggests that in high concentrations, such as in cartilage, proteoglycans can have a stabilizing effect on compact structures, such as collagen fibers. The exclusion phenomenon can also affect solubility where an increase in chemical activity due to steric exclusion can cause precipitation if a solubility limit is reached. The effect would be to accelerate precipitation reactions such as antibody complexes in disease states, the formation of collagen fibers or elastin fibers, and the deposition of amyloid in serum disease, lipids in atherosclerosis, amd uric acid in gout. Finally, the exclusion phenomenon can give rise to increased osmotic properties due to increased chemical activity of a compound (Comper and Laurent 1978). It is interesting to note that in all connective tissues, although hyaluronic acid and the proteoglycans may contribute to the exclusion phenomenon, collagen is by far the most predominant component in most tissue. For example, Comper and Laurent (1978) calculated that cartilage contains 680 mg of water, 190 mg of collagen, and 22 mg of proteoglycan. The collagen alone would have an exclusion effect on albumin on the order of $0.4 - 0.8$ cm^3/g tissue. Proteoglycans, if distributed within 50% of the cartilage volumes, since they cannot occupy the same space as collagen, would have a local concentration on the order of 50 mg/cm^3, which would be enough to completely exclude the remaining albumin. Indeed, Maroudas (1970) has found that molecules larger than hemoglobin do not enter cartilage. Similarly, one gram of human dermis contains approximately 650 mg water, 300 mg collagen, and 0.6 mg proteoglycan. In this case, the effect of collagen on albumin would be in order of $0.6 - 1.0$ cm^3/g tissue where the proteoglycan would contribute only 0.02 cm^3; the collagen excluded volume is an important factor in the dermis. Pearce and Grimmer (1970) have also shown that the dermis contains the protein equivalent to 0.2 cm^3 plasma protein in a gram of dermis, which is in agreement with this estimate.

Proteoglycan - Water Interaction

Proteoglycans have been commonly stated to bind water in connective tissue. However, Ogston (1966) has pointed out that water binding is an arbitrary term and should probably be aban-

doned. The actual number of water molecules bound by hydrogen and polar bonds to the hydroxyl groups and charged groups
of glycosaminoglycans is estimated at only 1-2.5 per repeat disaccharide (Bettelheim and Plessy 1975). In studies to date there
is no evidence that proteoglycans or hyaluronic acid can induce
any structuring of water, nor is there evidence of ice-like water
structures induced by these molecules (Laurent 1957; Balazs et
al. 1959). So the majority of interactions with the proteoglycans
in affecting the water content of a tissue are not related to their
specific binding or structuring of water. However, they apparently are related directly to the nature of a connective tissue in
that it is a network of collagen fibers filled with proteoglycan.

The interacting system of proteoglycan and collagen has been
described as a gel system that can generate a swelling pressure,
where the osmotic contributions from the glycosaminoglycans are
offset by the contributions from the contractability of the collagen fibers (Comper and Laurent 1978). The osmotic force tends
to imbibe the gel with water while the elastic force of the collagen network attempts to express the liquid from the system. At
equilibrium, these two forces balance one another and the swelling pressure is zero, i.e., the swelling pressure equals internal
osmotic contribution minus the elastic contribution. Swelling can
also be counteracted by external forces, such as mechanical force
applied to the gel. This system has been studied extensively
experimentally in model systems and intact tissues (Comper and
Laurent 1978). As would be expected for a system that includes
charged ions, swelling is also remarkably sensitive to pH, the
ions present, and the ionic strength. Also, in several systems,
such as cornea of the eye, there is an interplay between swelling
pressure and an active dehydration process (Hedbys and Mishima
1962).

The interactions between the collagen and the proteoglycan
network are also expected to have large effects on transportation
of nutrients and water. For example, such a network is responsible for the resistance to water flow through tissues and this

protects the tissue from deformation since water itself is incompressible. This has been demonstrated for cornea (Hedbys and Mishima 1962) and for the "creep" deformation of cartilage (Linn and Sokoloff 1965). The high resistance to solvent flow through departments containing immobilized proteoglycans is explained in terms of the highly entangled gel-like nature of the proteoglycan molecules. The transport of large molecules may depend to a high degree on the asymmetry of the molecule in that large molecules moving through a proteoglycan network frequently have free rotational movements, but the translation movement is markedly retarded, i.e., they find holes where they are trapped until they can find another hole to which they can move (Comper and Laurent 1978). There is some evidence that in some connective tissues there may be a two-phase system such as in the capillary system and lymphatic system. Wiederhielm (1972) suggested that there may be a colloid-rich water-poor phase and a water-rich colloid-poor phase, based on the fact that some large molecules equilibrate with tissues faster than smaller molecules. While there was no chemical evidence of the nature of these two phases, proteoglycans, hyaluronic acid, and collagen probably exclude large molecules from their area of localization in the tissue.

AORTA GLYCOSAMINOGLYCANS

The type and concentrations of glycosaminoglycans in aorta have been studied for a large number of species and under a wide variety of circumstances. In general, the glycosaminoglycans are hyaluronic acid, chondroitin-4- and 6-sulfate, dermatan sulfate, and heparan sulfate (Massaro et al. 1979; Stevens et al. 1976; Radhakrishnamurthy et al. 1978; Murata 1978 and references therein). Glycosaminoglycans are found in the highest concentration in the intima and decrease toward the adventitia. Some unusual glycosaminoglycans, such as oversulfated chondroitin sulfate, have been reported in the aorta (Stevens et al.

1977). There is an increase in chondroitin-6-sulfate with age in the human aorta (Toledo and Mauras 1979). There is an increase also in the percent of dermatan sulfate in developing atherosclerotic lesions (Stevens et al. 1979). In Rhesus monkeys with atherosclerotic lesions induced by diet, there is a positive correlation between aortic cholesterol content and dermatan sulfate content (Wagner and Salisbury 1978). In nonhuman primates, the heparan sulfate to chondroitin dermatan sulfate ratio may be related to susceptibility to atherosclerosis (Radhakrishnamurthy et al. 1978). These observations are coupled with the findings of Iverius (1972) that dermatan sulfate in vitro binds lipoproteins to form the basis of a hypothesis that early lesion formation and plaque progression may be related to changes in glycosaminoglycans. This is currently under investigation in many laboratories (Eisenstein 1979).

The effect of many experimental conditions on glycosaminoglycan synthesis by aorta cells has also been probed. For example, immunologic injury to the aorta increases collagen and glycosaminoglycan synthesis (Rokosova and Bentley 1979) and high-density lipoproteinemia inhibits [^{35}S]sulfate incorporation into aortic smooth muscle cells in culture (Tammi et al. 1979). Cortisol depresses hyaluronic acid synthesis, but not [^{35}S]sulfate glycosaminoglycan synthesis in aortic smooth muscle cell cultures (Larjava et al. 1980). Hormonal changes (Sirek et al. 1978), zinc deficiency (Philip and Kurup 1977), gravity (Merrilees et al. 1977), and ascorbic acid (Verlangieri and Stevens 1979) all influence aortic proteoglycan synthesis.

Some information has been presented on the structure, location, and function of the proteoglycan in aorta. Ultrastructurally, the major proteoglycan molecules localized are chondroitinase ABC sensitive. They are located in association with collagen and elastin fibers (Eisenstein and Kuettner 1976; Wight and Ross 1975; Wight 1980) and smooth muscle cell membranes. A class of ruthenium red positive matrix granules that are chondroitinase ABC resistent are localized in the basement membrane beneath

the endothelium and surrounding the smooth muscle cells (Wight
and Ross 1975). In culture, smooth muscle cells synthesize all
the glycosaminoglycans present in aorta (Burke and Ross 1979;
Gamse et al. 1978; Wight 1980). Endothelial cells produced more
heparan sulfate that is more N-sulfate than smooth muscle cells
(Gamse et al. 1978). Studies in aorta organ culture have shown
there are several glycosaminoglycan pools with considerable heterogeneity in their rate of turnover (Kresse et al. 1971; von
Figura et al. 1975; Deudon and Picard 1978; Vijayogopal et al.
1980).

In terms of specific interactions, aorta proteoglycans in vivo
are largely bound to elastin and collagen (see above, as well as
Junqueira et al. 1980; Radhakrishnamurthy et al. 1977; McMurtre
et al. 1974). Changes in glycosaminoglycan content with age
have not been correlated with changes in biomechanical properties, such as elasticity (Vogel 1978). The proteoglycan molecules are present in high enough concentrations to exert a significant exclusion volume effect in the tissue and effect transfer
rates (Glatz and Massaro 1976a,b). In vitro, the glycosaminoglycans inhibit partial thromboplastic time (Murata et al. 1978),
thrombin time, and platelet aggregation (Ts'ao et al. 1977; Eisenstein 1979).

AORTA PROTEOGLYCAN

Several attempts have been made to isolate aorta proteoglycans by means of various extraction techniques. Antonopoulos
et al. (1974) have reported the extraction of a molecule from
aortic proteoglycan using 4M guanidine hydrochloride extraction
followed by dialysis of the extracts into 6M urea and subsequent
chromatography on DEAE cellulose. This led to the isolation of a
chondroitin - dermatan proteoglycan that was partially excluded
on Sepharose CL-4B but did not interact with hyaluronic acid.
Kresse et al. (1971) reported the isolation of a large molecular
weight chondroitin dermatan proteoglycan containing about 28%

dermatan sulfate using an EDTA phosphate buffer extraction and ethanol fractionation. Although it was difficult to assess the overall yield, they recovered a fraction with an estimated molecular weight of about 2.5×10^6. Ehrlich and co-workers (1975) have isolated a low molecular weight (approximately 1×10^5) chondroitin sulfate – dermatan sulfate proteoglycan from bovine aortas. The molecule was extracted with 4M guanidine hydrochloride in the absence of protease inhibitors. A low-density proteoglycan has also been identified that is rich in protein complexed with hyaluronic acid (McMurtre et al. 1979); and using a sequential 0.15M NaCl, collagenase, elastase digestion method there was evidence that heparan sulfate is tightly associated with elastin (Radhakrishnamurthy et al. 1977a).

With this background, the extraction and purification of a large molecular weight proteoglycan from the aorta and also the detection of a small heparan sulfate proteoglycan from this tissue can be discussed. The large molecular weight proteoglycan has the ability to interact with hyaluronic acid. In recent studies, Gardell and co-workers (1980) have suggested that this complex also contains a link protein and hyaluronic acid binding regions that are immunologically similar to proteoglycan found in bovine nasal septum.

Initial purification process for the proteoglycan was similar to that used and previously reported by Eisenstein et al. (1975). Bovine aorta was obtained shortly after death and transported to the laboratory on ice in normal saline containing 0.1M 6-amino-hexanoic acid, 0.005M benzamidine hydrochloride, and 0.01M sodium EDTA at pH 7.0. The aorta was separated manually into the inner third, a more elastic tissue, and the outer two-thirds, a more muscular tissue. The inner third was coursely ground in the meat grinder and extracted with 5 volumes of 4M guanidine hydrochloride containing 0.1M 6-aminohexanoic acid, 0.005M benzamidine hydrochloride, 0.1M sodium EDTA, and 0.05M sodium acetate at pH 5.8 (Oegema et al. 1975) at 4°C overnight with shaking. These conditions are slightly less than optimum for the extraction of the proteoglycan but resulted in less proteoglycan breakdown (Eisenstein et al. 1975). Recently, Gardell et al. (1980) have reported that using microtome-thin slices of aorta will result in better extraction, and we have found that milling finely minced aorta fragments in the Spex mill at liquid nitrogen temperature will greatly improve the extractability of the molecules and the nature of the proteoglycan aggregate isolated. The extracts were clarified by centrifugation and 0.4 g cesium chloride was added per gram of extract to give an initial density of 1.40 g/ml. Samples were centrifuged at 40,000 rpm at 5°C for 40 hours in a Beckman 50-Ti rotor. The tubes were sliced into the top 3/5 and bottom 2/5 fraction. The bottom 2/5 fraction was dialyzed at 4°C against 6 changes of 4 liters each of 0.5M potassium chloride over a 48-hour period. The dialyzed sample was equilibrated at room temperature and 0.1 volume of 5% (wt/v) cetylpyridinium chloride (CPC) was added dropwise with stirring. The suspension was allowed to settle for several hours at room temperature, centrifuged at 1000 x gr for 5 - 10 minutes and the precipitate was washed with 0.5M potassium chloride containing 0.5% CPC. The pellet was dissolved in 4M guanidine hydrochloride in 0.05M sodium acetate, pH 7.0, and cesium chloride was added at the rate of 0.55 g/g to give it an initial density of 1.44 g/ml.

The second gradient was run for 48 hours at 40,000 rpm. The gradient tubes were cut into 10 equal fractions. The CPC was found in the top fraction of the gradient. The addition of CPC precipitation step and the second gradients were found to be necessary because of the more cellular nature of the aorta. In hyaline cartilage with a high matrix to cell ratio, very little DNA or RNA are detected in the extracts although some glycogen is found. The aorta extract apparently contains DNA and RNA as well as some glycogen and hyaluronic acid, and these are removed by this procedure. Additionally, it is noted that for good quantitation of the hexuronic acid in early extracts and in the tissues, the samples had to be digested with papain and precipitated sequentially with CPC and ethanol to prevent interference from other compounds, such as DNA. Aggregate preparations were made by dialyzing initial extract for 16 hr at 4°C against 6 volumes of extraction buffer without the guanidine hydrochloride but with the protease inhibitors. The extract was centrifuged in a cesium chloride density (1 g cesium chloride/g extract) for 40 hours at 8°C in a Ti-50 rotor. The bottom 2/5 were retained for further analysis (A1 fraction). A portion of the A1 fraction was refractionated in a dissociative gradient. Solid guanidine hydrochloride was added to a portion of the A1 fraction to a final concentration of 4M and 0.6 g cesium chloride added per gram of solution. Under these conditions, 24 hour extraction with 5 volumes of extract per gram of weight gave 35% of the total tissue hexuronic acid in the extract, 3.5 μg out of 10 μg of hexuronic acid/mg dry weight of aorta.

Over 60% of this hexuronic acid was found on the bottom fraction of the first gradient. The proteoglycans of the bottom 2/5 were precipitated with CPC, the pellet was dissolved and centrifuged in the second gradient with a slightly higher initial density gradient and cut into 10 fractions. Fractions 4 - 10 all contained dermatan and chondroitin sulfate with the hexuronic acid peak at fraction 8, which has a density of about 1.53. Dermatan sulfate and chondroitin sulfate were identified by cellulose acetate electrophoresis (Oegema et al. 1979) in all the fractions after digestion by papain. Fraction 10 also contained a different component that migrated to the same position as heparin and heparan sulfate. These bands were also resistant to chondroitinase ABC digestion.

Fractions 8 and 9 were used for extensive characterization of the chemical nature and some of the physical properties. Pooled fraction 8 and 9 gave a single symmetrical peak in the analytical ultracentrifuge in sedmentation velocity experiments with an extrapolated S_0 = 11 in 4M guanidine hydrochloride and 0.05M sodium acetate, pH 7.0. This value is substantially lower than the values found for proteoglycans from Swarm rat chondrosarcoma and bovine nasal septum where values on the order of 23S are found (Oegema et al. 1975). Yphantis meniscus depletion sedimentation equilibrium experiments were run on fraction 8 and 9; the plots obtained indicated that the proteoglycans were polydisperse with molecular weights estimated at 1.5×10^6 to 2.0×10^6. These are similar to the values found by light scattering techniques by Kresse et al. (1971) for an EDTA-extracted, ethanol-precipitated proteoglycan.

Fractions 6 - 10 were reduced and alkylated to prevent interaction with hyaluronic acid and then chromatographed on a gel exclusion column, Sepharose CL-2B. The proteoglycans were included in peaks with a K_{av} of about 0.26. This was compared to a value of 0.25 for the Swarm rat chondrosarcoma proteoglycan or nasal septa proteoglycan on the same column. Properties of this proteoglycan were then systematically examined.

Chondroitinase ABC was used to remove the majority of the glycosaminoglycans from the core protein; the sample was electrophoresed in 3% acrylamide gels in the presence of sodium dodecyl sulfate. Two major bands and several minor bands were determined. These bands had mobilities slightly slower than that found for the Swarm rat chondrosarcoma or bovine nasal proteoglycans, suggesting molecular weights for the core proteins of approximately the same order of magnitude. If undigested samples were electrophoresed in 1.2% acrylamide or 0.5% agarose, several bands with mobilities slightly slower than bovine nasal or chondrosarcoma proteoglycans were found (Oegema et al. 1979).

The type of glycosaminoglycans present were investigated using a combination of digestion with chondroitinase ABC, which will digest chondroitin-4- and 6-sulfate, and dermatan sulfate, and chondroitinase AC, which will not digest segments of dermatan sulfate. The results were assayed by chromatographing the mixtures after enzyme digestion and digestion with papain to obtain the free chains on Sepharose CL-6B columns.

After chondroitinase ABC digestion, all the uronic acid was found in the disaccharide peak on the Sepharose CL-6B column.

However, after digestion with chondroitinase AC, about 20% of the hexuronic acid chromatographed within the column, with sizes ranging from slightly smaller than the intact undigested chondroitin dermatan sulfate chains to small oligosaccharides. These results suggest that approximately 20% of the hexuronic acid is present as dermatan sulfate, as compared to a value of 7% found by colorimetric methods. From the elution profiles on Sepharose CL-6B, a molecular weight of 4.0×10^4 is estimated for the intact chain. After chondroitinase AC, few if any of the chains contain segments longer than 50% of the intact chains. The chondroitin - dermatan sulfate hybrid chain would then have an estimated length of approximately 80 repeat disaccharides. These values are in agreement with the values that were obtained by analysis of the galactosamine and xylose. Chondroitinase ABC digestion and quantitation of the sulfate isometric positions by paper chromatography gave a value of 54% chondroitin-4-sulfate and 46% for chondroitin-6-sulfate. Since dermatan occurs as the 4-sulfated isomer, this would give an overall composition of 47% chondroitin-4-sulfate, 7% dermatan sulfate, and 46% chondroitin-6-sulfate.

The amino acid composition of the proteoglycan is given in Table 1 in residues/1000 residues and compared with that of several other proteoglycans. There was a relatively high content of the aspartic acid, threonine, serine, glutamic acid, and glycine. These are consistent with these residues being in the attachment region of the chondroitin sulfate chain. Half-cysteine was present and these residues are believed to be localized in globular regions of proteoglycans, such as in the hyaluronic acid binding region. In the carbohydrate analysis of the proteoglycan, there was an excess of galactose over that which was expected for the linkage region of the chondroitin sulfate, and sialic acid as well as glucosamine were present (Table 1). This suggests the presence of oligosaccharides, possibly similar to those that have been recently found in the Swarm rat chondrosarcoma and

TABLE 1.   Chemical Composition of Selected Proteoglycans.

Amino acid	Bovine aorta[a]	Bovine nasal cartilage[b]	Rat chondrosarcoma[c]
Residues/1000 Residues			
Aspartic acid	103	67	73
Threonine	86	59	93
Serine	90	127	135
Glutamic acid	140	150	133
Proline	93	109	83
Half-cysteine	7	6	7
Glycine	67	123	138
Alanine	61	69	64
Valine	56	52	54
Methionine	11	3	5
Isoleucine	40	32	28
Leucine	88	74	74
Tyrosine	19	19	16
Phenylalanine	35	34	37
Histidine	24	21	24
Lysine	47	20	18
Arginine	33	33	29
Sugar residues/xylose			
Xylose	1.0		1.0
Glucosamine	5.8		0.7
Galactosamine	83		40
Galactose	12		2.1
Mannose	2.4		Trace
Sialic acid	2.4		0.7
Fucose	0.8		Trace

[a]Oegema et al. 1979
[b]Hascall and Sajdera 1970
[c]Oegema et al. 1975

chick limb bud system; their structure is currently being investigated.

The ability of the aorta proteoglycan to interact with hyaluronic acid and form aggregate complexes was investigated in two ways. Fractions 8 and 9 were chromatographed on Sepharose CL-2B columns in the presence and the absence of 0.7% wt/wt high molecular weight hyaluronic acid. Fig. 5A shows that there was a shift of about 9% of the proteoglycan to the excluded fraction. In subsequent experiments with the improved extraction technique, this fraction has been increased considerably. Also, direct isolation in an associative condition resulted in the isolation of the material seen in Fig. 5B. Molecules were then processed in a dissociative gradient and rerun on the same column. There was an approximately 25% shift in the molecules from the excluded volume or aggregate fraction to the included volume, suggesting that a large amount of molecules were present as aggregates.

This is further pointed out in recent work with rabbit aorta where the animals were labeled with 5 mCi [^{35}S]sulfate as a precursor for the dermatan sulfate proteoglycan. The molecules were isolated as described above under associative conditions except that the initial dialysis was against only 6 volumes of extraction instead of 7, thus causing less precipitation of extraneous protein and giving a clear solution (Gardell et al. 1980). The results obtained are shown in Fig. 5C. At least 70% of the molecules are now present as aggregate. The experiments then suggest very strongly that aorta proteoglycans can interact with hyaluronic acid and form aggregate structures.

These results have been recently confirmed by the work of Gardell et al. (1980). They made slices of bovine aorta with a microtome, extracted the tissues with 4M guanidine hydrochloride in the presence of protease inhibitors, dialyzed the extract to a final concentration of approximately 0.8M guanidine hydrochloride, and purified the material under associative conditions. They were able to demonstrate, using specific antibodies, the

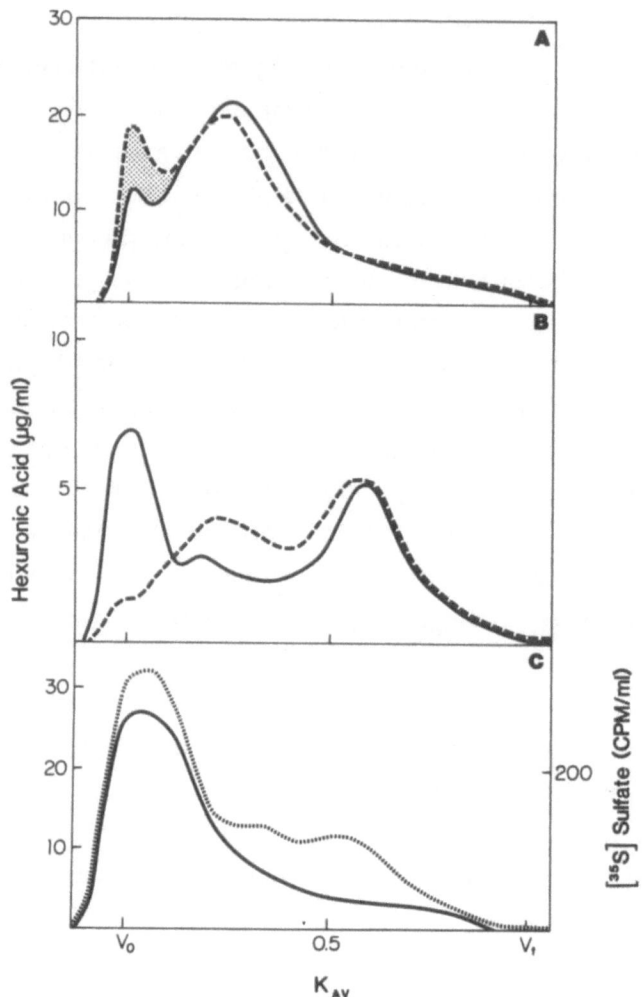

FIG. 5. Elution profile from Sepharose CL-2B of: A) Fraction 8-9 isolated from bovine aorta without (———), and with (- - -) 0.7% hyaluronic acid, B) A1 fraction isolated from bovine aorta before (———) and after (- - -) fractionation in a dissociative density gradient to remove hyaluronic acid and link protein, C) A1 fraction isolated from rabbit aorta, prelabeled in vivo with [^{35}S]sulfate; hexuronic acid (———), [^{35}S]sulfate (. . .).

presence of the link protein and hyaluronic acid binding region in the proteoglycan of the preparations. Taken together, these results would mean that the majority of the chondroitin sulfate –

dermatan sulfate proteoglycans present in the aorta are anchored in the tissue by a specific aggregation to hyaluronic acid, and stabilized by a link protein.

In recent work of Eisenstein, antibodies prepared against the aorta proteoglycan showed only partial cross-reactivity with cartilage proteoglycan (personal communication). Eisenstein and co-workers (Ts'ao et al. 1977) have gone on to investigate some of the biological properties of the aorta proteoglycan. They found that there were two anticoagulent activities present in the proteoglycan fractions. Fraction 10 contained a potent anticoagulant that was chondroitinase ABC and AC insensitive, which is presumably due to the heparan sulfate present in this fraction. Fractions 6 - 9 contained less potent anticoagulant activity that was chondroitinase ABC and AC sensitive and appeared to require a serum factor. The activity in fractions 6 - 9 was due to the dermatan sulfate chain alone since the anticoagulent activities were not affected by digestion with papain. The aorta chondroitin - dermatan sulfate proteoglycan has been localized by histologic techniques in the inner region layers of aorta where it coats collagen, is an antithrombin, and inhibits platelet aggregation induced by thrombin but not by agents such as collagen when used in similar concentrations. Ts'ao et al. (1977) has suggested that this proteoglycan will limit the aortic response to minor injury by allowing platelet aggregation while inhibiting extensive thrombus formation.

In fraction 10, there was an additional proteoglycan that contained heparan sulfate and migrated on Sepharose CL-2B with a K_{av} of 0.7. The molecule would be similar in size to the heparan sulfate proteoglycan isolated from liver membranes (Oldberg et al. 1979) and the lung proteoglycan isolated from rabbits (Oegema, unpublished results). The presence of large aggregating proteoglycan containing dermatan sulfate in aorta is not unique to this tissue. For example, Fig. 6A,B shows [^{35}S]sulfate proteoglycan isolated from skin fibroblast cultures in the presence and absence of hyaluronic acid. The results clearly show

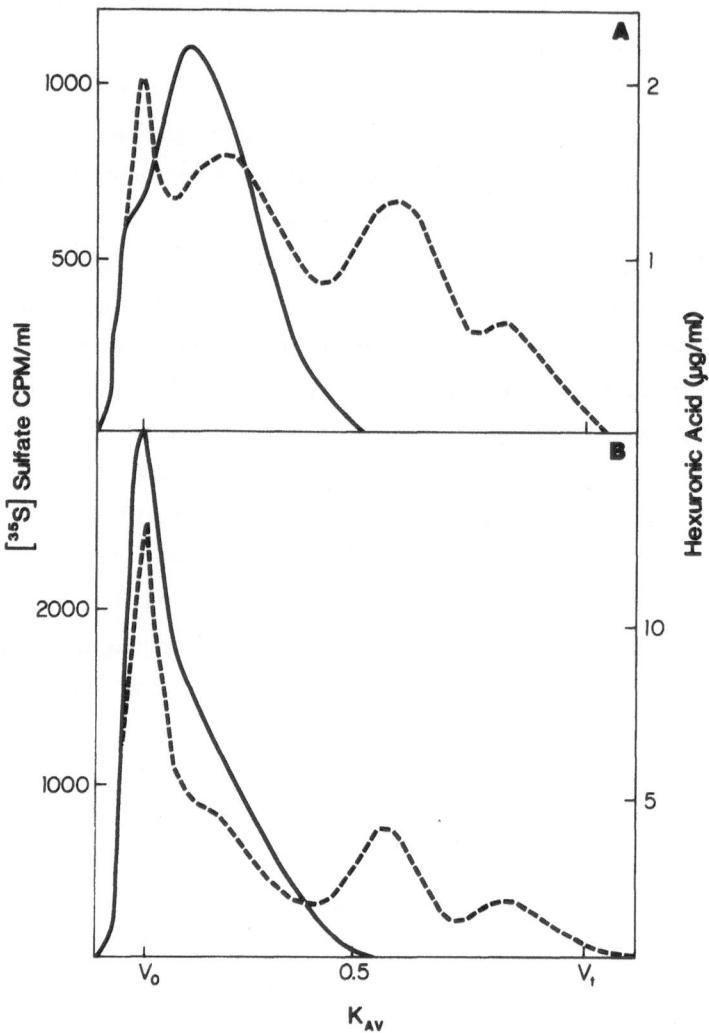

FIG. 6. Elution profile for Sepharose CL-2B of proteoglycan
isolated from skin fibroblast culture media in a dissociative density gradient. A) D1 fraction with 2 mg added rat chondrosarcoma carrier D1 proteoglycan. B) D1 fraction plus 1% added
hyaluronic acid in relation to 2 mg of carrier proteoglycan; carrier hexuronic acid, (————), [^{35}S]sulfate labeled proteoglycan,
(- - -). The cells were grown from tissue explants and maintained on RPMI-1640 with 10% fetal calf serum. Monolayer cultures of passage cells were labeled at confluence with [^{35}S]sul-
fate (100 μ Ci/ml) for 18 hr and the proteoglycans isolated in the
presence of protease inhibitors in a dissociative cesium chloride
density gradient.

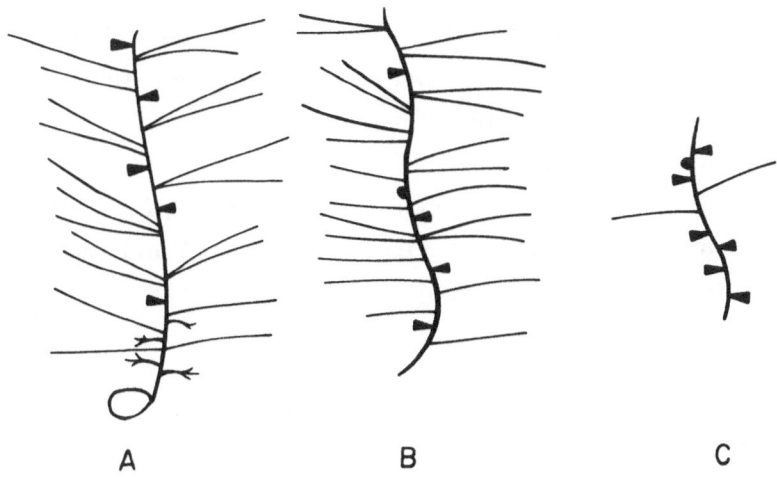

FIG. 7. Generalized model of proteoglycan structure. A) large aggregating proteoglycan, B) large nonaggregating proteoglycan, C) small nonaggregating proteoglycan.

an interaction with hyaluronic acid. These proteoglycan molecules contain about 30% dermatan sulfate and have densities similar to the aorta proteoglycan (Oegema, unpublished results). Fibroblasts from several sources, including meniscus, synovium, and lung, yield similar preparations. Dedifferentiated human chondrocytes also synthesized similar molecules (Oegema, unpublished results). This would mean the major proteoglycan of aorta may represent a more general class of molecules than those found in cartilage (Fig. 7). The aorta dermatan sulfate proteoglycan would have a molecular weight of 2×10^6 and contain a protein core of 1.5×10^5 to 2.0×10^5 with 19 - 25 dermatan sulfate chains per molecule present in the aggregating molecule. The heparan sulfate proteoglycan would be small and contain only a few glycosaminoglycan chains.

The basic knowledge of these structures should lead to experiments to delineate the rates of synthesis, localization, and other critical information that is not currently available but is much needed in this area.

Acknowledgments

The work was supported by grants from the National Cancer Institute, CA22558, the National Heart, Lung and Blood Institute, HL21612 and the National Arthritis, Metabolism and Digestion Disease Institute, AM 27262.

The author wishes to acknowledge the helpful collaboration with Reuben Eisenstein and Vincent C. Hascall and the preparation of the manuscript by Andrea Chatfield.

REFERENCES

Adams P, Muir H (1976) Quantitative changes with age of proteoglycans of human lumbar disc.   Ann Rheum Dis 35: 289-296

Antonopoulos CA, Axelsson I, Heinegård A, Gardell S (1974) Extraction and purification of proteoglycans from various types of connective tissue. Biochim Biophys Acta 338: 108-119

Axelsson I, Heinegård D (1978) Characterization of keratan sulfate proteoglycans from bovine corneal stroma. Biochem J 169: 517-530

Balazs EA, Bothner-By AA, Gergely J (1959) PMR studies on water in the presence of various macromolecular substances. J Mol Biol 1: 147-154

Baker JR, Caterson B (1977) The purification and cyanogen bromide cleavage of the "link proteins" from cartilage proteoglycans.   Biochem Biophys Res Commun 80: 496-503

Baker JR, Caterson B (1979) The isolation and characterization of the link proteins from proteoglycan aggregates of bovine nasal cartilage. J Biol Chem 254: 2387-2393

Baker JR, Cifonelli JA, Rodén L (1975) The linkage of corneal keratan sulfate to protein.   Connect Tiss Res 3: 149-156

Barber AJ, Kaser-Glanzmann R, Jakabova M, Luscher EF (1972) Characterization of a chondroitin-4-sulfate proteoglycan carrier for heparin neutralizing activity (platelet factor 4) released from human blood platelets. Biochim Biophys Acta 286: 312-329

Bettelheim FA, Plessy B (1975) The hydration of proteoglycans of bovine cornea. Biochim Biophys Acta 381:203-214

Bradford-White CJ (1978) Molecular organization of heparan sulfate proteoglycan from human dentine. Arch Oral Biol 23: 1141-1144

Burke JM, Ross R (1979) Synthesis of connective tissue macromolecules by smooth muscle. Int Rev Connect Tiss 8:119-157

Caterson B, Baker JR (1978) The interaction of link proteins with proteoglycan monomer in the absence of hyaluronic acid. Biochem Biophys Res Commun 80: 496-503

Chandrasekaran EV, Spolter L, Marx W (1975) Proteoglycans of soluble fraction of mouse mastocytoma. Prep Biochem 5: 281-303

Choi HO, Meyer K (1975) The structure of keratan sulfate from various sources. Biochem J 151: 543-553

Comper WD, Laurent TC (1978) Physiological function of connective tissue polysaccharides. Physiolog Rev 58: 255-315

Coster L, Carlstedt I, Malmström A (1979) Isolation of ^{35}S and ^{3}H-labeled proteoglycans from cultures of human embryonic skin fibroblasts. Biochem J 183: 669-681

Cuervo LA, Pita JC, Howell DS (1973) Inhibition of calcium phosphate mineral growth by proteoglycan aggregate fractions in a synthetic lymph. Calc Tiss Res 13: 1-10

Damle SP, Kieras FJ, Tzeng W-K, Gregory JD (1979) Isolation and characterization of proteochondroitin sulfate from pig skin. J Biol Chem 254: 1613-1620

Danielsson A, Bjole I (1978) The binding of low-affinity and high-affinity heparin to antithrombin. Eur J Biochem 90: 7-12

DeLuca S, Caplan AI, Hascall VC (1978) Biosynthesis of proteoglycans by chick limb bud chondrocytes. J Biol Chem 253: 4713-4720

DeLuca S, Lohmander LS, Nilsson B, Hascall VC, Caplan AI (1980) Proteoglycans from chick limb bud chondrocyte cultures. J Biol Chem 255: 6077-6083

Deudon E, Picard J (1978) Metabolic heterogeneity of proteoglycans from arterial wall. Int J Biochem 9: 19-26

Ehrlich KC, Radhakrishnamurthy B, Berenson GS (1975) Isolation of a chondroitin sulfate-dermatan sulfate proteoglycan from bovine aorta. Arch Biochem Biophys 171: 361-369

Eisenstein R (1979) Vascular extracellular tissue and atherosclerosis. Artery 5: 207-221

Eisenstein R, Kuettner KE (1976) The ground substance of arterial wall. Part 2, Electron microscopic studies. Atherosclerosis 24: 37-46

Eisenstein R, Larsson SE, Kuettner KE, Sorgente N, Hascall VC (1975) The ground substance of arterial wall. Part 1. Extractability of glycosaminoglycans and the isolation of a proteoglycan from bovine aorta. Atherosclerosis 22: 1-17

Emes JH, Pearce RH (1975) The proteoglycans of the human intervertebral disc. Biochem J 145: 549-556

Faltz LL, Caputo CB, Kimura JH, Schrode J, Hascall VC (1979) Structure of the complex between hyaluronic acid, the hyaluronic acid-binding region, and the link protein of proteoglycan aggregates from the Swarm rat chondrosarcoma. J Biol Chem 254: 1381-1387

Finne J, Krusius T, Margolis RK, Margolis RU (1979) Novel mannitol-containing oligosaccharides obtained by mild alkaline borohydride treatment of a chondroitin sulfated proteoglycan from brain. J Biol Chem 254: 10295-10300

Fransson LÅ (1976) Interactions between dermatan sulfate chains. I. Affinity chromatography of copolymeric galactosaminoglycans on dermatan sulfate-substituted agarose. Biochim Biophys Acta 437: 100-115

Gamse G, Fromme HG, Kresse H (1978) Metabolism of sulfated glycosaminoglycans in cultured endothelial cells and smooth muscle cell from bovine aorta. Biochim Biophys Acta 544: 514–528

Gardell S, Baker JR, Caterson B, Heinegard D, Roden L (1980) Link protein and hyaluronic acid-binding region on components of aorta proteoglycan. Biochem Biophys Res Commun (in press)

Gelman RA, Blackwell J (1974) Collagen-mucopolysaccharide interaction at acid pH. Biochim Biophys Acta 342: 254–261

Glaser JH, Conrad HE (1979) Chondroitin SO_4 catabolism in chick embryo chondrocytes. J Biol Chem 254: 2316–2325

Glatz CE, Massaro TA (1976a) Influence of glycosaminoglycan content on mass transfer behavior of porcine artery wall. Part 1. Diffusive transport of $^{45}Ca^{+2}$ and ^{3}H HO. Atherosclerosis 25: 153–163

Glatz CE, Massaro TA (1976b) Influence of glycosaminoglycan content on mass transfer behavior of porcine artery wall. Part 2. Differences in mass transfer rates related to variations in glycosaminoglycan content. Atherosclerosis 25: 165–173

Greenwald RA, Schwartz CE (1974) Complex formation between lysozyme and cartilage proteoglycans. Biochim Biophys Acta 359: 66–74

Hart GW, Lennartz WJ (1978) Effects of tunicamycin on the biosynthesis of glycosaminoglycans by embryonic chick cornea. J Biol Chem 253: 5795–5801

Hascall VC (1977) Interaction of cartilage proteoglycans with hyaluronic acid. J Supramol Struct 7: 101–120

Hascall VC, Oegema TR, Brown M, Caplan AI (1976) Isolation and characterization of proteoglycans from chick limb bud chondrocytes grown in vitro. J Biol Chem 251: 3511–3519

Hascall VC, Riolo RL (1972) Characterization of the protein-keratan sulfate core and keratan sulfate prepared from bovine nasal cartilage proteoglycan. J Biol Chem 247: 4529–4538

Hascall VC, Sajdera SW (1970) Physical properties and polydispersity of proteoglycan from bovine nasal cartilage. J Biol Chem 245: 4920-4930

Hassell JR, Newsome DA, Hascall VC (1979) Characterization and biosynthesis of proteoglycan of corneal stroma from Rhesus monkey. J Biol Chem 254: 12346-12354

Hedbys BO, Mishima S (1962) Flow of water in the corneal stroma. Exp Eye Res 1: 262-275

Heinegård D, Axelsson I (1977) The distribution of keratan sulfate in cartilage proteoglycans. J Biol Chem 252: 1971-1979

Heinegård D, Hascall VC (1974a) Aggregation of proteolgycans III. Characteristics of proteins isolated from trypsin digests of aggregates. J Biol Chem 249: 4250-4256

Heinegård D, Hascall VC (1974b) Characterization of chondroitin sulfate isolated from trypsin-chymotrypsin digests of cartilage proteoglycans. Arch Biochem Biophys 165: 424-441

Heinegård D, Hascall VC (1979a) Characteristics of the nonaggregating proteoglycans isolated from bovine nasal cartilage. J Biol Chem 254: 927-934

Heinegård D, Hascall VC (1979b) The effects of dansylation and acetylation on the interaction between hyaluronic acid and the hyaluronic acid-binding region of cartilage proteoglycan. J Biol Chem 254: 921-926

Iverius PH (1972) The interaction between human plasma lipoproteins and connective tissue glycosaminoglycans. J Biol Chem 247: 2607-2613

Junqueira LCU, Bignolas G, Maurao PAS, Bonetti SS (1980) Quantitation of collagen-proteoglycan interaction in tissue sections. Connect Tiss Res 7: 91-96

Kieras FJ (1974) The linkage regions of cartilage keratan sulfate protein. J Biol Chem 249: 7506-7513

Kimata K, Oike Y, Ito K, Karasaw K, Suzuki S (1978) The occurrence of low buoyant density proteoglycan in embryonic chick cartilage. Biochem Biophys Res Commun 85: 1431-1439

Kimura JH, Hardingham TE, Hascall VC, Solursh M (1979) Biosynthesis of proteoglycans and their assembly into aggregates in cultures of chondrocytes from the Swarm rat chondrosarcoma. J Biol Chem 254: 2600-2609

Kimura JH, Osdoby P, Caplan AI, Hascall VC (1978) Electron miscroscopic and biochemical studies of proteoglycan polydispersity in chick limb bud chondrocyte cultures. J Biol Chem 253: 4721-4729

Kresse H, Heidel H, Buddecke E (1971) Chemical and metabolic heterogeneity of a bovine aorta chondroitin sulfate dermatan sulfate proteoglycan. Eur J Biochem 22: 557-562

Larjava H, Saarni H, Tammi M, Penttinen R, Rönnemaa T (1980) Cortisol decreases the synthesis of hyaluronic acid by human aortic smooth muscle cells in culture. Athersclerosis 35: 135-143

Laurent TC (1957) On the hydration of macromolecules, x-ray diffraction studies on aqueous solutions of hyaluronic acid. Arkiv Kemi 11: 503-512

Laurent TC, Tengblad A, Thunberg L, Höök M, Lindahl U (1978) The molecular-weight-dependence of the anti-coagulent activity of heparin. Biochem J 175: 691-701

Linn CF, Sokoloff L (1965) Movement and composition of interstitial fluid of cartilage. Arth and Rheum 8: 481-494

Lohmander LS, DeLuca S, Nilsson B, Hascall VC, Caputo CB, Kimura JH, Heinegård D (1980) Oligosaccharides on proteoglycans from the Swarm rat chondrosarcoma. J Biol Chem 255: 6084-6091

Lohmander LS, Hascall VC, Caplan AI (1979) Effects of 4-methyl-umbelliferyl-β-D-xylopyranoside on chondrogenesis and proteoglycan synthesis in chick limb bud mesenchymal cell cultures. J Biol Chem 254: 10551-10561

MacGregor EA, Bowness JM (1971) Interactions of proteoglycans and chondroitin sulfate with calcium or phosphate ions. Can J Biochem 49: 417-425

Malmström A, Rodén L, Feingold DS, Jacobsson I, Backstrom G, Lindahl U (1980) Biosynthesis of heparin partical purification of a uronosyl C-5 epimerase. J Biol Chem 255: 3878-3883

Margolis RU, Lalley K, Kiang W-L, Crockett C, Margolis RK (1976) Isolation and properties of a soluble chondroitin sulfate proteoglycan from brain. Biochem Biophys Res Comm 73: 1018-1024

Maroudas A (1970) Distribution and diffusion of solutes in articular cartilage. Biophys J 10: 365-379

Massaro TA, Glatz CE, Peppas NA, Chisolm GM, Colton CK (1979) Distribution of glycosaminoglycans in consecutive layers of the rabbit aorta. Artery 5: 1-13

Mathews MB (1970) Binding of calcium to proteoglycan of chondroitin sulfate. In: Bulazs EA (ed) Chemistry and Molecular Biology of the Intracellular Matrix. Academic Press, New York, pp. 1121-1123

McMurtre J, Radharishnamurthy B, Dalenes ER, Berenson GS, Gregory JD (1979) Isolation of proteoglycan-hyaluronate complexes from bovine aorta. J Biol Chem 254: 1621-1626

Merrilees MJ, Merrilees MA, Birnbaum PS, Scott PJ, Flint MH (1977) The effect of centrifugal force on glycosaminoglycan production by aortic smooth cells in culture. Atherosclerosis 27: 259-264

Murata K (1978) Differences in the constitution and distribution of acidic glycosaminoglycans in the intimal and adventitial layers of bovine aorta. Connect Tiss Res 6: 131-138

Murata K, Izuka K, Nakazawa K (1978) Effects of acidic glycosaminoglycans in human aortic inner and outer layers on partial thromboplastin time. Atherosclerosis 29: 95-104

Mutoh S, Funakoski I, Yamashina I (1978) Isolation and characterization of proteoheparan sulfate from plasma membranes of an ascites hepatoma AH66. J Biochem Tokyo 84: 483-489

Nakamura H, Nagai Y (1979) Isolation and partial characterization of low sulfated chondroitin 4-sulfate-proteoglycan in bovine blood. Biochim Biophys Acta 579: 361-371

Norling B, Glimerius B, Westermark B, Wasteson Å (1978) A chondroitin sulfate proteoglycan from human cultured glial cell aggregates with hyaluronic acid. Biochem Biophys Res Comm 84: 914-921

Öbrink B (1972) Isolation and partial characterization of a dermatan sulfate proteoglycan from pig skin. Biochim Biophys Acta 264: 354-361

Öbrink B (1973) A study of the interactions between monomeric trophocollagen and glycosaminoglycans. Eur J Biochem 33: 387-400

Öbrink B, Laurent TC, Carlsson B (1975) The binding of chondroitin sulfate to collagen. Fed Eur Biochem Soc Lett 56: 166-169

Öbrink B, Sundelöf L-O (1973) Light-scattering in the study of associating macromolecules. The binding of glycosaminoglycan to collagen. Eur J Biochem 37: 226-232

Oegema TR, Bradford DS, Cooper KM (1979) Aggregated proteoglycan synthesis in organ cultures of human nucleus pulposis. J Biol Chem 254: 10579-10581

Oegema TR, Brown M, Dziewiatkowski DD (1977) The link protein in proteoglycan aggregates from the Swarm rat chondrosarcoma. J Biol Chem 252: 6470-6477

Oegema TR, Hascall VC, Dziewiatkowski DD (1975) Isolation and characterization of proteoglycans from the Swarm rat chondrosarcoma. J Biol Chem 250: 6151-6159

Oegema TR, Hascall VC, Eisenstein R (1979) Characteristics of bovine aorta proteoglycan extracted with guanidine hydrochloride in the presence of protease inhibitors. J Biol Chem 254: 1312-1318

Oegema TR, Laidlaw J, Hascall VC, Dziewiatkowski DD (1975) The effects of proteoglycans on the formation of fibrils from collagen solutions. Arch Biochem Biophys 170: 698-709

Ogston AG (1966) On water binding. Fed Proc 25: 986-989

Oldberg Å, Kjellen L, Höök M (1979) Cell-surface heparan sulfate isolation and characterization of a proteoglycan from rat liver membrane. J Biol Chem 254: 8505-9510

Pearce RH, Grimmer RJ (1970) The nature of ground substances. In: Montagna W, Bentley JP, Dobson RL (eds) Advances in Biology of Skin, Appleton, New York, Vol. X, pp 89-101

Philip B, Kurup PA (1977) Zinc and metabolism of glycosamino-glycans in normal and atherosclerosic rats. Ind J Biochem Biophys 14: 354-358

Pita JC, Muller FJ, Morales SM, Alarcon EJ (1979) Ultracentri-fugal characterization of proteoglycans from rat growth carti-lages. J Biol Chem 254: 10313-10320

Radhakrishnamurthy B, Ruiz H, Berenson GS (1977a) Interac-tions of glycosaminoglycans with collagenase elastin in bovine aorta. Adv Exp Med Biol 82: 160-163

Radhakrishnamurthy B, Ruiz HA, Berenson GS (1977b) Isolation and characterization of proteolgycans from bovine aorta. J Biol Chem 252: 4831-4841

Radhakrishnamurthy B, Ruiz HA, Dalferes ER, Friedman M, Seethanathan P, Berenson GS (1978) Connective tissue com-position of aortas from non-human primates: a comparative study. Atherosclerosis 29: 25-38

Richmond ME, DeLuca S, Silbert JE (1973) Biosynthesis of chon-droitin sulfate, microsomal acceptor of sulfate, glucuronic acid and N-acetylgalactosamine. Biochem 12: 3898-3903

Robinson HC, Horner AA, Höök M, Ogren S, Lindahl U (1978) A proteoglycan form of heparin and it's degradation to single-chain molecules. J Biol Chem 253: 6687-6693

Rodén L, Baker JR, Helting T, Schwartz NB, Stoolmiller AC, Yamagata S, Yamagata T (1972) Biosynthesis of chondroitin sulfate. Methods of Enzymol 28: 638-676

Rodén L, Horowitz MI (1978) Structure and biosynthesis of con-nective tissue proteoglycans. In: Horowitz MI, Pigman W (eds) The Glycoconjugates, Academic Press, New York, Vol. II, pp 3-71

Rokosova B, Bentley JP (1979) Biosynthesis of aorta collagen and glycosaminoglycans following immunological injury. Atherosclerosis 32: 359-365

Sandy JD, Brown HLG, Lowther DA (1978) Degradation of proteoglycans in articular cartilage. Biochim Biophys Acta 543: 536-544

Sheehan JK, Nieduskynaki IA, Phelps CF, Muir H, Hardingham TE (1978) Self-association of proteoglycan subunits from pig larynegeal cartilage. Biochem J 171: 109-114

Sirek OV, Cukerman E, Sirek A (1978) The relationship of hormones to arterial glycosaminoglycans and atherosclerosis. Med Hypothesis 4: 531-539

Stevens RL, Binette JP, Kimura A, Nimberg RB, Schmid K (1977) A low molecular weight glycosaminoglycan from the human aorta. Experientia 33: 1282-1283

Stevens RL, Colombo M, Gonzales JJ, Hollander W, Schmid K (1976) The glycosaminoglycan of the human artery and their changes in atherosclerosis. J Clin Invest 58: 470-481

Stevens RL, Ewins RJF, Revell PA, Muir H (1979) Proteoglycans of the intervertebral disc: Homology of structure with laryngeal proteoglycans. Biochem J 179: 561-572

Tammi M, Ronnema A, Vihersaari T, Lehtonen A, Vhkari J (1979) High density lipoproteinemia due to vigorous physical work inhibits the incorporation of [^{3}H]thymidine and synthesis of glycosaminoglycans by human aortic smooth muscle cells in culture. Atherosclerosis 32: 23-32

Toledo OMS, Mauras PAS (1979) Sulfated glycosaminoglycans of human aorta; chondroitin 6-sulfate increase with age. Biochem Biophys Res Commun 89: 50-55

Toole BP, Lowther DA (1968) Dermatan sulfate-protein: Isolation from and interaction with collagen. Arch Biochem Biophys 128: 567-578

Truppe W, Kresse H (1978) Uptake of proteoglycans and sulfated glycosaminoglycans by cultured skin fibroblasts. Eur J Biochem 85: 351-358

Ts'ao C-H, Eisenstein R, Schumacker B (1977) Effect of an aortic proteoglycan on platelet aggregation and thrombin time: Plasma requirement and active moieties. Proc Soc Expt'l Biol Med 156: 162-167

Upholt WB, Vertel BM, Dorfman A (1979) Characterization of messenger RNA's in differentiating chicken cartilage. Proc Natl Acad Sci USA 79: 4847-4851

Verlangieri AJ, Stevens JW (1979) L ascorbic acid: Effects on aortic glycosaminoglycan ^{35}S incorporation in rabbit induced atherogenesis. Blood Vessels 16: 177-185

Vijayagopal P, Radhakrishnamurthy B, Srinivasan SR, McMurtney J, Berenson GS (1980) Proteoglycan synthesis and secretion by bovine aorta tissue in organ culture. Artery 6: 458-470

Vogel HG (1978) Influence of maturation and age on mechanical and biochemical parameters of connective tissue of various organs in rat. Connect Tiss Res 6: 161-166

von Figura K, Kioloski W, Buddeke E (1975) Metabolic characteristics of different types of chondroitin sulfate-dermatan sulfate hybrids in arterial tissue. Hoppe Seyler Z Physiol Chem 356: 1517-1525

Wagner WD, Salisbury BGJ (1978) Aortic total glycosaminoglycan and dermatan sulfate changes in atherosclerotic rhesus monkeys. Lab Invest 39: 322-328

Wiederhielm CA (1972) The interstitial space. In: Fung YC, Perrone N, Anliker M, (eds) Biomechanics in Foundation and Objectives. Prentice Hall, Englewood Cliff, New Jersey, pp 273-286

Wight TN (1980) Vessel proteoglycans and thrombogenesis. In: Spaet TH (ed) Progress in Hemostasis and Thrombosis. Grune and Stratton, Inc. Vol. 5: 1-39

Wight TN, Ross R (1975) Proteoglycans in primate arteries. I. ultrastructural localization and distribution in the intima. J Cell Biol 67: 660-674

Yanagishita M, Hascall VC (1979) Biosynthesis of proteoglycans
by rat granulosa cell culture in vitro. J Biol Chem 254:
12355-12364

Yanagishita M, Rodhand D, Hascall VC (1979) Isolation and characterization of proteoglycans from porcine ovarian follicular
fluid. J Biol Chem 254: 911-920

Discussion

Chandler. Beta lipoprotein and fibrinogen are present in virtually 100% of fatty streaks. You showed how beta lipoprotein
tended to bind to proteoglycans. Is there any information on
the binding of fibrinogen to proteoglycans, and might this have
an effect on stimulating the proliferative response in atherosclerosis?

Oegema. As far as I know, there is no information about
binding of fibrinogen or fibrin to proteoglycans. However, the
hypothesis that proteoglycans are involved primarily in progression of atherosclerosis is a controversial one and one I have
tried to avoid since it is just at the hypothetical stage. If there
were injury to the arterial wall, perhaps there would be only
limited thrombus formation because the proteoglycan, which is
probably made by the smooth muscle, would be a dermatan sulfate type and would allow a small thrombus to accumulate, but
would not promote large thrombus formation and platelet aggregation (Ts'ao C-H, Eisenstein R, Schumacker B [1977] Effect of an
aortic proteoglycan on platelet aggregation and thrombin time:
plasma requirement and active moieties. Proc Soc Expt'l Biol
Med 156: 162-167). This would be an ideal protecting mechanism
for the organism. Wight (Wight TN, Ross R [1975] Proteoglycans in primate arteries. I. Ultrastructural localization and distribution in the intima. J Cell Biol 67: 660-674) who used bal-
loon catheters to denude arteries, has watched the repair process as endothelial cells grow back again. Histochemically he
does not see early plaque formation with the denuded smooth

muscle, but rather finds it after the endothelial cells have over-grown the area. Apparently the seat of this problem is a whole new set of reactions that haven't been defined yet.

McDonald. You showed us the biochemical aspects of how proteoglycan molecules are synthesized and aggregated. Would you comment on the role of the cell in this process?

Oegema. This is obviously of great interest. Hascall and Kimura (Kimura JH, Hardingham TE, Hascall VC, Solursh M [1979] Biosynthesis of proteoglycans and their assembly into aggregates in cultures of chondrocytes from the Swarm rat chondrosarcoma. J Biol Chem 254: 2600-2609) and others have some interesting results in chondrocyte culture, mostly with the Swarm rat chondrosarcoma system. Apparently, the aggregating proteoglycan monomer is secreted and bound to the link protein but is not attached to hyaluronic acid. In other words, it is not an aggregate. These molecules, over a period of time, assemble themselves outside the cell in the matrix on the hyaluronic acid molecule. Proteoglycan researchers are just becoming aware of how you localize or place proteoglycans in the tissue after you get them out of the cell. For example, we found recently in some disease states, such as steroid-induced avascular necrosis, that there may be a delay in aggregation and assembly in the matrix.

Snider. In talking about the functions of proteoglycans, you referred to their role in the microenvironment. Please comment on what role proteoglycans might play in the mechanical behavior of the entire aorta.

Oegema. I think this is an area for a lot of research in the future. Proteoglycans may act as a lubricant to prevent collagen fibers from rubbing against each other and mechanically degrading each other, or they may exclude some molecules from an area and greatly alter the microenvironment. This means that you would find regions in the tissue where, although the overall proteoglycan concentration of the tissue would be low, the proteoglycans would effectively function as if they were present in high concentrations. Since there are also different classes of proteoglycans, such as nonaggregating heparan sulfate proteoglycans, they may have very specialized functions.

Glagov. On that same line, both cells and matrix fibers are highly oriented and aligned structures in normally distended arteries, and several investigators have shown that proteoglycan structures are arranged in a very regular array between collagen fibrils in relation to the collagen bands. Considering that proteoglycans are polar molecules forming an extensive interstitial continuum among artery wall cells and fibers, is it not likely that these molecules play some role in organizing and aligning collagen fibers along lines of mechanical stress?

Oegema. I think we are going to have to look at two different things -- first, at the initial development of the organ as function begins and, second, at the maintenance of that matrix after the organ is functioning. There is some suggestion, for example, that in corneal development the proteoglycans may function in the alignment of collagen fibers in the initial organ development. However, they might serve an entirely different function after the organ is functional. I don't think proteoglycans in aorta would affect collagen orientation relative to the strain, but they may affect its alignment relative to other collagen fibers. Even though there is only a small amount of proteoglycans present, they may well affect the alignment and perhaps allow movement past one another of the fibers without rubbing.

Kramsch. I have a question about the proteoglycans that are associated with elastin. Do you have any recent information on their composition? It has been said that the proteoglycans that coat the elastin may protect it from enzymatic degradation.

Oegema. I don't have any recent evidence for the organization of elastin and proteoglycans. Work in which the aorta is sequentially extracted with different chemicals and enzymes, suggests that heparan sulfate proteoglycan may be tightly bound to elastin (Radhakrishnamurthy B, Ruiz H, Berenson GS [1977] Interactions of glycosaminoglycans with collagenase elastin in

bovine aorta.   Adv Exp Med Biol 82: 160-163).   However, this is
only suggestive and there has not been any definitive work in
this area.

Quantitation of Cells and Fibers in Histologic Sections of Arterial Walls: Advantages of Contour Tracing on a Digitizing Plate

SEYMOUR GLAGOV, JOSEPH GRANDE,
DRAGA VESSELINOVITCH, and CHRISTOPHER K. ZARINS

A major objective of the study of histologic sections is the elucidation of the relation of structure to function under normal and abnormal conditions. Utilizing appropriate staining procedures for identification of specific components, comparisons of sections taken in orthogonal planes and reconstructions from serial sections have provided insights into details of microarchitecture (Bernimoulin and Schroeder 1977; Elias and Henning 1967; Takahashi and Suwa 1978; Underwood 1970). Morphometric techniques may also be applied to individual histologic sections in order to derive quantitative estimates of tissue composition and to establish the shape, dimensions, and orientation of cell and tissue components. Extrapolations of volume and surface features of these components from measurements on cross-sectional profiles are based on a series of geometric considerations and measurement procedures that comprise the analytical method known as stereology.

For clinical purposes, estimates of tissue composition and architecture from histologic preparations are usually sufficient for assessment of tissue response or diagnosis of disease without recourse to numerical determinations. Principles of stereologic analysis are nevertheless implicit in such examinations, for cells, organelles, connective tissue fibers, and other microscopic struc-

tures are reduced to 2-dimensional profiles on tissue sections
and the observer makes a number of assumptions that permit
comparisons with previously studied material. These include the
conviction that the section under study is representative of the
tissue from which it was taken, that the structural relationships
were maintained or modified in some consistent manner throughout
processing, and that sectioning and staining procedures are more
or less uniform from section to section. The observer has also
learned by experience the stereologic principal that it is not possible to determine the 3-dimensional shape or size of a component
from a single profile. A circular profile, for example, may result from section of an ellipsoidal, cylindrical, conical, or irregular volume as well as from section of a spherical volume (Weibel
1973). Thus, even an approximate estimate of the shape and/or
size of a repeated tissue structure requires inspection of many
of its profiles.

Although most diagnostic criteria can be established on the
basis of impressions derived from thorough inspection of more or
less standard preparations by an experienced observer, application of stereologic morphometric methods for the precise quantitative determination of tissue composition from tissue sections offers several advantages over pattern recognition or chemical
analysis. Subtle changes in number, configuration, or size of
cells, organelles, fibers, and other tissue structures may reflect
profound changes in function even when their relative sizes and
concentrations are not markedly altered. Significant differences
may become apparent only after computations are made from careful measurements on many cross sections. Contiguous or closely
associated structures such as microscopic lesions or tissue components distributed in spatial gradients of size or concentration
are not readily isolated for chemical analysis, while specific areas
for study can be identified and quantitated readily on sections.
Samples or sections available for study may be inadequate or
unsuitable for chemical analysis but determinations from a single
tissue section may provide quantitative information which reflects

chemical composition. Finally, quantitative relationships can be established among overall dimensions, microarchitectural details, and chemical composition in the same tissue section.

We have been preoccupied for a number of years with the relation of structure to function in arterial walls and have applied a number of histometric techniques to such studies. These studies have resulted in an improved view of the functional architecture of arterial walls (Wolinsky and Glagov 1964, 1967a, 1967b, 1969; Clark and Glagov 1979). We have also wished to apply stereologic methods to artery sections to determine quantitative differences in mural composition and component orientation which correspond to altered hemodynamic states and to anatomically defined locations, and to assess the composition of arterial lesions in relation to lesion size, shape, and location. If such determinations are to be used to establish differences related to a variety of experimental conditions or to clinical data of individual patients, evidence must be furnished that fixation, sampling and sectioning methods are sufficiently uniform to produce comparable specimens, that staining or other component enhancing methods are sensitive and specific enough to correspond to chemically or morphologically distinct structures, that differences due to experimentally induced changes are distinguishable from differences related to the location of the field used for measurement, that the morphometric methods employed are suited to the size, shape, and configuration of the component to be measured, and that measurements are not only accurate and reproducible but obtainable on a large series of specimens in a reasonable time.

Differential staining of components of artery walls and arterial lesions can be accomplished by any of several methods. We have found the Weigert - Van Gieson technique particularly useful for connective tissue fibers, especially since Dr. Puchtler and her associates (Sweat et al. 1964) taught us several years ago to utilize sirius red for sharp and relatively uniform identification of collagen with minimal subsequent fading. We have also been able to reduce the tedium and improve the accuracy of stereologic measurements, improve data storage and retrievability, and accelerate computation. These improvements have been achieved by projecting microscopic images onto the surface of a digitizing plate and utilizing signals produced by a tracing cursor or stylus to record data on tape in conjunction with suitable computer programs which process the data rapidly. Such advances greatly enhance the feasibility of applying quantitative methods to large numbers of specimens. We have presented the methods we now use to quantitate that size, shape, and occlusiveness of experimental atherosclerotic lesions elsewhere (Wissler et al. 1980).

In preparation for extensive studies of the composition of vessels and lesions which now appear to be possible, we have undertaken a series of studies designed to establish standard methods of sampling, processing, and measuring. Data obtained from aortas fixed by controlled pressure perfusion are being compared with those obtained from aortas fixed by excision and immersion in order to determine the effects of spatial distortion. The contributions of section thickness and staining techniques to differences in volume fraction determinations are under study. The relative merits and problems related to contour tracing, line segment measurement, and point counting are being investigated. The reproducibility of measurements are being tested with respect to identification of components and with respect to selection of fields. It is our intent in this report to present illustrative data that indicate that tracing and analysis of contours by means of a projector - digitizer - computer system provides an accurate and efficient method for determining lesion, cell and structural fiber composition of arteries and to identify some of the precautions that should be considered before definite conclusions can be reached.

Materials and Methods

Stereologic Principles and Determinations

The basis for stereologic determinations was established by Delesse when he found that the volume density of constituents of rocks could be estimated from measurements of the relative areas occupied by their profiles on random cross sections. Other early contributors of basic and seminal concepts for determining volume fractions from surface measurements, such as Rosiwal, Glagolev, and Chalkley, have been acknowledged by more recent investigators who have contributed to the development of these methods (Weibel 1969). Delesse showed that A_a, the relative area occupied by a constituent on a cross section, is equal to V_v, the relative volume of the component in the specimen. There are several techniques by which measurements can be made on cross-sectional surfaces in order to arrive at estimates of V_v. These include a) tracing of the profile contours, b) measurement of line segments which traverse the profiles, and c) counting points which fall on the profiles.

With the contour method, profiles of the component i to be measured, are traced. The areas delineated by the tracings are summed to give A_i and compared to the total test area A_t. The ratio A_i/A_t is A_a. The total area occupied by a component can, for example, be estimated simply by tracing the contours onto paper, cutting them out, and weighing them. The contours can also be fitted to a suitable geometric figure whose area is easily determined or else analyzed by means of a numerical integration.

The line method reduces the measurement procedure by one dimension. A series of random test line segments are superimposed on the section. The ratio of the total length of the test line segments falling on the component i to the total length of the superimposed test lines is L_i/L_t. This ratio L_l can be shown to be equal to A_a and therefore to V_v.

The point counting technique is based on the idea that the number of random points falling on the profiles, divided by the total number of points on the test area, i.e., P_i/P_t, also gives an estimate of A_a and therefore of V_v. This method may be rationalized as follows: To find A_a by the contour method as described above, the area of all contours of the component i would be summed. If the test area were divided into small squares of side length l, A_i could be approximated by counting the squares lying inside the profiles of the component i and multiplying the total number of squares by the area of each square, $P_i l^2$. The total area A_t may be calculated as $P_t L^2$. Therefore, A_a, which is equal to A_i/A_t, is given by $P_i l^2/P_t L^2$ or P_i/P_t. Both the point counting and line methods have been utilized by superimposing suitable grids on photographed or projected images and by viewing microscopic preparations through optical systems with suitable reticles mounted in the eyepiece plane of focus (Henning 1958). Variations include the utilization of moveable cross hairs coupled to micrometer spindles for measurement of line segment lengths which traverse profiles.

Statistical analysis has shown that the contour method is more accurate than point counting for determining the area of an individual profile, but that point counting is at least as accurate as contour tracing for summing areas of large numbers of profiles. Since an individual profile may not be representative of the population of profiles and many profiles must be measured when point counting is used, ease of data aquisition becomes an important criterion for selecting the optimal test system for a given problem. Point counting might be the method of choice based upon ease of direct numerical determination, but could be excessively time consuming. The number of points required for analysis may be estimated from formula $P_t=0.453(1-V_v)/V_v E^2(V_v)$, where $E^2(V_v)$ is the error and V_v is the estimated volume fraction (Weibel and Bolender 1973). It can also be shown that the total length of all profile boundaries per unit area of section B_a, may be used to estimate the surface density S_v of a component using the relation $S_v=4/\pi B_a$ (Weibel 1969). The number of objects in a unit volume N_v, may also be obtained by counting the objects

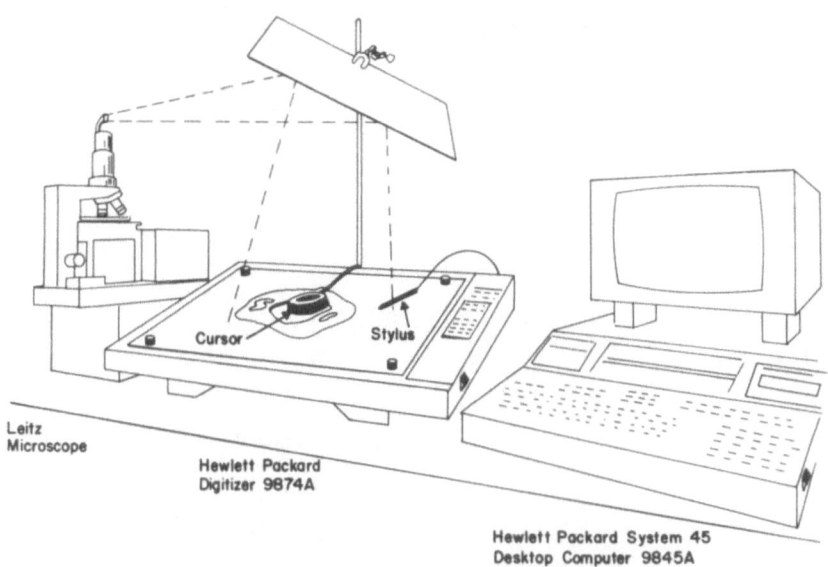

FIG. 1. Semidiagramatic drawing of equipment used for stereo-logic determination. At the left is a microprojector mounted on a moveable and adjustable frame. The image is reflected onto the digitizer plate in the center by means of an adjustable mirror. The contours, lines, or points are traced or counted by means of a cursor or stylus, and the data is processed by the desk top computer at the right. (From A. Gotto, L. Smith, B. Allen Atherosclerosis V, International Symposium on Atherosclerosis. New York, Springer-Verlag, 1980)

in a unit area, N_a. $N_v = N_a/D$, where D is the mean diameter of the object. Object size may be estimated from the relation $D = kL_3$, where L_3 is the mean length of chords of linear intercepts formed by random test lines. $L_3 = 4$ v/s, where v/s is the volume to surface ratio. For spheres, $K = 3/2$ (Underwood 1970).

The data which form the basis of the present report were obtained by utilizing the contour, line, and point counting methods to analyze projected images of histologic sections. The images were projected onto the plate of a Hewlett-Packard 9878 Digitizer by means of a Neo-Promar projecting microscope (Leitz). Data were stored and analyzed by means of a Hewlett-Packard 9845A computer. This digitizer - computer combination is known as the Hewlett-Packard System 45. A semidiagramatic drawing of our

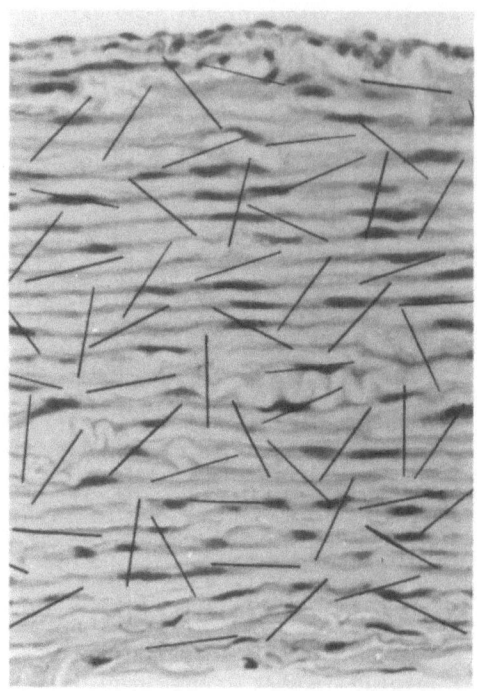

FIG. 2. For determinations of volume fractions by the line measurement method, the artery wall image is superimposed on an array of randomly oriented line segments. The section is that of an incompletely distended rabbit aorta. Stained with hematoxylin and eosin. X 340

apparatus is shown in Fig. 1. An adjustable mirror was used to reflect the microscopic image onto the digitizing plate. The projector was mounted on a rigid but moveable frame so that image magnification could be varied not only by changing microscope objectives but also by varying the distance between projector and mirror. Projector, mirror, and digitizing plate orientation could be adjusted to minimize image distortion. The distance between selected points on a calibrating slide with an engraved scale was entered into the computer at the start of each determination. Programs were written to enable recording, storage, and analysis of contours, lines, and points. The system provides for the display on a cathode ray screen and for printing on

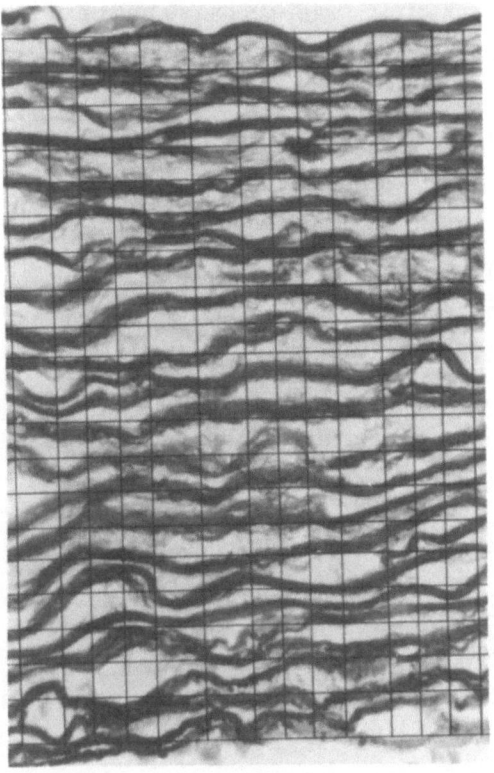

FIG. 3. For determinations of volume fraction by point counting, the artery wall image is superimposed on a grid of two sets of mutually perpendicular randomly spaced lines, the intersections of which are the points to be counted. The section is of a proximal sample of an undistended rabbit aorta stained by the Weigert – Van Gieson method. X 340

paper of the contours, lines or points as well as the computations associated with each determination.

The contour method was applied by tracing the contours of nuclei, elastin fibers, collagen fibers, and total field of examination with a cursor furnished with cross hairs and equipped with signaling switches to identify the beginning and end of each trace and to store a sequence of traces for future analysis. For the line method, images were projected onto an array of random line segments (Fig. 2) drawn on a sheet of paper mounted on the digitizer plate; line segments were measured by means of the cursor. Point counting was accomplished by projecting images onto a grid of randomly spaced mutually perpendicular parallel lines (Fig. 3) generated by a computer program and counting the intersections as points by means of a stylus. For most of the point counting a grid of 400 random points was used. A random array was used in order to minimize errors associated with the anisotropic arrangement of artery wall structures. Each determination was repeated at least four times. Statistical significance of differences was determined by means of Student's t test. Programs developed for both measurements and analysis will be presented elsewhere. It is the purpose of this communication to present data dealing with problems of validation and standardization of stereologic methods as applied to vessels.

Effects of Section Thickness and Stains

The fact that a histologic section is not a simple surface of transection but is instead a slice of finite thickness introduces measurement errors. Opaque constituents tend to be overestimated while translucent structures may be underestimated. In general, the ratio of section thickness T to object diameter D determines the extent of overestimation of opaque objects due to section thickness; the greater the ratio, the greater the overestimation. Correction factors have been provided for spheres, $V_v = V_{vo}/1 + 3T/2D$; and for plates, $V_v = V_{vo}/1 + T/2D$, where V_{vo} is the volume fraction determined by an appropriate method (Weibel and Bolender 1973). Translucent, lightly stained, or relatively small objects are underestimated because they tend to be masked by dense, intensely stained, and relatively large objects when polychromatic staining procedures are used.

In order to assess the closely related effects of section thickness, and element size, we prepared 3-, 4-, and 7-μm thick sections of the same vessel blocks and compared the effects on volume fraction determinations of nuclei, elastin fibers, and collagen fibers. Nuclei are well-circumscribed objects, easily distinguished and usually encompassed within the thickness of the section. Elastin fibers are more or less distinct, depending on fiber size; although their lateral margins are discernable, their limits in the direction of maximum length are difficult to identify. Collagen fibers are the least clearly defined in all dimensions, and many are too fine to be identified with certainty. The effect of staining intensity and overlap was investigated by applying two different polychromatic stains, the Weigert - Van Gieson and the Gomori trichrome aldehyde - fuchsin methods, and by utilizing separately the agents that identify the various components. The Weigert - Van Gieson stains elastin intensely and collagen moderately well, while the Gomori trichrome aldehyde - fuchsin stains elastin moderately and is not entirely specific for collagen. Nuclei were best studied on standard hematoxylin and eosin preparations.

Effects of Fixation and Processing

Although section shrinkage due to processing will not affect volume fraction determinations if all components are equally shrunken or compressed, this condition may not hold in many cases. Fixation of tissues by simple immersion of excised samples may also result in estimates that are different from those made on tissues fixed by controlled pressure perfusion. The relative volume of tissue interstices is, in general, increased by perfusion, especially when the interstices consist of relatively loose connective tissue and total tissue volume expands due to perfusion. In highly organized, dense tissues, such as artery walls, configuration of medial and intimal components are greatly altered when distending pressures are absent or lower than normal. Although total volume of an arterial wall may be unchanged by intraluminal distention, the increase in radius and circumference associated with increasing distending pressures from zero to normal levels is accompanied by thinning of the wall, elongation and circumferential orientation of cells and fibers, and closer radial approximation of the fibroelastic elements (Wolinsky and

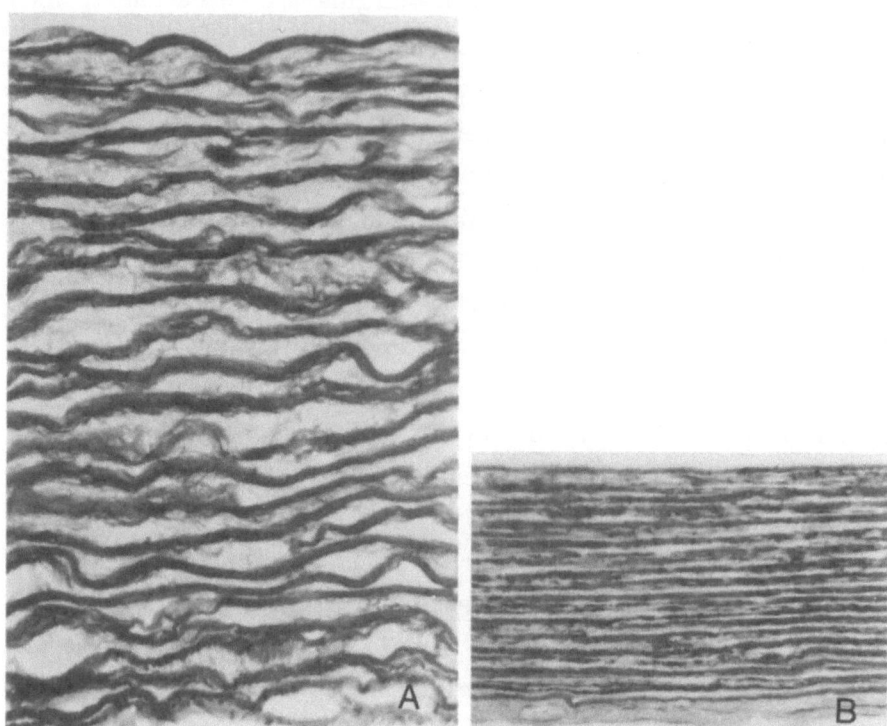

FIG. 4.   Comparison of configuration of the aortic media sampled
from undistended (A) and distended (B) vessels. Each section
is from the proximal thoracic aorta of an animal weighing approximately 1500 g.   Controlled pressure distention during fixation
results in a much thinner wall, straightened and somewhat narrowed elastin lamellae, and markedly reduced interlamellar distances.   Both sections are stained by the Weigert - Van Gieson
method.   X 340

Glagov 1964).   Thus, interstices in the media are less prominent
in cross sections when normal distending pressures are maintained during fixation than when excised specimens are immersion
fixed (Fig. 4).

Volume fractions of components may therefore be quite different in perfused and nonperfused material, depending on the tissue under study.   Rigid structures may be expected to maintain

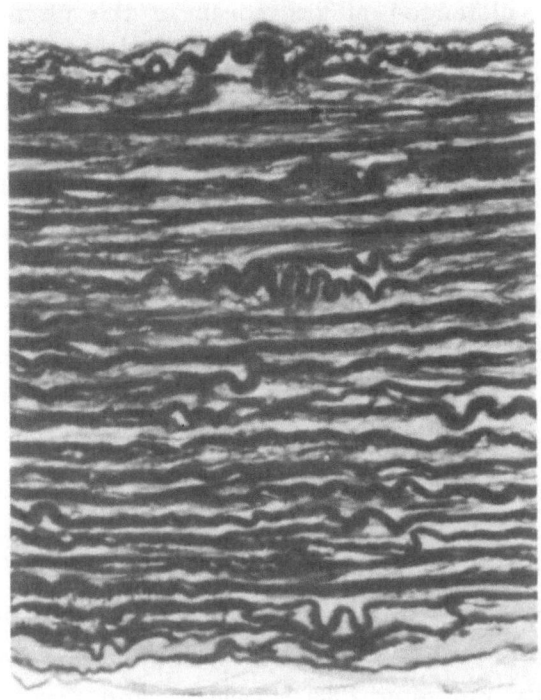

FIG 5.   Incompletely distended aorta shows thinning of media intermediate between the vessels shown in Figs. 4A and 4B, persistence of wavy elastin lamellae, and variation in interlamellar
distances. Weigert - Van Gieson.   X 390

the same volume whether fixed by perfusion or immersion, but
deformability in any dimension would be expected to alter configurations, curvatures, and relative positions of components. De-
formations of relatively plastic structures by fixation and processing techniques would not usually affect determinations of
component surface areas, but would create marked differences in
volume fraction determinations and surface to volume ratios.

For the aorta, one may also expect to find gradients in the
distribution and concentration of structural materials with respect
to distance across the wall from the lumen (Feldman and Glagov
1971), with respect to position about the circumference, and with
respect to distance along the aorta from the heart (Cleary 1963).

To determine the effects of distention, some vessels were fixed in situ while distended at pressures in the physiologic range, while others were removed before fixation and fixed by immersion of excised segments. Histologic examination sometimes revealed incomplete distention during controlled pressure fixation as judged by incomplete straightening of elastin lamellae (Fig. 5). Samples were removed from several standard sites to assess the effects on different locations along the aorta. Measurements were made at four arbitrary positions 90° apart on circular sections to evaluate differences related to circumferential position. Determinations were made in the inner half and in the outer half of the media at each of the four circumferential positions to reveal effects of transmural gradients.

Fixation and Sampling Procedures

The material presented here was obtained from a group of four New Zealand white rabbits weighing 1550 - 1620 g, a group of four rabbits weighing 2200 - 2400 g, and from a cynomolgous monkey weighing 4.25 kg. Two rabbits of each group were used to obtain controlled pressure perfusion fixed aortas while two were used to obtain unperfused aortas and material for chemical analysis. The monkey aorta was not fixed by perfusion.

Controlled pressure perfusion fixation of the aorta in situ was performed utilizing procedures described in detail elsewhere (Clark and Glagov 1979). In brief, animals were anesthetized with sodium pentobarbital (50/mg/kg body wt). The right carotid and femoral arteries and the left iliac vein were then cannulated. The arterial cannulae were passed into the thoracic and abdominal aortic segments just beyond the branch orifices. The femoral artery cannula was connected to a strain gauge in order to monitor intra-aortic pressure, and the carotid cannula was connected to the manifold of a pressure system. Pressure was regulated by means of a Nullmatic pressure control valve (Model 40-7; Moore, Inc.) connected to a pressure reservoir. The reservoir was connected to flasks containing buffered normal saline or 2.5% buffered glutaraldehyde; the outflow of each was connected to the outlet manifold. The perfusion mixture could therefore be switched from saline solution to fixative without any drop in pressure. Saline and fixative solutions were maintained at 37°C and monitored pressure was maintained at 90 mmHg by control of the pressure valve and the venous efflux. Normal saline was introduced initially until the efflux from the venous catheter was clear of blood and the manifold control was then switched to the fixative. Perfusion fixation was carried out for 30 minutes.

Upon completion of fixation, the abdomen and thorax were opened and sutures placed in the periaortic tissue at points one-fourth and three-fourths of the distance between the ligamentum arteriosum and the superior mesenteric artery. The aorta was then removed carefully and circular samples removed at three standard positions: at the suture markings (proximal and distal thoracic), and between the superior mesenteric and renal arteries (abdominal). The sections were stored in 2.5% glutaraldehyde and subsequently processed through graded alcohol and xylene solutions and embedded in paraffin. Sequential sections of each sample, cut at thicknesses of 3, 5, and 7 μm, were stained by means of the Weigert – Van Gieson procedure, utilizing sirius red as the collagen stain (Sweat et al. 1964), by the Gomori trichrome – aldehyde fuchsin (Gomori 1950) method, and also sirius red alone for collagen and aldehyde fuchsin alone for elastin. Separate sections were stained by standard hematoxylin and eosin procedures.

Aortas prepared for study without controlled pressure perfusion fixation were obtained from animals killed by an overdose of anesthetic. The sampling positions were marked in situ, the aorta removed, and the sections processed and stained in the same manner as those obtained from perfusion fixed animals. In addition, the remaining unfixed proximal and distal aortic segments from the unperfused animals were stored for chemical determinations.

Chemical Determinations

The aortic segments obtained for chemical determinations were
not pooled. Each of the two segments from each animal were analyzed separately for DNA, elastin, and collagen content. Adventitia was removed by sharp dissection according to the method
of Wolinsky and Daly (1970). The resulting intima - media preparation was then minced and delipidated by extraction with a
3:1 absolute ethanol:anhydrous ether mixture. The tissue was
then extracted in anhydrous ether for 1 day and dried in a
vacuum oven at 50C° for 3 days. The material was then weighed
and divided into two portions for DNA analysis and collagen-elas-
tin determination.

DNA. The tissue set aside for DNA analysis was digested in
1N NaOH for 1 day in a 37°C water bath. The solutions were
then neutralized with HCl, and trichloroacetic acid (TCA) was
added at 0°C to make a 5% solution of TCA. BSA (0.25 mg/ml)
was added to facilitate the precipitation of DNA and protein.
The TCA precipitation was repeated followed by chilling for 30
minutes in ice. DNA was solubilized and thereby separated from
the protein pellet by adding 5N perchloric acid and heating in a
70°C water bath twice for 10 minutes; the pellet was resuspended
between the two 70°C solubilizations. DNA concentrations were
determined by the diphenylamine method of Burton (1956) modified by Richards (1974).

Collagen and Elastin. Analysis for collagen and elastin was
carried out by the method of Lansing et al. (1952). Samples
were suspended in 0.1N NaOH and heated in a 98°C water bath
for 50 minutes. The alkali extract was separated from the insoluble residue. The insoluble residue was washed twice with 0.1N
NaOH and once with distilled water. The alkali and distilled
water washes were pooled with the alkali extract. Two ml 6N
HCl was added to the insoluble residue. The extract and pool
washes were adjusted to 6N HCl with concentrated HCl. Both
the elastin and collagen extract and the elastin residue were hy-
drolized in a glycerol bath at 105°C for 40 hours. One milliliter

aliquots of the hydrolyzates were taken and dried under a vacuum with phosphorus pentoxide and solid sodium hydroxide. Elastin was determined by a modification of the Kjeldahl procedure for nitrogen (Ballentine 1957). A nitrogen content of 14.8% was used for elastin. Collagen was determined by a modification (Martin and Axelrod 1953) of the method of Newman and Logan (1950) for hydroxyproline. A hydroxyproline content of 14.4% was assumed for collagen.

Results and Comments

Comparison Contour Tracing, Line Measurement, and Point Counting Techniques

Determinations by the three surface measurement methods were usually comparable with respect to standard deviation when obtained from measurements repeated on the same field with the identical line-array or point-grid left in the same position each time. Table 1 shows typical volume fractions obtained in this manner on a thoracic aorta section, for nuclei utilizing hematoxylin and eosin stain, for elastin using the aldehyde fuchsin method, and for collagen utilizing sirius red only. The line array consisted of 26 random line segments 1.25 cm long on the projection surface, corresponding to 7.44 μm on the specimen field; the point counting grid consisted of 400 points/field. For the number of lines, points, and contours used, determinations for nuclei and elastin by line measurement or point counting took two to three times longer than by contour tracing; for collagen, time consumed was about the same by all methods. The findings give some indication of standard deviations to be expected for a given set of conditions due to problems encountered by the observer in identifying and delineating the elements to be measured and in performing the measurement operations. The relatively low standard deviations for all of the methods may be attributable in part to observer recognition of identical details seen and repetition of identical measurement decisions.

TABLE 1.   Comparison of Volume Fractions Obtained by Different
Methods of Surface Measurement: Fixed Field and
Grid Orientation[a]

Method	Elastin	Collagen	Nuclei
Contour tracing	31.8 ± 0.77%	8.95 ± 1.17%	5.4 ± 0.50%
Line intersections	34.8 ± 1.98%	8.70 ± 1.42%	6.8 ± 0.48%
Point counting	34.4 ± 1.09%	9.41 ± 1.00%	7.4 ± 0.30%

[a]All determinations are of proximal thoracic aortic sections.

Standard deviations were always lowest for elastin determinations by the contour method and were similar or lower by the
contour method than by line or point counting for nuclei or collagen.   Standard deviations were consistently higher for collagen
determinations regardless of the method used.   Mean values consistently showed the greatest range among the methods for the
nuclear determinations, and mean values obtained by line method
or point counting were overall somewhat higher than by contour
tracing.   Increasing the number of randomized lines or points
resulted in closer approximation of mean values obtained by the
various methods, but there was little change in standard deviations.

The relatively high standard deviation for collagen estimation
probably corresponds to the difficulty in delineating collagen
fibers even in repeated examinations of the same portions of the
same fibers by the same observer.   This is due to the considerable range of fiber size, relative irregularity of fiber distribution, and the variable degree of approximation of individual fine
fibrils into distinct bundles (Fig. 6).   Although mean values of
nuclear volume fraction were similar for the line or point methods
and were greater than those obtained by contour determination,
determinations utilizing denser arrays of random lines and points
always produced values closer to those obtained by the contour
method but were far more tedious and time consuming, taking on

FIG. 6. Section of aorta stained with sirius red only. Collagen fibers are identifiable, but there is great variation in size, prominence, and discreteness of fibers. Proximal thoracic aorta of rabbit, undistended during fixation. X 340

the average 3 - 4 times as long as contour tracing. Since nuclei were easily identified, discrete, of relatively uniform size, and far enough apart to present few overlaps due to section thickness, one would expect the contour method to be the most accurate and reproducible method for determining total nuclear area.

When lines or points were superimposed for repeat measurements on the same field, but with a different random orientation of the measuring grid each time, results similar to those shown in Table 2 were obtained for nuclei (proximal aortic segment), elastin (proximal segment), and collagen (distal segment). Standard deviations for the contour tracing method remain low while the standard deviations for the point method for nuclei, and for the line and point methods for elastin and collagen, are elevated.

TABLE 2.   Comparison of Volume Fractions Obtained by Different
          Methods of Surface Measurement: Fixed Field and
                    Varied Grid Orientation[a]

Method	Elastin	Collagen	Nuclei
Contour tracing	31.8 ± 0.77%	15.8 ± 0.91%	4.0 ± 0.43%
Line intersections	38.4 ± 3.60%	17.9 ± 2.90%	6.5 ± 0.26%
Point counting	32.3 ± 2.63%	18.7 ± 3.12%	6.1 ± 1.23%

[a]Elastin and nuclei determinations were on proximal thoracic aortic sections; collagen determined were on distal thoracic aortic
segment.

The range of mean values remained relatively narrow for collagen
regardless of method, while the contour method for nuclei again
gave a lower mean value than the line or point method.   Thus,
if random, repeated superimpositions are used for each determination of a given field, the increased number of observer decisions results in increased standard deviations.   A larger number
of determinations with more lines or points also reduced the
standard deviation for these methods at the expense of measurement time, but did not affect the mean or standard deviation
determined by contour tracing, for the same contours were
traced each time and no new decisions were needed.   For a single field, contour tracing under the conditions provided by the
digitizer - computer combination was both accurate and efficient.
    It should be emphasized that for a highly oriented structure
such as the aortic media, line segments and points used for
stereologic determinations should be in random arrays (Weibel
and Bolender 1973).   An underlying assumption of stereologic
methodology is that the components to be measured on cross sections are discrete and randomly distributed.   In the aortic media,
nuclei meet one of these criteria in that they are sharply delineated, but nuclei are not randomly distributed, being centrally
located in cells of fairly uniform size arranged in successive lay-

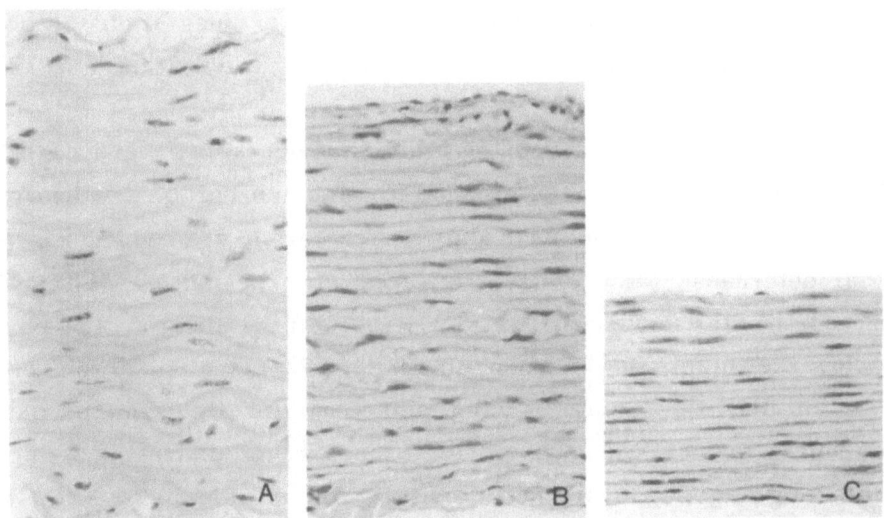

FIG. 7. Changes in nuclear size, orientation, and distribution related to distention. A. Nuclei appear almost randomly distributed in undistended vessel wall. B. Partial distention orients most of the nuclei circumferentially so that most are sectioned in oval or elongated profiles. C. Complete distention elongates and orients all of the nuclei in successive parallel layers. Hematoxylin and eosin stain. All magnifications X 250

ers (Fig. 7). Neither elastin nor collagen fibers are entirely "discrete" for they form a complex 3-dimensional series of branching or interlacing elements both within fibroelastic layers and about cells (Figs. 4 and 6). This feature presents special difficulties in determining an optimal grid size for point counting analysis, for an optimal grid size consists of about one intersection per discrete particle (Underwood 1970). If point counting is desired for elastin or collagen, optimum grid size is best determined by trial and error, i.e., a number of grid sizes should be tried in order to ascertain the conditions necessary to produce an acceptable standard deviation in a reasonable time. This would require a plot of standard deviation for given numbers of measurements against grid size, subjectively weighted for the amount of time available. For the line method, the use of many short line segments in a random orientation is recommended. As with point counting, the optimal number of lines would be obtained by considering the required standard deviation and the time needed to obtain it.

In contrast, the number of individual operations needed with the underline contour method is determined by the number of profiles on the cross section, and it is only the error of observer decision that determines the standard deviation and the number of repeat measurements required. For arteries, the more discrete the particle, the fewer the number of repeat determinations required. Use of digitizer - plate tracing and computer treatment of data obviously avoids the cumbersome procedure of tracing, cutting, and weighing paper profiles or fitting the profile to a geometric figure. For these reasons contour tracing presents a decided advantage over the other methods. The number of measurements needed to arrive at the minimal standard deviation due to observer error is easily determined simply and directly by computing a new mean after each determination. On a given section we have found that sequential contour determination produced a minimal standard deviation for nuclei in most instances by the third measurement; for elastin, four or five determinations were usually sufficient, and for collagen, about eight. Although collagen presents special problems for contour tracing for the reasons given above and may be better suited at first consideration to point counting, we feel that the greater time efficiency of contour tracing and immediate computer processing compensates for the possible greater accuracy of repeated point counts. The use of yellow paper on the digitizer surface greatly enhanced visualization of the red stained collagen fibrils, providing further facilitation for contour tracing.

Tracing of contours on a digitizing plate in conjunction with immediate computer storage and treatment of data has additional advantages. In addition to accuracy and speed, determination of contours on a cross section provides all the information needed to derive not only the volume fraction of the component in the

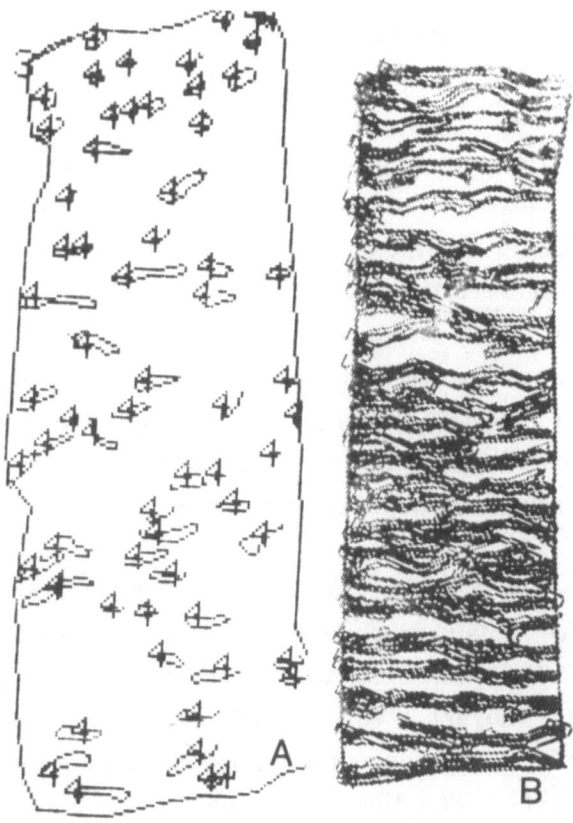

FIG. 8. Sample print-out copy produced from recorded images of contour tracings. A. Nuclear profiles traced on a field from the same section shown in Fig. 7. The superimposed numbers ("4") correspond to a component identification code. B. Elastin profiles traced on a field of the same section shown in Fig. 4A.

tissue, but such features as perimeter, shape, and surface to volume ratio, as well as gradient, distribution, and orientation of the components in the tissue section. The data are also stored for future recall and a "printout" copy of the recorded contours and computations is provided. This copy provides an immediately comprehensible recorded image of the components measured for further visual qualitative comparison (Fig. 8).

Effects of Staining Procedures

Sectioning and fixation techniques proved to have a much larger effect on collagen and elastin determination than did choice of stains. With the staining procedures used, we found that for elastin, staining by the complete Weigert - Van Gieson or Gomori trichrome - aldehyde - fuchsin method or staining only by the reagents in these polychrome stains that color elastin gave the same results. For example, elastin determined from a Gomori trichrome stain of a proximal thoracic segment with all elements stained was 37.5±2.44%; the estimation from an immediately adjacent section stained for elastin alone was 37.9±5.5%. Staining of elastin was sufficiently intense and elastin fibers sufficiently prominent not to be masked or eclipsed by other components.

This was not the case for collagen. The highest values for collagen were obtained when collagen was determined from the trichrome stained sections, the lowest from those processed by the complete Weigert - Van Gieson procedure. Determinations utilizing sirius red alone were close to those obtained from a complete Weigert - Van Gieson but tended to be somewhat higher. For example, a determination from a complete trichrome stained section gave a value of 15.9±3.61% while the immediately adjacent section stained by sirius red alone gave a value of 8.80±2.42%. The complete Weigert - Van Gieson yielded a value of 8.75±2.22% for collagen. Collagen stained with sirius red was more easily distinguished from the green-blue stained elastin and other tissue components in the complete Weigert - Van Gieson stain, but was paler than elastin and therefore obviously masked to some degree and therefore distinguished with difficulty in some instances. Collagen stained with fast green could be distinguished from elastin in the combined trichrome stain, but only with difficulty from other materials in the blue-green counterstained background; the relatively high value noted above was obtained by counting all material stained like collagen and decisions by the observer were made on the basis mainly of color rather than fiber identification.

Our findings therefore indicated that quantitative estimates of elastin can be made effectively with either of the complete connective tissue staining procedures used by us, but that collagen determinations are best made by means of sirius red stains, which distinguishes collagen from background, and preferably on sections not stained for elastin as well (Fig. 6).

In stereology, as in usual histologic studies, an ideal stain of a particular constituent differentiates the constituent from all other tissue components. The criteria for an adequate histologic stain are therefore specificity, intensity, and clarity of image. Resolution of architectural detail is the major requirement if the effects of different staining intensities are to be minimized for stereologic analysis. Stain intensities that delineate architectural detail are therefore, in general, preferable to those which color intensely. For complicated microstructures of variable thickness such as collagen, slides stained by a specific stain such as a sirius red should be used and visualization should be further enhanced by projecting on a suitably contrasting background. Background stains that stain a component but are not specific for the component should be avoided. Standardization of staining technique, based on trial determinations, should be done prior to establishment of an experimental protocol. It may also be useful to prepare a set of standard slides for periodic rechecking, especially if different observers are making determinations. Projection onto the digitizer plate entails the use of an intense light source which may bleach stains. The use of filters may reduce this effect but may also reduce intensity of the image. Complete darkness of the facility and the use of contrasting projection backgrounds may also be used to reduce light intensity requirements.

TABLE 3.   Comparison of Volume Fractions Obtained From
          Sections of Undistended and Distended Aortas and
          at Different Section Thickness[a]

| | Section Thickness | | |
Elastin	4 μm	5 μm	7 μm
Undistended	38.5 ± 5.89%	37.9 ± 5.5%	45.0 ± 2.50%
Distended	51.5 ± 4.29%	55.2 ± 2.4%	54.8 ± 6.75%
Nuclei			
Undistended	4.7 ± 0.22%	5.7 ± 0.36%	7.0 ± 0.77%
Distended	7.7 ± 1.02%	7.8 ± 1.17%	11.0 ± 1.01%

[a]All determinations were on sections of proximal thoracic aorta.

Effect of Section Thickness and Component Configuration

Section thickness had a marked effect on stereologic estimates of medial components, but this effect was not independent of the mode of fixation.   The configuration of wall elements associated with controlled pressure distention or nondistention during fixation influenced the effect of section thickness.   Illustrative results, shown in Table 3, were taken from the proximal thoracic location of a rabbit aorta.   There was no significant difference in calculated volume percent composition of elastin estimated from 4 or 5 μm sections stained with aldehyde fuchsin and obtained from nondistended aortas, but determinations made from 7 μm sections of nondistended aortas were much higher.   There was, however, no significant effect of section thickness on determinations of elastin from distended aortas stained by aldehyde fuchsin.   For nuclei, 7 μm sections gave higher values regardless of fixation procedure, but the values obtained from perfusion fixed specimens cut at 7 μm were highest.

An implicit assumption of stereologic analysis is that section thickness is negligible when compared to the diameters of the objects of interest.   Since sections do have a finite thickness, increased section thickness leads to an increased number of intercepts or profiles of tissue constituents per unit test area. The larger number of intercepts due to section thickness will therefore lead to a systematic overestimation of a constituent. This is known as the Holmes effect (Weibel and Elias 1967). If the section thickness to object diameter ratio (T/D) is greater than 0.1, the calculated volume fraction should be corrected for section thickness if an absolute volume fraction is desired. To calculate a correction factor for a given element, determinations of average particle diameter and shape must be made. As noted above, these data can be obtained and a suitable corrective factor can be computed directly from contour determinations utilizing suitable computer programs without recourse to additional measurements. Correlations between section thickness and calculated volume fractions of elastin and collagen are being determined and will be presented elsewhere. For quantitative studies now in progress we section all tissues at 4 - 5 µm.

At all section thicknesses studied, perfusion fixation gave rise to higher calculated volume fractions of components than determinations made from undistended specimens of the same thickness (Table 3). It has been shown repeatedly that normal distention of aortas during fixation narrows the distance between the fibrous layers more than it decreases the thickness of the fibrous layers, that elastin layers become straightened, and that cells become circumferentially oriented (Wolinsky and Glagov 1964). One would therefore expect the volume fraction of fibers noted in distended material to be greater than those seen with immersion fixed specimens. Nuclear shape is moderately altered by distention, but cell bodies became markedly elongated, narrowed, and oriented as the intervals between elastin lamellae decrease, accounting for the increase in nuclear volume fraction. When distention during fixation is incomplete, the spacing between fibrous layers is narrower than in nonperfused vessels, but elastin fibers are still focally wavy (Fig. 7). The calculated volume fraction of nuclei in such a vessel was, for example, 6.5% compared to the volume fraction for nuclei of 5.7% from an analo-

gous sample of a nonperfused aorta, and 7.8% for a fully perfused aorta sampled at the same anatomic location. Nuclei in
partly perfused vessels were somewhat elongated compared to
those in nondistended vessels and became oriented more or less
circumferentially. In completely distended vessels, nuclei appeared to be even more oriented but not markedly narrower than
in partially distended vessels (Fig. 7). Linear orientation of a
partially oriented system of surfaces in space can be estimated
by determining the number of intersections of a test arrays of
lines oriented perpendicular and parallel to the long axis of the
structure under study (Underwood 1970). Utilizing a suitable
computer program this can be computed from the contour measurements recorded for the volume determinations. The average
degree of nuclear orientation for nonperfused specimens was
33.38±12.86%. The average degree of orientation for the partially
distended specimens was 76.31±8.94%.

Sampling of Aortas and Selection Fields

It is evident from the determinations shown in Tables 1 and 2
that samples taken from different locations of the aortas with respect to clearly defined anatomic landmarks yielded different
mean values for connective tissue content. It has been shown
repeatedly by means of chemical determinations that percent concentration of aortic elastin generally decreases, while the percent
composition of collagen generally increases with distance from the
heart (Cleary 1963). Nuclear volume fraction changes much less.
Arteries also show marked differences related both to age (Leung
et al. 1977; McCloskey and Cleary 1974) and to different vascular beds (Fischer and Llaurado 1966). Chemical determinations
have revealed that there are transmural gradients (Feldman and
Glagov 1971) of aortic connective tissue in man. This was also
readily demonstrable in rabbits by stereologic methods used in
conjunction with our equipment. For example, utilizing the medial cross sectional test area measured to provide the collagen
data shown in Table 2, we found that the inner, subintimal half

of the media gave a value of 13.3±0.63%, while the value for the outer half was 18.5±1.05%. The value obtained for the wall as a whole was 15.8±0.91%. The contour method may be utilized to detect such gradients, since the standard deviation for the determinations was much smaller than the observed difference. It is also possible to obtain a graphic representation of such a gradient from the contour data as well as a pictorial display. Such information cannot be obtained readily from chemical determinations of aortas, particularly in small animals.

In establishing a protocol for the quantitative analysis of arterial wall constituents, standard deviations obtained from multiple determinations of the same test field, which estimate visualization and measuring errors, should be compared with the standard deviations obtained from multiple determinations from different areas of the samples to be compared. The difference between these sets of standard deviations will provide an estimate of the uniformity of distribution of the constituent of interest. This difference can be used to provide an estimate of the number of different sample areas that must be measured in order to characterize the tissue. If, for example, no attention is paid to position across the wall or to radial position around the wall, standard deviations may be expected to remain relatively elevated; even with 24 determinations on a section of monkey proximal thoracic aorta, random positions gave values of 38.9±3.35% for elastin and 12.3±2.68% for collagen. With the contour method, all profiles of the constituent of interest are considered in the test area. Assuming that the contours are accurately traced, most of the error from this method will then be due to inadequate field selection from the tissue and/or section. A suitable program can be used to establish the necessary sampling level. With the line and point counting methods, not all contours are intercepted and two randomization procedures are necessary, i.e., the selection of the test areas, as in the contour method, and the selection of an appropriate test lattice.

TABLE 4.   Comparison of Stereologic and Chemical Determinations

| | Volume Fractions[a] | | |
	Undistended	Distended	Chemical analysis[b]
Elastin(E)	37.9 ± 5.5%	55.2 ± 2.4%	45.6
Collagen(C)	8.8 ± 2.4%	16.2 ± 2.47%	13.1
E/C[c]	4.31	3.42	3.48
Nuclei	4.11 ± 0.43%	7.8 ± 1.17%	4.57[d]
Cellularity[e]	10.1 ± 0.4	19.1 ± 0.6	

[a]Determinations on proximal thoracic aorta
[b]mg/100 mg
[c]Ratio of mean values of elastin and collagen
[d]DNA (μg/mg)
[e]Nuclei per 1000 μm^2

Comparisons with Chemical Determination

Elastin.   Volume fraction estimates for elastin fibers, determined from sections of undistended vessels, gave lower values than chemical determinations expressed as percent of dry weight, while volume fractions of elastin determined from sections of distended vessels were higher than the gravimetric values obtained by chemical analysis.   Results are shown in Table 4 for the proximal portion of a rabbit aorta.   The histologic sections were stained with aldehyde fuchsin.

Collagen.   The volume fraction of collagen determined by stereologic methods always tended to be lower than the chemical determinations expressed as percent dry weight, particularly when stains for other medial constituents were present.   Volume fractions were determined from sections stained with sirius red (Table 4).

Nuclei.   There was no consistent pattern of correlation between volume fraction determinations of nuclei from distended or undistended vessel sections and chemical estimates of DNA.   Nuclear content could also be expressed as the number of nuclear contours per unit test area. These values paralleled the difference between volume fraction determinations related to distention and were also a function of section thickness (Table 4).

Comparisons of morphometric with chemical data are difficult to interpret. Histologic sections used for volume fraction estimates reflect composition at a plane of cross section, while chemical data were obtained from relatively large tissue segments pooled from above and below the histologic sample sites. There is no basis at this time for assuming that the composition at the plane of transection represents the average of the composition above and below the histologic sampling site. Furthermore, chemical determinations were made only on the aortas which were not fixed before sampling, i.e., on the undistended specimens shown in Table 4. The distended aortas used for the stereologic determinations shown in Table 4 were from other animals of the same weight. The differences in volume fraction between undistended and distended vessels were, however, sufficiently great compared to difference between animals treated in the same manner to indicate that gravimetric values expressed as percent dry weight lie somewhere between values of volume fraction obtained from distended and undistended specimens.

Values of volume fractions obtained from stereologic determinations would be expected to correlate best with chemical concentrations expressed as percent wet weight, since histologic sections are processed from fixation through staining and mounting with wet volumes maintained throughout. Yet, tissue wet weights are notoriously inaccurate, and the shrinkage of tissue components during histologic processing is not uniform. If corrections were made for shrinkage, it might be useful to utilize the density of collagen (1.29) or of elastin (1.42) to convert volume fraction determinations to weights. Better standardization of volume and weight relationships in aortas may also be forthcoming if interval sections along the aorta are compared to chemical determinations of the intervening segments on vessels derived

from large animals in order to provide sufficient tissue for repli-
cate chemical analysis. For many purposes, establishment of
elastin to collagen ratios from stereologic determinations may be
quite adequate, and even these may be rendered more comparable
to ratios obtained from chemical determinations by multiplying by
the ratio of the densities (0.91). Ratios obtained from determinations on distended aortas were remarkably close to those
obtained from chemical determinations (Table 4).

Conclusions

Volume fractions and orientation of artery wall components can
be determined by applying principles of stereology. Several
surface measurement methods are available. These include contour tracing, line segment measurement, and point counting. All
of these require repeated measurements in order to establish and
assure levels of reproducibility and accuracy necessary for determination of significant changes related to experimental or clinical conditions. Contour tracing, particularly on profiles of easily identified, discrete elements is the most reproducible measuring operation and requires the fewest repeated measurements to
establish an acceptable standard deviation. Estimations of volume
fractions from tracings of component contours may require manip-
ulations and processing that may be excessively tedious and may
introduce additional variation. Use of direct computer analysis
of contours traced on a digitizing plate from projected images
eliminates many of these problems and renders contour tracing
both more accurate and more time efficient than do the other
procedures for a given number of measurement operations. Contour tracing also includes the information necessary to compute
features such as perimeter, diameter, shape, orientation, and
distribution directly by means of suitable computer programs and
without necessitating additional measurements.

Contour tracing from projected images is well suited to studies
of arterial lesions and arterial wall composition. Relationships

among lesion size, configuration and composition, lumenal shape and diameter, and medial composition and dimensions are readily established; available systems provide data storage and printed images for further evaluation. Precision obtainable is, however, related to component measured, section thickness, staining procedure, and conditions of fixation as well as to choice of sample site and field. The method is most accurate for measurements of nuclei and elastin and least accurate for collagen fibers. Collagen fiber measurements are nevertheless almost as effective by contour tracing as by means of suitable grids used for point counting. Most consistent results are obtained from 4 - 5 µm sections stained specifically for one element.

Volume fractions obtained from fields of vessel walls fixed by excision and immersion contrast markedly with values obtained from vessels distended at physiologic pressures during fixation. Although chemical determinations of aortic medial components did not correspond in any simple manner to values obtained by stereology, ratios of elastin to collagen obtained by chemical methods appeared to correspond best to ratios obtained morphometrically from distended vessel specimens. Random field selection with respect to position around the vessel circumference or across the wall introduces considerable variation; even greater variation is introduced by random sampling along the aorta. Although analytical programs can be developed to provide useful data on component distribution with respect to anatomic location, investigations designed to correlate changes in vessel wall composition with experimental conditions should utilize precisely defined standard sampling and field selection sites. The application of contour tracing to projected images of arterial sections in conjunction with storage and processing of data by an on-line minicomputer promises to permit detailed studies of large numbers of experimental and human specimens and furnish new insights into the relation of composition and structure to function in normal and abnormal vessels.

Acknowledgments

The work was supported by United States Public Health Service Grant HL 15062-08.

The work by Joseph Grande was done during the tenure of a Medical Scientist Training Program Grant (PHS # 2T32 GM07281).

REFERENCES

Ballentine R (1957) Determination of total nitrogen and ammonia. Methods Enzymol 3: 984-995

Bernimoulin JP, Schroeder HE (1977) Quantitative electron microscopic analysis of the epithelium of normal human alveolar mucosa. Cell Tiss Res 180: 383-401

Burton K (1956) A study of the conditions and mechanisms of the diphenylamine reaction for the colorimetric estimation of deoxyribonucleic acid. Biochem J 62: 315-323

Clark JM, Glagov S (1979) Structural integration of the arterial wall: I. Relationships and attachments of medial smooth muscle cells in normally distended and hyperdistended aortas. Laboratory Investigation 40: 587-602

Cleary EG (1963) A correlative and comparative study of the non-uniform arterial wall. PhD dissertation, University of Sydney

Elias H, Henning A (1967) Stereology of the human renal glomerulus. In: Weiber E, Elias H (eds) Quantitative methods in morphology. Springer-Verlag, New York

Feldman SA, Glagov S (1971) Transmedial collagen and elastin gradients in human aortas: reversal with age. Atherosclerosis 13: 385-394

Fischer GM, Llaurado JG (1966) Collagen and elastin content in canine arteries from functionally different vascular beds. Circ Res 19: 394-399

Gomori G (1950) Aldehyde fuchsin: A new stain for elastic tissue. Am J Clin Path 20: 665-669

Henning A (1958) A critical survey of volume and surface measurement in microscopy. Zeiss Werkzeitschrift 30: 78

Lansing AI, Rosenthal TB, Dempsey EW (1952) The structure and chemical characterization of elastic fibers as revealed by elastase and electron microscopy. Anat Rec 114: 555-575

Leung YM, Glagov S, Mathews MB (1977) Elastin and collagen accumulation in rabbit ascending aorta and pulmonary trunk during postnatal growth. Circ Res 41: 316-323

Martin CJ, Axelrod AE (1953) A modified method for determination of hydroxyproline. Proc Soc Exp Biol Med 83: 461-462

McCloskey IM, Cleary EG (1974) Chemical composition of rabbit aorta during development. Circ Res 34: 828-835

Newman RE, Logan MA (1956) Determination of hydroxyproline. J Biol Chem 184: 299-305

Richards GM (1974) Modifications of the diphenylamine reaction giving increased sensitivity and simplicity in the estimation of DNA. Anal Biochem 57: 369-376

Sweat F, Puchtler H, Rosenthal SI (1964) Sirius red F3BA as a stain for connective tissue. Arch Path 78: 69-72

Takahashi T, Suwa N (1978) Stereological and topological analysis of cirrhotic livers as a linkage of regenerative nodules multiply connected in the form of a 3-dimensional network. In: Miles E, Bue J (eds) Buffon bicentenary symposium on geometrical probability image analysis, mathematical stereology, and their relevance to the determination of biological structures. Springer-Verlag, New York

Underwood EE (1970) Quantitative stereology. Addison-Wesley Publishing Co

Weibel ER (1969) Stereological principles for morphometry in electron microscopic cytology. Int Rev Cyt 235-302

Weibel ER, Bolender RP (1973) Stereological techniques for electron microscopic morphometry. In: Hayat MA (ed) Principles and techniques of electron microscopic morphometry. Van Nostrand Reinhold Co, Vol. 3, pp. 237-296

Weibel ER, Elias H (eds) (1967) Quantitative methods in morphology. Proceedings of the symposium of quantitative methods in morphology. Springer-Verlag, New York

Wissler RW, Vesselinovitch D, Schaffner TJ, Glagov S (1980) Quantitating rhesus monkey atherosclerosis progression and regression with time. In: Gotto AM, Smith LC, Allen B (eds) Atherosclerosis V, Proceedings of the Fifth International Symposium, Springer-Verlag, New York

Wolinsky H, Daly MM (1970) A method for the isolation of intima-media samples from arteries. Proc Soc Exp Biol Med 135: 364-368

Wolinsky H, Glagov S (1964) Structural basis for the static mechanical properties of the aortic media. Circ Res 14: 400-413

Wolinsky H, Glagov S (1967a) A lamellar unit of aortic medial structure and function in mammals. Circ Res 20: 99-111

Wolinsky H, Glagov S (1967b) Nature of species differences in the medial distribution of aortic vasa vasorum in mammals. Circ Res 20: 409-421

Wolinsky H, Glagov S (1969) Comparison of abdominal and thoracic aortic medial structure in mammals: Deviaton from the usual pattern in man. Circ Res 25: 677-686

Discussion

Kramsch. I like the way you relate structure to hemodynamic function of blood vessels. I have a question about the way you relate pressure to elastic lamellar units of arteries. I think it is plausible for the aorta, but I am somewhat puzzled as to other arteries, for example, the renal, coronary, in fact, all of the systemic and organ arteries that are exposed to some pressure but have far less elastic lamellar units. Do you think it may have something to do with the pulse pressure, which is greatest in the thoracic aorta, because even the abdominal aorta has far less elastic lamellar units?

Glagov. For any given homologous vessel in mammals, the number of medial lamellae, or layers, seems to correspond to the tangential tension in the wall rather than to the intraluminal pressure. The tension of course is a function of both the pressure and the radius of the vessel. For the mammalian adult aorta, for example, the number of lamellae at a given location corresponds to the total tension. Since the mean pressure is about the same for most mammals, the number of lamellae therefore is a function of the radius. In general, for each additional 2000 dynes per centimeter of tension an additional layer is present, and these layers are quite uniform in thickness and in general configuration regardless of species. Similarly, when mammalian pulmonary trunks, coronary arteries or renal arteries are sampled at standard locations, the number of medial layers corresponds to the radius of the vessel. Each homologous vessel, however, has its own characteristic medial structural organization and is unlike that of the aorta or other specific arteries. The pulmonary trunk, for example, has layers which are quite different in structure from those of the aorta, and each layer corresponds to an increase of about 1000 dynes per centimeter. Thus the medial microarchitecture of an adult mammalian artery is governed by its anatomical position and is independent of species and diameter, while the number of its layers, relative to other homologous vessels, is governed by its diameter. Simply stated, all aortas tend to be alike, all pulmonary arteries tend to be alike, all coronary arteries tend to be alike, et cetera, and for each homologous vessel, the number of layers is linearly related to radius.

Biochemical Changes of the Arterial Wall in Atherosclerosis with Special Reference to Connective Tissue: Promising Experimental Avenues for their Prevention

DIETER M. KRAMSCH

In man atherosclerosis generally involves the large and medium sized arteries in which connective tissue proteins comprise more than half the dry weight. Connective tissue contributes to some of the most important alterations in the significant human lesion, the fibrous plaque. It is this lesion that poses the most serious threat to health and life. As recently reviewed by Smith and Smith (1976), it is still open to debate whether or not fibrous plaques, or at least some of them, develop from fatty streaks. We, therefore, will restrict our discussion to fibrous lesions. Fibrous lesions begin to develop in the second to third decade of life in almost all individuals of our type of society. However, it takes decades of slow growth before they produce clinical symptoms.

As recently summarized by Ross and Glomset (1976a,b), the main processes leading to the formation of atherosclerotic plaques appear to be: 1) increased permeability of arterial endothelium to macromolecules such as lipoproteins; 2) migration of smooth muscle cells (SMCs) from the media into the intima; 3) proliferation of these cells by mitosis; 4) secretion by the increased SMCs of excessive amounts of collagen, elastin, and glycosaminoglycans; as well as 5) endocytosis (phagocytosis) of lipids and/or lipoproteins by intimal cells. Calcium mineralization, espe-

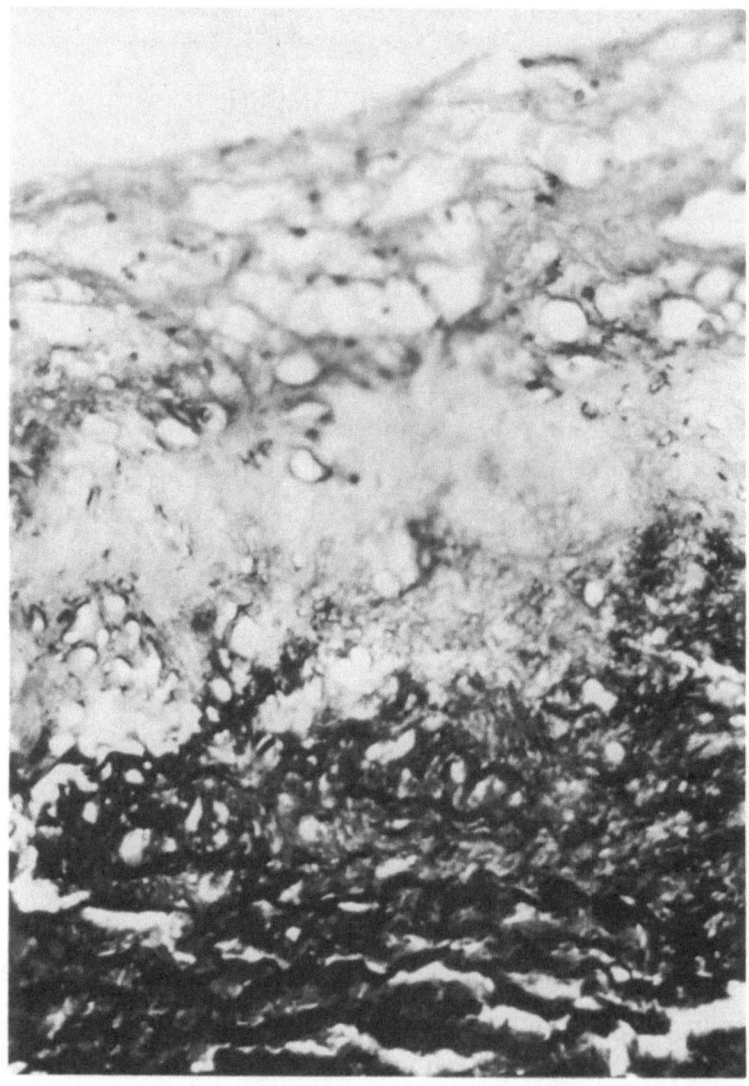

FIG. 1. Human fibrous plaque of aorta. Note fibrous cap (top) with some lipid-filled "foam cells" overlying a necrotic core (middle). The intimo-medial elastica (bottom black) was fragmented and deranged. Verhoeff's - Van Geison, X 90

cially of arterial elastin, also appears to be a frequent integral part of atherogenesis (Yu and Blumenthal 1963).

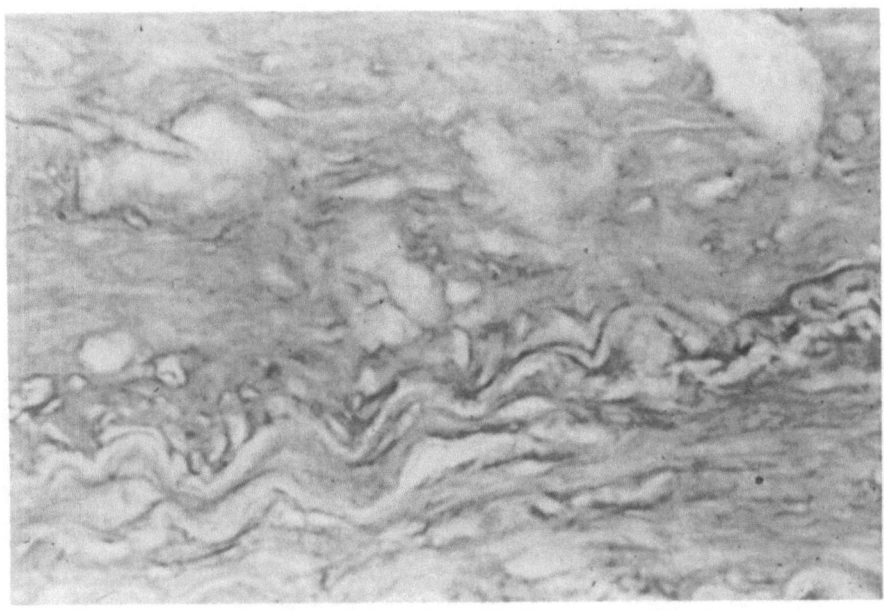

FIG. 2. Sequential section of the same plaque as in Fig. 1. Alcian Blue staining material indicating glycosaminoglycans (dark grey) is on the deranged elastica (light undulating bands) and in "lakes" in the raised intima. Also note the PAS-staining material (light grey) in close association with the duplicated elastica and in the overlying intima (top half). PAS - Alcian Blue, X 140

The importance of the connective tissue changes is that the alterations seriously impair arterial function by raising the intima to the point of stenosis, by loss of elasticity, and by increased rigidity and brittleness (calcium), leading to harmful sequellae such as insufficiency of blood flow, hypertension, aneurysms, vessel rupture, and thrombosis. Another important fact about the connective tissue alterations of plaques is that they may resist attempts at their reversal once they have been established. It is true that there may be ways to prevent or at least retard these connective tissue damages in man by appropriate diet and/or drug treatment. However, it is equally true that all attempts to cause regression of established connective tissue lesions by initiation of therapeutic diets and/or restoring blood

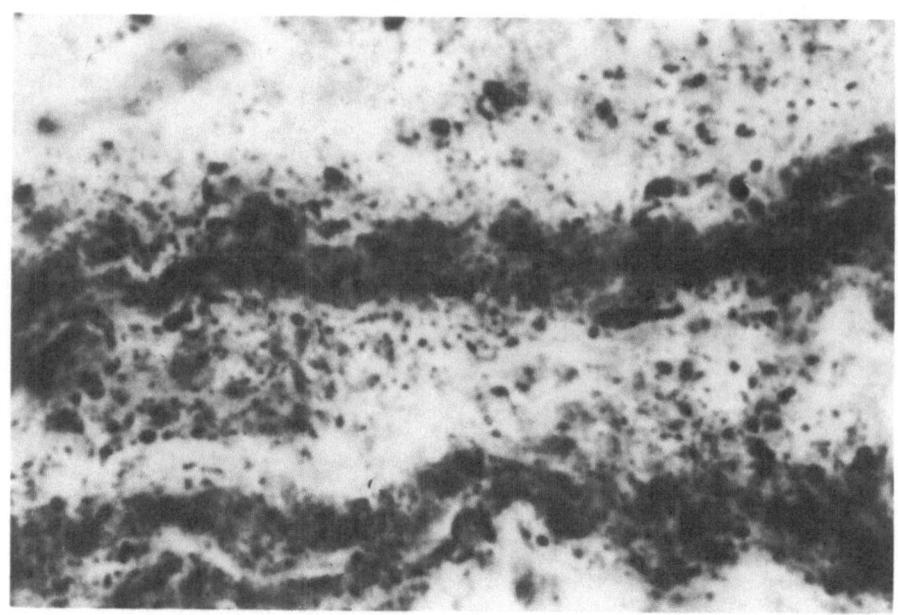

FIG. 3. Sequential section of the same plaque as in Fig. 1.
Lipid droplets (black, red in the original) were on and around
the duplicated internal elastica and in cells (top). Oil Red 0,
X 180

lipids to normal by drugs have failed in man and in experimental
animals, including in nonhuman primates as in our own studies.
It should be kept in mind that all that has been shown in so-
called regression experiments by even the most drastic diet re-
striction (complete cessation of the dietary stimuli) is that lipid-
filled cells may disappear from the established lesions. Substantial accumulations of lipids, and equally important of calcium,
remain in established lesions after long periods of normalization
of serum lipids and lipoproteins. These remaining lipids and
calcium appear to be associated with the accumulated plaque connective tissue which shows little if any potential of regression.

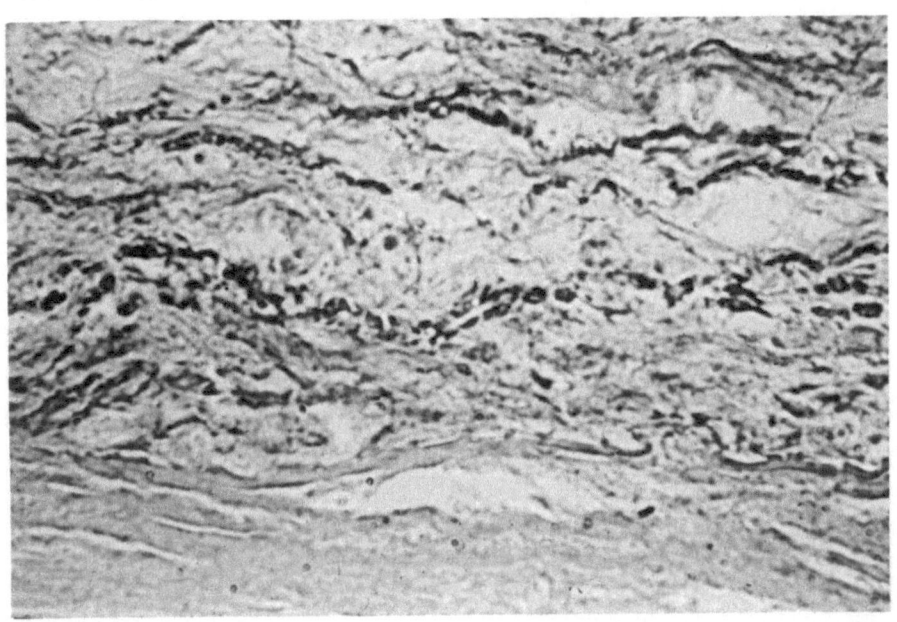

FIG. 4. Mild human fibrous plaque of aorta without necrotic core. Calcium (black) was deposited on the fragmented and deranged intimo-medial elastica (top two thirds). Alizarin Red – Light Green, X 90

Composition of Fibrous Plaques

Morphologic Aspects

Let us briefly review some of the morphologic features of fibrous lesions. The raised intima of the fully developed fibrous plaque (Fig. 1) consists of a fibrocellular cap with or without an underlying lipid-rich necrotic core. The cap contains massive depositions of collagen, cells (sometimes filled with lipid), and frequently some fine elastic elements. The intimo-medial elastica of most plaques is fragmented and deranged, often deep into the media. Accumulations of glycosaminoglycans (acid mucopolysaccharides) (Fig. 2) frequently can be demonstrated enveloping the deranged or duplicated elastica and in "lakes" over the collagenous part of the cap. PAS-staining material, perhaps glycoproteins, also may be seen deposited in close association with duplicated elastica and with what appears to be collagen of the fibrous cap. Depositions of stainable lipids, if present, often are associated (Fig. 3) with duplicated and/or fragmented elastic laminae, their coat of glycosaminoglycans, or with collagenous areas of the cap. Finally, calcium may be deposited in fibrous lesions. In mild plaques (Fig. 4), the calcium is deposited predominantly on the deranged elastica. In advanced lesions, collagen areas or the entire plaque can calcify, rendering it impossible to differentiate the structural plaque elements with which the calcium minerals are associated. Calcification of advanced plaques is often so massive as to be grossly recognizable as a stone-hard plate.

The connective tissue alterations sometimes may involve only the elastica. Figure 5 shows a split internal elastica with deposition of stainable lipids in an otherwise normal human coronary artery. Lillie et al. (1976) recently also have observed selective lipid staining of human arterial elastica, apparently preceding the appearance of fibrous plaques by some years. These and other authors (Lansing et al. 1950; Moon and Rinehart 1952; Zugibe and Brown 1960; Parker 1960; Adams and Tuqan 1961; Osborn 1963; Friedman 1963; Smith et al. 1967; Kramsch and Hollander 1968) have advanced the concept that elastica changes may be the earliest alterations in atherosclerosis.

Figure 6 shows an autoradiograph of an advanced encapsulated plaque of aorta from a moribund patient who had been intravenously injected with a tracer dose of tritiated cholesterol 4 months prior to death. It is of interest that the injected radioactive cholesterol was mainly deposited in the plaque capsule: in cells, over collagen and especially over the elastica at the border of the plaque. It is also noteworthy that very little, if any, cholesterol radioactivity was found over the lipid-rich core of the plaque. This finding suggests that the cholesterol contained in the necrotic core of encapsulated plaques may not exchange readily with the cholesterol circulating in the blood stream.

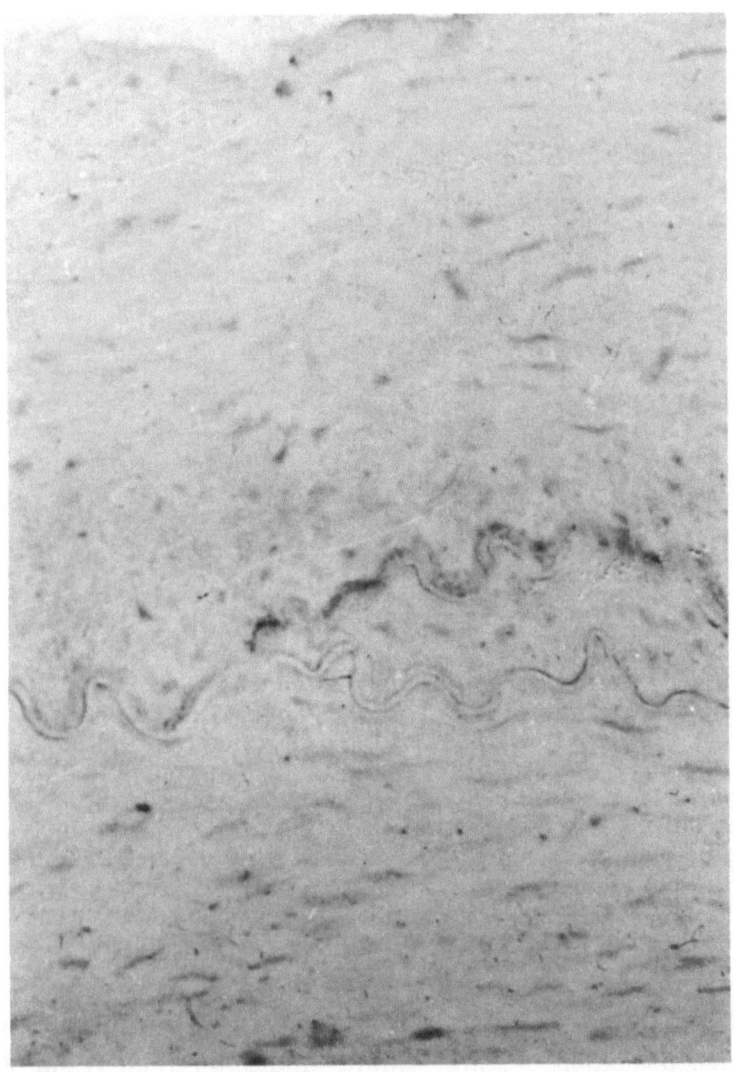

FIG. 5. Human coronary artery showing splitting (or reduplication) of the internal elastica (undulating bands) with lipid droplets (black) on the upper strand of the duplicated elastica. Note the paucity of lipid deposition in cells of the intima and media. Oil Red 0, X 85

Figure 7A shows a micrograph of a fibrous plaque of femoral artery from the same patient. Although no lipid was detectable

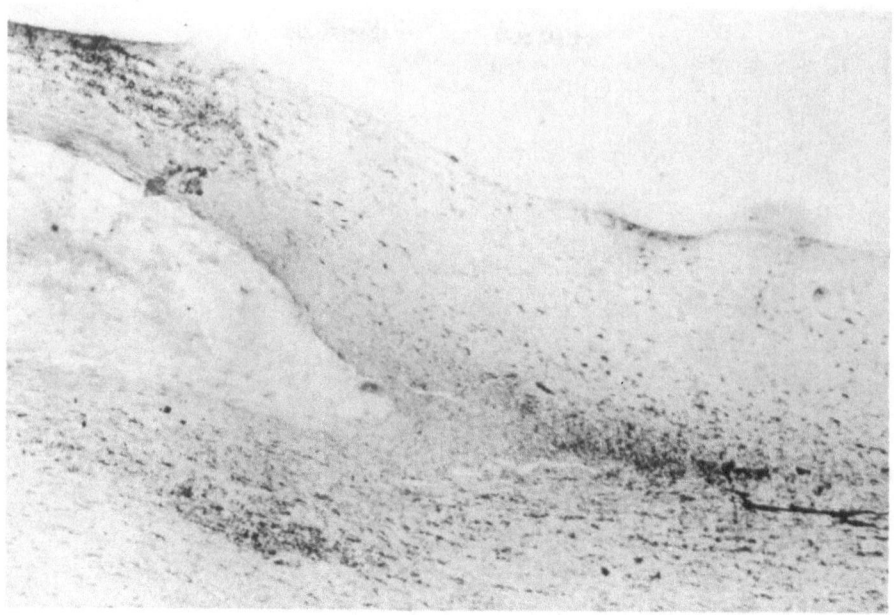

FIG. 6. Autoradiograph of an advanced encapsulated fibrous plaque of human aorta. The intravenously injected tritiated cholesterol radioactivity (black dots) was seen deposited over collagen areas of the plaque capsule and on duplicated intimo-medial elastica (black bands) at the border of the plaque. Note the virtual absence of cholesterol radioactivity over the encapsulated necrotic (lipid-rich) core. Hematoxylin - Van Gieson, X 70

in this lesion by Oil Red 0 staining, the radioautograph of a sequential section (Fig. 7B) revealed marked deposition of radioactive cholesterol on the fragmented elastica and in areas of collagen accumulation. This finding indicates that if no lipid is detectable by staining, as in many fibrous plaques, it does not necessarily mean that none is present. It may be masked, for example, by other proteins or proteoglycans that are associated with the connective tissue proteins.

These observations indicate that fibrous plaques appear to have several pools of lipid deposition: small amounts contained in cells and larger amounts associated with the connective tissue or contained in the necrotic core and in the extracellular choles-

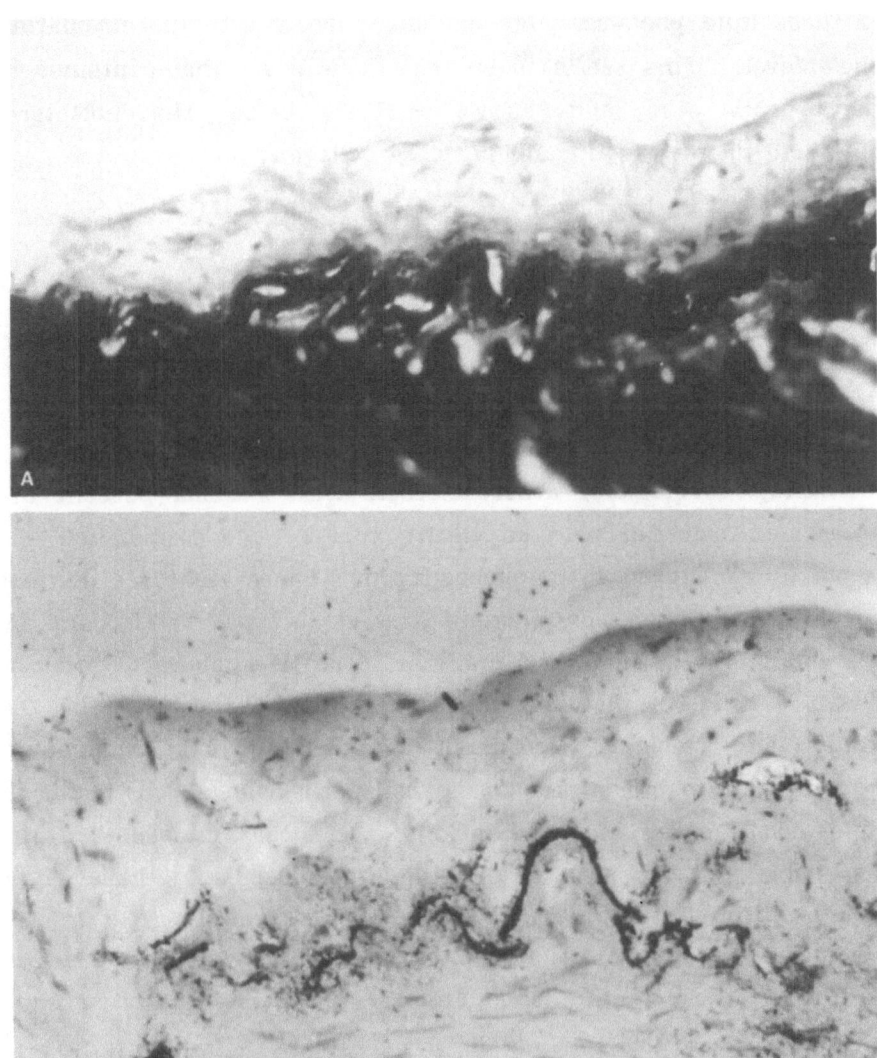

FIG. 7. Sequential sections through a small fibrous plaque of human femoral artery. A. The intima is mildly raised by an accumulation of collagen and proliferation of cells; the internal elastica was duplicated. Verhoeff's - Van Gieson, X 70. Oil Red 0 staining of a sequential section did not reveal the presence of lipids in the lesion. B. Autoradiograph showing the presence of intravenously injected tritiated cholesterol on and around the split elastica as well as in areas of collagen deposition but not in intimal cells.

terol clefts. It appears that the cholesterol contained in several
of these lipid pools may not exchange freely with the circulating
cholesterol. This seems to be true at least for that contained in
the necrotic core, and, as we shall see below, the cholesterol
bound to plaque elastin and possibly collagen.

Biochemical Aspects

Fibrous plaques are biochemically characterized by focal accumulations of four classes of extracellular macromolecules: collagen, elastin, glycosaminoglycans, and glycoproteins.

Collagen. The largest component of these accumulated macromolecules obviously is collagen, which is known to increase with
increasing severity of atherosclerosis with maximal percent increases in calcified plaques (Smith 1974). The composition appears to be altered in plaque collagen. There are three distinct
species of collagen contained in arteries: types I, III, and IV
(Trelstad 1974). In normal arteries, type III appears to predominate. In human plaques, however, type I appears to be the
predominant collagen (McCullagh and Balian 1975), changes in
type IV (the basement membrane collagen) have as yet not been
reported to occur in these lesions. Of great interest are the
immunohistochemical studies showing that the subendothelial layer
of the fibrous cap appears to contain predominantly type III collagen (Gay and Balleisen 1977). Type III collagen is, at least in
vitro, the most potent stimulator of platelet aggregation and,
potentially of thrombosis (Barnes et al. 1976).

Collagen normally has a marked affinity for lipids which may
be structural components of the collagen protein (Nikkari and
Heikkinnen 1968). In atherosclerosis, this association appears to
be increased since about 8% - 10% of the total cholesterol of
human fibrous plaques can be contained in the insoluble plaque
collagen (Kramsch and Hollander 1973; Hollander et al. 1974a).
Furthermore, collagen from plaques but not from adjacent normal
intima appears to have especially pronounced antigenic properties
which could represent autoantigenicity (Hollander et al. 1974a).

Immunoglobulins G(IgG) and A(IgA) as well as compliment are extractable with the acid soluble tissue-bound collagen fractions, as well as with collagenase. A small amount of collagen-bound IgG appears to be synthetized locally in plaques.

Elastin. Elastin appears to be quantitatively the second major extracellular macromolecule of fibrous plaques. Although no exact data on the content of elastin in human fibrous lesions are available, there is no question from many animal experiments (Kramsch et al. 1974; Armstrong and Megan 1975; Wolinsky et al. 1975) that arteries with induced fibrous-type atherosclerosis have an increased content of elastin (as well as of collagen) if expressed in absolute amounts per length-defined artery.

In atherosclerotic lesions, elastin, the backbone protein of elastic lamellae, was shown to be qualitatively altered in man (Kramsch et al. 1971; Yu 1971; Keeley and Partridge 1974; Kramsch et al. 1974a) as well as in rabbits and monkeys (Kramsch et al. 1974b). The amino acid composition of normal elastin from normal arteries or normal areas of diseased arteries was remarkably similar in adult animals and humans and did not appear to change markedly with increasing age. However, the alkali-isolated elastin fraction from atherosclerotic lesions had a much greater content of polar amino acids (Table 1), an abnormality which increased with increasing severity of the disease. Similar increases in polar amino acids of alkali-isolated elastin have been found in atherosclerotic arteries of monkeys and rabbits (Table 1). There were no significant changes in the remaining amino acids of these elastin fractions.

The compositional abnormality of plaque elastin may be due to a close binding of one or more other proteins to the original elastin, such as the normally closely associated microfibrillar glycoprotein (Ross and Bornstein 1969) or the likewise associated proteoglycans (Gotte et al. 1965; John and Thomas 1972; Moczar and Robert 1970), as well as elastase or lysyl oxydase, both of which are known to bind to elastin (Gertler 1971; Kagan et al. 1974). Robert et al. (1971) have shown that solubilized peptides

TABLE 1. Changes in the Amino Acid Composition of Alkali-Insoluble Aortic "Elastins" in Human and Experimental Atherosclerosis (Residues/1000 Residues; Means ± S.D.)

Amino acid	Normal aorta[a]	Fatty streak	Moderate fibrous plaque	Severe fibrous plaque	Macaca fascicularis,[b] no drugs	Rabbit[c] without drugs
Oh-pro	10.5 ± 1.5	13.2 ± 4.0	14.5 ± 4.6	15.2 ± 0.6	13.0 ± 2.5	13.5 ± 2.5
Asp	5.6 ± 1.6	14.6 ± 4.7[d]	21.5 ± 2.7[d]	22.7 ± 3.9[d]	13.1 ± 4.2[d]	8.2 ± 2.0[d]
Thre	12.5 ± 2.4	16.8 ± 2.2	16.9 ± 1.6[e]	18.0 ± 1.8[d]	10.2 ± 2.8	9.9 ± 3.4
Ser	9.5 ± 1.1	14.8 ± 3.1[d]	16.9 ± 2.6[d]	18.1 ± 1.8[d]	13.6 ± 1.4[d]	12.6 ± 2.3
Glu	21.2 ± 2.3	33.1 ± 5.2[d]	39.2 ± 6.2[d]	40.7 ± 2.7[d]	31.0 ± 6.9[d]	27.3 ± 2.8[d]
Ly	6.0 ± 1.2	12.2 ± 2.3[d]	14.9 ± 2.2[d]	12.4 ± 1.2[d]	9.3 ± 1.6[c]	8.3 ± 1.0[e]
His	1.9 ± 1.1	4.4 ± 1.1[d]	5.4 ± 0.9[d]	5.0 ± 0.6[d]	2.3 ± 1.3	1.0 ± 0.8
Arg	4.9 ± 0.9	11.5 ± 3.6[d]	14.7 ± 1.1[d]	14.2 ± 1.2[d]	8.9 ± 2.1[d]	7.9 ± 1.4[d]

[a] Normal elastin
[b] Cholesterol and butter
[c] Cholesterol and peanut oil
[d] $P < 0.01$ from normal values
[e] $P < 0.05$ from normal values

of arterial elastin are antigenic and that the microfibrillar glyco-protein of elastic tissue has one of the most powerful antigenic properties. It therefore is possible that antimicrofibrillar and/or antielastin immunoglobulins may become tightly bound to the elas-tin. Still another possibility is that at least part of these sec-ondary proteins may be derived from low-density (LDL) and very-low-density lipoproteins (VLDL), both of which have been shown by immunohistochemical techniques to associate with plaque elastica (and collagen) (Walton and Williamson 1968; Hoff and Glaubatz 1977). Finally, a small portion of these secondary pro-teins of plaque elastin could be collagen (Keeley and Partridge 1974).

On the other hand, it may be that the newly synthesized elas-tin has an altered composition, possibly by close association with one or more of the above-listed proteins (especially the microfi-brillar proteins and proteoglycans) that cannot be removed by hot alkali. It is of interest in this context that Dr. Franzblau's group have shown (Faris et al. 1976) that newly synthesized alkali-isolated elastin at certain stages in arterial smooth muscle cell cultures also is rich in acidic (polar) amino acids, reminis-cent of the abnormal elastin from lesions.

As reported in our studies and by others (Kramsch et al. 1971; Kramsch et al. 1974b; Szigeti et al. 1972; Robert et al. 1972; Wagner and Clarkson 1973; Noma et al. 1979), normal arte-rial elastin as well as elastin from plaques appears to be a pro-tein -lipid complex with the lipids presumably bound by hydro-phobic stacking to hydrophobic sites of the elastin molecule (Jacotot el al. 1973). While the lipid moiety of normal elastin is small, it increases markedly, especially ester cholesterol, in the abnormal elastin from plaques in man (Kramsch et al. 1971) as well as in atherosclerotic arteries from monkeys and rabbits (Kramsch et al. 1974b). In uncomplicated fibrous plaques of man, about 30% of the total cholesterol can be contained in the altered plaque elastin (Kramsch and Hollander 1973). Whether the fatty acid composition of the cholesterol esters associated with this abnormal protein complex is similar to that reported for "perifibrous" lipids (Smith et al. 1976) is not known.

The prerequisite for the increased lipid binding appears to be the altered amino acid composition of the plaque elastin protein, and the mechanism of binding appears to be a transfer, predominantly cholesterol, from serum and/or arterial LDL and VLDL but not from high-density lipoproteins (HDL) or chylomicrons to the abnormal protein, at least as shown in vitro (Kramsch and Hollander 1973). In vivo binding of radioactive cholesterol to arterial elastin has been demonstrated in man (Kramsch and Hollander 1973) and rats (Jacotot et al. 1971). The ester cholesterol transferred in vitro from lipoproteins to plaque elastin protein was firmly bound to the elastin and could not be removed by subsequent incubations with apo-LDL, apo-VLDL, apo-HDL, intact HDL, or treatment with trypsin and hot alkali (Kramsch and Hollander 1973). These findings suggest that the lipid pool associated with plaque elastica may be rather stagnant and not easily removed. Wagner and Clarkson (1973) arrived at a similar conclusion from regression experiments in animals with induced atherosclerosis.

Glycosaminoglycans. A third major component of the extracellular matrix that is increased in fibrous plaques of arteries is the glycosaminoglycans (GAGs). Stevens et al. (1976) at Dr. Karl Schmidt's laboratory have unequivocally shown that the GAGs increase in human lesions with increasing severity of atherosclerosis when their content was expressed per square centimeter of intima instead of in gram per dry defatted tissue. There was approximately a tenfold increase of these macromolecules in advanced fibrous plaques. This increase was mainly due to large increases in dermatan sulfate, while heparan sulfate decreased slightly and classical chondroitin-4-sulfate (chondroitin sulfate A) was not detectable in diseased or normal aortic intima. However, hyaluronic acid was present in the intima of lesions and nonlesions in agreement with the small amounts required for the aggregation of proteoglycans. The increase of dermatan sulfate in lesions is of great interest since it is this GAG which has been shown in vitro to bind most avidly but reversibly LDL and VLDL.

Except for hyaluronic acid, all GAGs are bound to proteins of various composition to form proteoglycans. It is noteworthy that according to Radhakrishnamurthy et al. (1977) the protein moieties of all arterial proteoglycans contain large amounts of the polar amino acids, glutamic acid, and aspartic acid. These authors also reported that in normal bovine aorta a fairly large amount of proteoglycans are soluble and can be extracted with 0.15M NaCl. These proteoglycans contain about 50% of the total aortic content of chondroitin-4- and 6-sulfates and almost all chondroitin. About 75% of hyaluronic acid also is extractable by saline solutions. The soluble proteoglycans and hyaluronic acid presumably constitute the major portion of the so-called ground substance as well as proteoglycans bound to soluble collagen. Most of the remaining proteoglycans and GAGs not extractable by saline appear to be bound to the arterial connective tissue protein elastin (which per se is an insoluble protein) and the insoluble collagen. The insoluble collagen is mainly associated with proteoglycans containing large amounts of chondroitin-6-sulfate as well as smaller amounts of chondroitin-4-sulfate, dermatan sulfate and hyaluronic acid, while the proteoglycans associated with elastin contain exclusively heparan sulfate.

However, it is of interest that elastase solutions (containing inhibitors of nonspecific proteolytic activity) solubilized large amounts of dermatan sulfate along with the elastin from the NaCl-extracted aortic tissue (Radhakrishnamurthy et al. 1977). This finding suggests that protein-free dermatan sulfate may be bound to arterial elastin and it could also explain the deposition of LDL and VLDL seen on plaque elastica by immunohistochemical techniques (Walton and Williamson 1968; Hoff and Glaubatz 1977). One could speculate that an increase in the GAGs bound to elastin of plaques could, in turn, facilitate an increase deposition of LDL and VLDL from which an increased transfer of cholesterol esters to plaque elastin could occur in vivo. Unfortunately, it was not technically possible to demonstrate any such role of GAGs in our own studies (Kramsch et al. 1971; Kramsch and Hollander 1973) since the hot alkali used to isolate an elastin protein - lipid complex with a reasonably collagen-free protein moiety was so drastic that virtually all GAGs were destroyed and none were detectable in the purified elastin fraction. However, the protein moiety of the proteoglycans associated with plaque elastin may not have been destroyed completely by the alkali and may in part account for the high content of glutamic and aspartic acid in the elastin.

In contrast to our lack of knowledge of the quantity of GAGs bound to the elastin fraction of plaques, it is known (Hollander et al. 1974a) that about 18% of the total GAGs in plaques are bound to the insoluble collagen. These GAGs could play a role in the direct or indirect binding of lipoproteins and lipids to the collagen of lesions.

Glycoproteins. The fourth class of extracellular macromolecules is the glycoproteins. As opposed to proteoglycans in which the protein moiety is small and the bulk of the macromolecules consists of acidic polysaccharides, glycoproteins are predominantly proteins in nature, bearing a small number of branched oligosaccharide units. According to a recent review by Anderson (1976), the presence of four distinct varieties of glycoproteins in arteries has definitely been established. They are: 1) glycoproteins that are closely associated with collagen, 2) the microfibrillar glycoproteins of elastin, 3) glycoproteins that are covalently bound to the basement membrane, and 4) glycoproteins concerned with the aggregation of proteoglycans. Many of these glycoproteins are soluble, such as those linked with NaCl-soluble collagen and proteoglycans. The glycoproteins that are tightly bound to insoluble arterial components, such as elastin, insoluble collagen, or basement membranes, or are associated with the proteoglycans bound to these insoluble structures also are insoluble in NaCl and can be broadly termed structural glycoproteins.

It has been proposed by Robert and Robert (1973) that these structural intercellular matrix macromolecules direct the oriented formation of collagen fibers, elastic laminae, and basement membranes. Because of this capacity, any alterations of glycoproteins in plaques would play a major role in atherosclerosis. However, little is known about quantitative or qualitative changes of glycoproteins in plaques. The only exception is the probable role of structural glycoproteins as autoantigenic factors in the formation of atherosclerotic lesions (Robert et al. 1971) and their apparent overproduction in plaques, especially their presumed increase in the elastin fraction, as a result of tissue degradation in the original lesion (Ouzilou et al. 1973). It is also of interest that very acidic glycoproteins are known to be involved in the calcification of collagen (Zamoscianik and Veis 1966; Anderson 1976).

Formation and Degradation of Connective Tissue in Plaques

The cells responsible for the synthesis of connective tissue macromolecules in arteries appear to be mainly the arterial smooth muscle cells, although cultured endothelial cells (Macarak et al. 1976) also have been reported to synthesize collagen. Arterial smooth muscle cells in culture have been shown to synthesize crosslinked collagen (Ross and Glomset 1973), including type I and type III collagen (Layman et al. 1977), the microfibrillar glycoprotein of elastin (Ross and Glomset 1973), other glycoproteins (Robert and Robert 1974), crosslinked elastin (Faris et al. 1976), and the GAGs dermatan sulfate, the chondroitin sulfates, and hyaluronic acid (Wight and Ross 1973).

Collagen and elastin appear to be extruded from the cells in the form of soluble procollagen and tropoelastin via, at least in part, a system which includes microtubules and the Golgi apparatus. This has been demonstrated with certainty for collagen (Ehrlich et al. 1974); elastin possibly is extruded in a similar manner. Before extrusion, procollagen is hydroxylated at certain proline and lysine residues by the enzymes prolyl and lysl hydroxylase. Unhydroxylated procollagen is not secreted by the cells (Grant and Prockop 1972). A sensitive method for detecting early increases in collagen synthesis is the determination of prolyl hydroxylase (Fuller and Langner 1970). Crosslinking of soluble precursors occurs extracellularly, resulting in the extracellular deposition of collagen and elastin fibers. The mechanisms for the synthesis and secretion of GAGs and glycoproteins by arterial smooth muscle cells are less well understood. Furthermore, GAGs are known to circulate in the blood stream (Calatroni et al. 1969) and plasma GAGs also could be a source for the GAG increase in plaques.

Little is known about factors that might trigger the sclerogenic response of arteries leading to the formation of fibrous plaques. As recently reviewed in part by Armstrong (1976), an arterial fibrogenic effect could result from dietary factors such as cholesterol, saturated fats in general, peanut oil, as well as monounsaturated and transpolyunsaturated cholesterol esters. Diabetes, immune reactions, hypertension, and various chemical and mechanical injuries to the arterial wall or just its endothelial layer also appear to be fibrogenic.

The turnover rate of arterial collagen in normal adults is believed to be slow. Similarly, the half-life of normal mature elastin is considered to approximate the life span of the animal (Slack 1954). And yet, as recently shown by Yu and Yoshida (1977), most of the ^{14}C-labeled elastin implanted into the peritoneal cavity of normal rats was degraded between 6 and 15 days by macrophages present in large numbers at the implantation site.

In experimental atherosclerosis, however, the turnover of arterial collagen appears to be accelerated with the synthesis outweighing degradation (Wartman et al. 1967; Lindner 1974; McCullagh and Page 1974), leading to a net increase of collagen in advanced lesions (Lindner 1974). The arterial wall was found to have a marked collagenolytic activity, at least in rabbits

(Lindner 1974); collagenases also are thought to be contained in the serum (Lindner 1974), in platelets and polymorphnuclear leucocytes (Mustard et al. 1974), as well as in macrophages (Wahl et al. 1974). Macrophages are known to be actively engaged in the resorption of tissue collagen (Schwarz and Guldner 1967; Parakkal 1969).

No exact data are available on the turnover rate of elastin, GAGs, or glycoproteins in atherosclerosis. It is of interest, however, that our laboratory (Kramsch and Chan 1976) was able to show that the in vivo synthesis of elastin appeared to be increased in atherosclerosis. It is possible that the doubling of elastica seen by microscopy in lesions may result from new formation of elastic tissue (reduplication).

On the other hand, the doubling of lesion elastica also may be caused by degradation (splitting). There is good evidence (Jordan et al. 1974) that naturally occurring hydrophobic ligands such as free fatty acids bind to isolated elastin in vitro, presumably to hydrophobic sites, increasing elastolysis by pancreatic elastase up to 25-fold with linoleic acid being the most effective. Studies by Kagan and Lerch (1976) revealed that approximately 70% of the potentially anionic dicarboxylic residue of elastin, glutamic, and aspartic acid are amidated, rendering the intrinsic negative charge of elastin considerably lower than previously suspected. The positively charged enzyme elastase, however, needs negative charges on elastin in order to attach to its substrate and unfold its elastolytic activity. This would explain why anionic hydrophobic ligands, such as fatty acids bound to elastin, could attract elastase and increase its elastolytic effect so dramatically. In recent studies by Kagan and ourselves (1979), we have shown that in perfused intact rabbit aortae, linoleic acid also increased markedly the effect of elastase in degrading the intimo-medial elastic lamellae of normal aortae. An increased amount of free fatty acids has been observed in lesion elastin with increasing severity of atherosclerosis (Jacotot 1974).

It has been advanced that elastase, presumably of pancreatic origin, circulates in the blood stream (Loewen 1969) where it is inhibited by α_1-antitrypsin and presumably α_2-macroglobulin (Baumstark 1967). Proteases with elastolytic activities have been obtained from human spleen (Franzblau 1971) and from granules of circulating neutrophil granulocytes (Janoff and Scherer 1968) and platelets (Legrand et al. 1973; Mustard et al. 1974). Since platelets also contain other proteolytic enzymes (such as cathepsin) and polysaccharide-degrading enzymes (Mustard et al. 1974), it seems possible that proteolytic and mucolytic enzymes released from platelet thrombi forming on elastic laminae after endothelial (or other arterial) injury (Bjorkerud 1969; Stemerman and Ross 1972) can destroy the protective proteoglycan coat of elastin (Partridge and Keeley 1974), exposing it to elastolysis by elastase. However, elastase from neutrophil granulocytes appears to be different from pancreatic elastase. Its effect on elastin is not increased but inhibited by unsaturated fatty acids (Ashe and Zimmerman 1977).

It is of particular interest that an especially active form of elastase has been found in macrophages (Werb and Gordon 1975), which also are known to contain many other proteolytic and mucolytic enzymes. Glagov (1977) and also Schwartz (1977) recently have demonstrated that monocytes, the circulating precursors of macrophages, can be found in experimental animals deep in the arterial media in areas of endothelial injury. A substantial number of monocyte-derived macrophages have recently been detected in diet-induced lesions of nonhuman primates (Schaffner et al. 1977). It is very possible that these macrophages are involved in the degradation of arterial elastica. Presumably, both processes, degradation and de novo synthesis of elastin, occur simultaneously in athersclerosis, with synthesis outweighing degradation. As shown by Clark and Glagov (1977) elastic branch fascicles are attached to arterial smooth muscle cells and form one functional unit. One can imagine what deleterious effect the destruction of large segments of elastica must have on the functional integrity of the arterial walls.

Calcium in the Pathobiochemistry of Connective Tissue

Calcium appears to play an important role in the pathobiochemistry of the intercellular matrix macromolecules. Calcium ions are required for the complexing of LDL and VLDL to GAGs in the serum (Srinivasan et al. 1970) as well as to GAGs in arteries (Radhakrishnamurthy et al. 1977). Ca^{++}-dependent mechanisms may be responsible for excessive degradation of arterial elastin. At the appropriate concentration and appropriate ionic strength, Ca^{++} has been shown to significantly increase elastolysis by pancreatic elastase in vitro (Kagan 1977, unpublished work). The calcium chelator EDTA inhibits the elastolytic activity of macrophage elastase (Werb and Gordon 1975). Since the elastolytic, collagenolytic, and mucolytic properties of enzymes contained in platelets also may play a role in the connective tissue alterations in atherosclerosis, it is of particular interest that Packham et al. (1978) have demonstrated that the adherence of platelets to collagen, their aggregation, and their release reaction require Ca^{++}; all these phenomena can be prevented by EDTA or citrate. The reactions of platelets to arterial collagen are thought to be important factors in the initiation of atherogenesis (Ross and Glomset 1976a,b) as well as in the thrombotic complications of late atherosclerosis (Mustard and Packham 1970).

Calcium ions also appear to mediate cellular functions operative in the synthesis and secretions of connective tissue. The anticalcific agent ethanehydroxy diphosphate has been shown to inhibit proline hydroxylation in collagen (Minkin et al. 1974), a necessary step for the secretion of procollagen from collagen synthetizing cells (Grant and Prockop 1972). Likewise, the addition of increasing concentrations of the direct Ca^{++}-antagonist lanthanum to arterial smooth muscle cells in culture has recently been shown to increasingly inhibit the secretion but not the synthesis of collagen and presumably elastin (Kramsch and Allam, unpublished work).

In addition, calcium appears to play an important part in the binding of secondary proteins to lesion elastin either through Ca^{++} bridges or simply by incrustation of the whole elastic fiber with calcium minerals (Keeley and Partridge 1974). Proposed possible nucleation sites for calcium mineralization include the polar microfibrillar glycoprotein associated with the elastin (Ross and Bornstein 1969) or the likewise closely associated GAGs (Weissman and Weissman 1960; Yu and Blumenthal 1963), or neutral peptide groups of the elastin itself (Urry et al. 1973). Acid phospholipids also have been shown to bind Ca^{++} (Vogel and Boylan-Salyers 1976). It is noteworthy that the phospholipid content of the elastin fraction from plaques, though small, may be increased tenfold as compared to that of normal arterial elastin. Calcium and phosphorus have been shown to bind to arterial elastin purified with formic acid (Seligman et al. 1975). Binding of Ca^{++} to normal arterial elastin in vitro has been shown to cause configurational changes in this protein, exposing more hydrophic sites and giving rise to an increased absorption of other hydrophobic molecules such as cholesterol (Hornebeck and Partridge 1975).

The principal target tissue for calcification of arteries in atherosclerosis and aging appears to be the elastica (Weissman and Weissman 1960; Yu and Blumenthal 1963; Haust and Geer 1970; Keeley and Partridge 1974). Calcium mineralization of aortic elastica in preference to collagen also has been demonstrated in vitro (Bladen and Martin 1962). The main constituents of the minerals associated with elastins appeared to be calcium and phosphorus (Yu and Blumenthal 1963; Yu 1971), which appeared to be present, at least at later stages, in the form of hydroxy-appatite crystals (Bladen and Martin 1962; Yu and Blumenthal 1963; Serafini-Fracassini 1963) as indicated by x-ray diffraction and electron microscopy.

Plaque collagen also can calcify presumably with associated glycoproteins serving as nucleation sites (Anderson 1976). But there are several examples of calcified tissues that contain proteins other than collagen, indicating that collagen is not essential for calcification (Anderson 1976). An α-carboxyglutamic acid-containing noncollagenous protein that binds Ca^{++} and phospholipids has been detected in calcified plaques but not in the tissue from normal areas of human aortae (Lian et al. 1976). However, the plaque components that this protein is associated with is still unknown.

It also should be recognized that all processes leading to the formation of fibrous plaques: the biosynthesis of connective tissue macromolecules, their secretion, and their degradation require energy in the form of Ca^{++}- (and Mg^{++}-) dependent high-energy phosphates.

Suppression of Connective Tissue Alterations

Since it is the alterations of the arterial connective tissue that render atherosclerosis so dangerous, it has become imperative to search for means to prevent, reverse, or at least arrest these changes.

Recent reports (Walker 1977; Levy 1980) have shown that morbidity and mortality from cardiovascular disease has declined slightly in the United States during the last decade. However, it appears still too early to say whether this is the result of less pronounced atherosclerosis or a diminishing and/or better treatment of its sequellae, notably thrombosis and cardiac complications. With some notable exceptions (Buchwald et al. 1974; Blankenhorn 1977), all means to lower elevated serum cholesterol levels in Western man have resulted in serum cholesterol levels still above the level that would be atherogenic in nonhuman primates (Kramsch and Hollander 1968; Armstrong 1976; Wissler and Vesselinovitch 1976). Even if the serum cholesterol levels in our population were lowered to nonatherogenic levels, which is considered by several investigators (Lee et al. 1963; Geerdink et al. 1973; Armstrong 1976; Wissler and Vesselinovitch 1976) to be around 150 - 160 mg/100 ml, regression of fibrous lesions might be extremely slow, if one can extrapolate from several pertinent experiments in nonhuman primates (Armstrong and Megan 1975; Wissler and Vesselinovitch 1976). Heavily calcified human plaques may not regress at all.

Since it still appears uncertain whether serum cholesterol levels in our society generally can be lowered to the required nonatherogenic levels, it seems reasonable to test agents that might inhibit or prevent the disease despite continued high serum cholesterol levels. Several such studies already have been performed using rabbits and pigeons on various atherogenic regimens. For example, Wartman et al. (1967) reported diminished accumulation of aortic collagen and elastin after treatment with Mg-EDTA; Hollander et al. (1974b) reported complete prevention of collagen and elastin accumulation by treatment with the microtubular disruptive drug colchicine and the copper chelator penicillamine; Rosenblum et al. (1975) reported inhibition of lesion formation and calcium mineralization in rabbits by treatment with relatively low dosages (up to 5 mg/kg body wt/day) of ethane-1-hydroxy-1,1-diphosphonic acid (EHDP); and Wagner et al. (1977) recently suppressed the usually occurring calcium mineralization of lesions during regression from induced atherosclerosis in pigeons, also with small doses of EHDP.

In our laboratory we have been experimenting to achieve these goals in rabbits and monkeys on fibrogenic atherogenic diets. The animals were treated with EHDP, an agent which is known to prevent the deposition of calcium into soft tissue (Fleisch et al. 1970; Rosenblum et al. 1975; Wagner et al. 1977). EHDP also has been shown to inhibit the proline hydroxylation of procollagen (Minkin et al. 1974). Other diphosphonates employed were the disodium salts of amino-1-hydroxy-propane-1,1-diphosphonic acid (APDP) and azacycloheptane-2,2-diphosphonic acids (AHDP). These newer diphosphonates have been shown to have anticalcific properties similar to EHDP (Potokar and Schmidt-Dunker 1978). Other animals on the atherogenic diet were treated with the methylated derivative of 2-thiophene carboxylic acid (Methyl-ThCA). Thiophene carboxylic acid is thought to exert a thyrocalcitonin-like effect on maintaining calcium homeostasis (Lloyd et al. 1969). Successful treatment with these calcium-regulating agents suggested that atherogenesis may be beneficially influenced by regulating the availability of ionic calcium. We therefore treated atherogenic animals with the direct calcium ion antagonist, lanthanum, at different dosage levels. Other animals were treated with the microtubular disruptive drug (Yin et al. 1972) n-acetyl-n-methyl-colchicine (Colcemid), which probably, like its parent compound, colchicine, increases the biosynthesis of collagenase (Harris and Krane 1971). Still other animals received the antimicrotubular drug Vinblastine or a combination of a microtubular disruptive drug (Colcemid) and an anticalcium agent (EHDP).

The fibrogenic atherogenic diet for rabbits contained 8% peanut oil and 2% cholesterol according to a slight modification of the method of Kritchevsky et al. (1971); that for monkeys contained 10% unsalted butter and 0.1% cholesterol as previously described (Kramsch et al. 1973). The control diets were Purina Rabbit and Monkey Chow with banana mash added to the ground monkey chow.

Altogether, 12 groups of 10 New Zealand White Rabbits each and 8 groups of generally 8 adult male Macaca fascicularis (cynomolgus) monkeys each were fed the atherogenic diets or the control diets: rabbits for 8 weeks, monkeys for 18 months. One group of rabbits was fed the control diet and one group the atherogenic diet alone, while 10 groups were given the atherogenic diet plus EHDP, APDP, AHDP, Methyl-ThCA, $LaCl_3$ (at three dosage levels), Colcemid, Vinblastine, and Colcemid, and EHDP combined, respectively. Likewise, one group of monkeys was fed the control diet and one group the atherogenic diet alone while three groups were given the atherogenic diet plus EHDP,

$LaCl_3$ (8 monkeys each), and Colcemid (3 monkeys), respectively. In addition, two groups of 4 monkeys each were exercised
in a tread-mill by having them run 1 hour/day every other day
at a speed of 3 km/hour. One of these groups of monkeys was
fed the control diet and the other the atherogenic diet without
drugs. In animals receiving drugs, the daily oral dosages per
kilogram body weight were: EHDP, APDP, and AHDP = 40 mg
for rabbits; EHDP for monkeys = 120 mg for 6 months and 40 mg
thereafter (EHDP as the calculated substance of the hexahy-
drate); $LaCl_3$ = 20, 30, and 40 mg for rabbits and for monkeys
120 mg followed by 40 mg as with EHDP; Colcemid and Vinblastine = 0.06 mg for both species. In exercising monkeys the
heart rates at rest and during exercise were reduced to 70% -
75% of the untrained rates, indicating exercise conditioning.

In all animals on the atherogenic diet, the serum cholesterol
was markedly elevated to about the same levels within each animal species regardless of whether or not any of the drugs were
given; exercise likewise had no influence on the raised cholesterol levels in monkeys on the atherogenic diet (Table 2). The
serum calcium content remained normal in both species regardless
of diet, drug treatment, or exercise, with the exception of rabbits treated with either dose of lanthanum or with Colcemid, in
which it was elevated.

As compared to animals on the control diet, rabbits (Table 3)
and monkeys (Table 4) on the atherogenic diets revealed drastic
increases in the content of the following components of the aortic
intima-media: collagen, elastin, cholesterol, calcium, and non-
lipid phosphorus. As mentioned before, the arterial elastin fraction of untreated atherogenic animals of both species also was
markedly altered, revealing marked increases in its content of
polar amino acids (Table 1) as well as cholesterol, calcium and
phosphorus (elastin constituents for monkeys: Table 5).

In rabbits (Table 3), simultaneous treatment with any of the
drugs resulted in marked reductions in the atherogenic changes
despite continued presence of the atherogenic stimulus of unmiti-

TABLE 2. Serum Components of Animals on Control Diets and on Atherogenic Diets with and without Treatment

rabbits = 8 weeks, monkeys = 18 months, values in mg/100 ml (mean ± s.d.)

Experimental groups	Rabbits		Monkeys	
	Cholesterol	Calcium	Cholesterol	Calcium
Control diet	82 ± 23	13.2 ± 1.1	136 ± 42[a]	11.0 ± 2.3[a]
Atherogenic diet, untreated	2573 ± 568[d]	13.3 ± 1.2	539 ± 157[a,d]	10.8 ± 1.8[a]
Atherogenic diet + EHDP	3535 ± 738[d]	13.4 ± 0.6	492 ± 183[a,d]	9.7 ± 1.6[a]
Atherogenic diet + APDP	2488 ± 534[d]	14.5 ± 0.9	--	--
Atherogenic diet + AHDP	2283 ± 664[d]	14.7 ± 0.7	--	--
Atherogenic diet + Methyl ThCA	3324 ± 716[d]	13.4 ± 0.7	488[a,b]	10.8[a,b]
Atherogenic diet + LaCl$_3$ (20 mg)	2431 ± 489[d]	14.8 ± 1.0[e]	--	--
Atherogenic diet + LaCl$_3$ (30 mg)	2035 ± 921[d]	15.3 ± 1.3[d]	--	--
Atherogenic diet + LaCl$_3$ (40 mg)	2537 ± 621[d]	16.0 ± 1.2[d]	513 ± 108[a]	9.5 ± 2.0[a]
Atherogenic diet + Colcemid	3841 ± 938[d]	13.9 ± 0.6[d]	583[a,b]	11.5[a,b]
Atherogenic diet + Vinblastine	3181 ± 896[d]	13.2 ± 1.0	--	--
Atherogenic diet + Colcemid + EHDP	2973 ± 865[d]	13.2 ± 0.8	--	--
Atherogenic diet + exercise	--	--	602[c]	10.9[c]
Control diet + exercise	--	--	128[c]	11.3[c]

[a] "Sedentary" monkeys   [b] Average values from 3 monkeys   [c] Average values from 4 monkeys
[d] Highly significant changes from controls (P<0.01)   [e] Significant changes from controls (P<0.05)

TABLE 3. Components of Intima-Media from Rabbits on Control Diets and Atherogenic Diets with and without Treatment

(absolute amounts in mg/whole aorta/kg body weight; mean ± s.d.)

Experimental groups	Collagen	"Elastin"	Cholesterol	Calcium	Nonlipid phosphorus
Control diet	2.8 ± 0.5	10.3 ± 2.8	0.3 ± 0.2	0.03 ± 0.007	0.04 ± 0.02
Atherogenic diet, untreated	6.5 ± 1.3[a]	27.1 ± 1.7[a]	3.5 ± 1.2[a]	0.08 ± 0.012[a]	0.15 ± 0.03[a]
Atherogenic diet + EHDP	4.3 ± 1.1[b]	21.5 ± 1.6[a]	1.3 ± 0.5[a]	0.06 ± 0.013[a]	0.11 ± 0.06[b]
Atherogenic diet + APDP	3.7 ± 0.4[b]	15.3 ± 1.6[a]	0.7 ± 0.3[b]	0.06 ± 0.015[b]	0.13 ± 0.08
Atherogenic diet + AHDP	2.9 ± 0.8	12.4 ± 1.4	0.5 ± 0.1[b]	0.04 ± 0.017	0.11 ± 0.05
Atherogenic diet + Methyl ThCA	3.2 ± 0.8	12.8 ± 2.7	0.7 ± 0.3[b]	0.02 ± 0.010	0.05 ± 0.02
Atherogenic diet + LaCl$_3$ (20 mg)	4.2 ± 0.6[a]	17.3 ± 1.9[a]	1.9 ± 1.0[a]	0.04 ± 0.010[b]	0.06 ± 0.01[b]
Atherogenic diet + LaCl$_3$ (30 mg)	3.6 ± 0.6[b]	14.4 ± 0.7[a]	1.4 ± 0.7[a]	0.03 ± 0.010	0.04 ± 0.03
Atherogenic diet + LaCl$_3$ (40 mg)	2.9 ± 0.8	13.6 ± 4.7	0.6 ± 0.1[b]	0.03 ± 0.008	0.05 ± 0.02
Atherogenic diet + Colcemid	3.8 ± 0.5[b]	16.4 ± 1.8[a]	0.6 ± 0.2[b]	0.04 ± 0.009[b]	0.03 ± 0.01
Atherogenic diet + Vinblastine	4.3 ± 1.2[b]	17.2 ± 2.2[a]	0.9 ± 0.4[b]	0.03 ± 0.004	0.04 ± 0.03
Atherogenic diet and Colcemid + EHDP	3.2 ± 1.2	14.4 ± 4.3	0.8 ± 0.3[b]	0.03 ± 0.009	0.06 ± 0.03

[a]Highly significant changes from control values (P<0.01).
[b]Significant changes from control values (P<0.05).

TABLE 4. Components of Aortic Intima-media from Monkeys on Control Diets and Atherogenic Diets with and without Treatment (m/cm length in situ/kg body weight; mean ± s.d.)

Aortic segment and treatment	Collagen	"Elastin"	Cholesterol	Calcium	Nonlipid phosphorus
Thoracic aorta					
Control diet[a]	217 ± 31	544 ± 39	22 ± 8	4 ± 2	3 ± 2
Atherogenic diet, untreated[a]	782 ± 183[d]	912 ± 165[d]	347 ± 127[d]	82 ± 29[d]	49 ± 14[d]
Atherogenic diet + Colcemid[a]	675[b]	967[b]	328[b]	73[b]	64[b]
Atherogenic diet + EHDP	307 ± 97	633 ± 46[e]	156 ± 75[d]	5 ± 2	4 ± 2
Atherogenic diet + LaCl$_3$ (40 mg)[a]	388 ± 112[d]	771 ± 199[d]	178 ± 83[d]	6 ± 1[e]	5 ± 1[e]
Atherogenic diet + exercise	321[c]	516[c]	110[c]	10[c]	12[c]
Control diet + exercise	298[c]	354[c]	20[c]	2[c]	2[c]
Abdominal aorta					
Control diet[a]	308 ± 46	312 ± 29	10 ± 3	2 ± 1	1 ± 1
Atherogenic diet, untreated[a]	963 ± 105[d]	474 ± 102[d]	457 ± 198[d]	46 ± 18[d]	34 ± 12[d]
Atherogenic diet + Colcemid[a]	812[b]	524[b]	396[b]	42[b]	40[b]
Atherogenic diet + EHDP[a]	262 ± 88	267 ± 52	122 ± 62[d]	3 ± 1	3 ± 2
Atherogenic diet + LaCl$_3$ (40 mg)[a]	225 ± 75	242 ± 80	143 ± 71[d]	2 ± 1	2 ± 1
Atherogenic diet + exercise	413[c]	320[c]	98[c]	4[c]	3[c]
Control diet + exercise	223[c]	129[c]	7[c]	1[c]	1[c]

[a]"Sedentary" monkeys   [b]Average values from three monkeys   [c]Average values from four monkeys

[d]Highly significant changes from control values (P<0.02)   [e]Significant changes from controls (P<0.05)

TABLE 5. Constituents of Elastin from Control Monkeys and Monkeys on the Atherogenic Diet with and without Drugs (μg/g elastin; mean ± s.d.)

Arteries	Calcium				Nonlipid phosphorus			
	Control diet	Athero diet	Athero + La^{3+}	Athero + EHDP	Control diet	Athero diet	Athero + La^{3+}	Athero + EHDP
Thorac. aorta	3.6 ± 0.3	97.1 ± 21.3[a]	5.9 ± 0.4[a]	7.0 ± 0.5[a]	3.1 ± 1.5	50.7 ± 16.3[a]	3.5 ± 0.9	3.0 ± 1.1
Abdom. aorta	2.8 ± 1.1	77.4 ± 19.0[a]	3.2 ± 1.3	4.2 ± 1.6	3.7 ± 1.3	14.0 ± 3.8[a]	2.2 ± 1.5	3.2 ± 0.8
Subclavian	3.9 ± 0.8	22.9 ± 6.5[a]	2.0 ± 1.2	5.3 ± 0.6[b]	2.8 ± 0.7	8.3 ± 2.2[a]	3.5 ± 1.4	4.5 ± 1.1
Carotid	3.7 ± 1.2	22.5 ± 7.7[a]	3.8 ± 0.4	5.4 ± 1.2	1.2 ± 0.4	10.2 ± 4.1[a]	1.2 ± 0.2	1.4 ± 0.3
Iliac	4.3 ± 1.5	16.9 ± 4.9[a]	3.8 ± 0.5	7.7 ± 2.6	5.3 ± 1.6	11.9 ± 2.6[a]	3.2 ± 1.7	5.4 ± 1.4
Femoral	2.6 ± 0.7	6.4 ± 1.8[a]	3.1 ± 0.6	3.9 ± 1.3	--	--	--	--

[a]Highly significant changes from control values (P<0.01)
[b]Significant changes from control values (P<0.15)

gated hypercholesterolemia. Best results were obtained by treatment with AHDP, Methyl-ThCa, La Cl$_3$ (40 mg), and the combination of Colcemid with EHDP. Treatment with these drugs completely suppressed the aortic accumulation of collagen, elastin, calcium, and phosphorus. Also, the accumulation of aortic cholesterol was drastically reduced. Lipid, presumably contained in the thin layer of intimal foam cells (Fig. 9A), was the only atherogenic alteration observed in these animals. The amino acid, calcium, and lipid composition of elastin also was normal in rabbits treated with this four-drug regimen.

In monkeys (Table 4), treatment with Colcemid alone did not inhibit the biochemical arterial changes elicited by the atherogenic diet, at least not at the dosage level given. But treatment with EHDP, LaCl$_3$, and exercise did result in marked reductions in the biochemical arterial alterations, with the atherogenic changes of collagen, elastin, calcium and phosphorus being completely suppressed in the abdominal aorta. The exception again was the arterial cholesterol content, which was greatly reduced but not to normal, with residual lipids presumably being contained mainly in the intimal cells of the few and small cellular lesions present in the intima in all of these three treatment groups. Treatment with EHDP and LaCl$_3$ also suppressed the atherogenic calcium and phosphorus changes of elastin in the abdominal aorta as well as in other systemic arteries (Table 5). The arterial elastin composition in exercised monkeys has as yet not been analyzed.

It is noteworthy that, with the exception of the collagen content of thoracic aorta, the contents of all aortic components measured (collagen, elastin, cholesterol, calcium, and phosphorus) was lower in exercising monkeys on the control diet than in sedentary control monkeys on the same diet, including collagen in the abdominal aorta. These results indicate a direct effect of conditioning exercise on these arterial components even in normal animals. On the other hand, no effect of drug treatment has been observed on the normal arterial components measured in

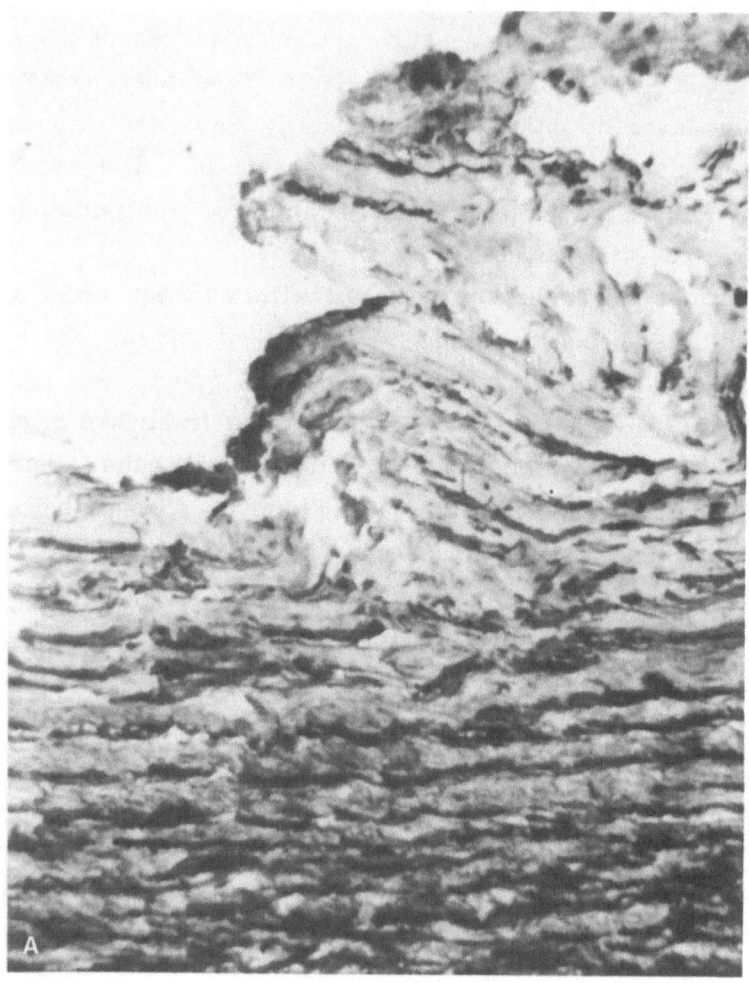

FIG. 8. A (above) and B (facing page) are sequential sections through a characteristic lesion of thoracic aorta of rabbit on the fibrogenic atherogenic diet for 8 weeks without drugs. A. Note proliferated intimal foam cells (top), accumlation of collagen (grey) and deranged and fragmented elastica (black) in the intimo-medial area. Gomori trichrome - aniline blue, X 85. B. Note calcium deposition (black) on the deranged elastica. Yasue's - light green, X 85

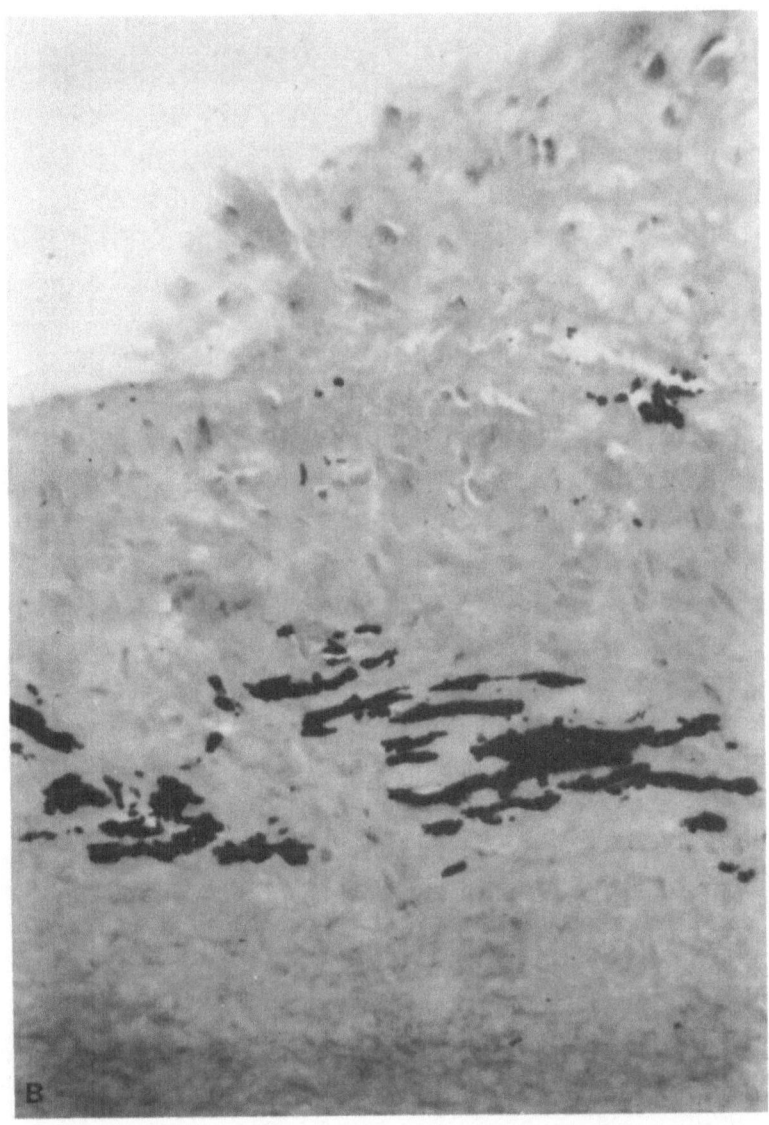

control-diet animals, at least not in the lanthanum, EHDP, and Colcemid treated rabbits where it has been tested (Kramsch et al. 1980; Kramsch, unpublished observations).

The histologic results were in agreement with the biochemical findings. Figure 8A shows a section through a typical lesion of aorta in a rabbit on the atherogenic diet for 8 weeks without

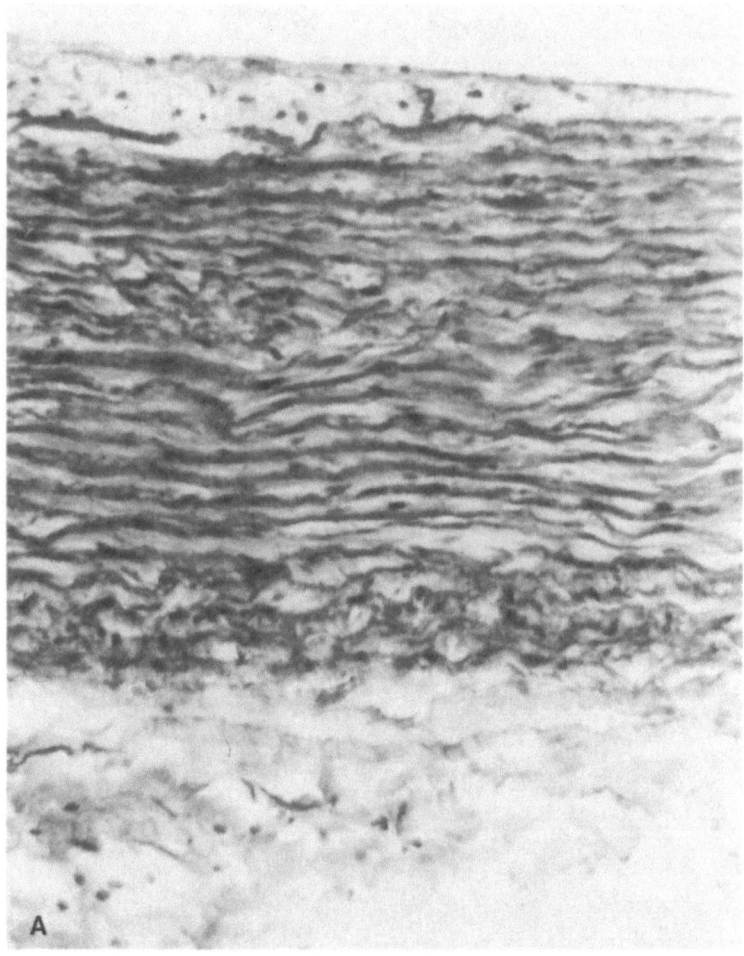

FIG. 9. A (above) and B (facing page) are sequential sections
through a lesion of thoracic aorta of a rabbit on the atherogenic
diet and treated with lanthanum. A. Note absence of collagen
accumulation, normal arterial elastica, raising of the intima by a
thin layer of (lipid-rich) foam cells. Gomori trichrome - aniline
blue, X 85 B. No calcium deposition was detectable in a sequential section. Yasue's - light green, X 85

drug treatment. The markedly raised lesion contained proliferated (lipid-rich) foam cells, marked accumulations of collagen,
fragmented and deranged elastica, as well as (Fig. 8B) deposi-

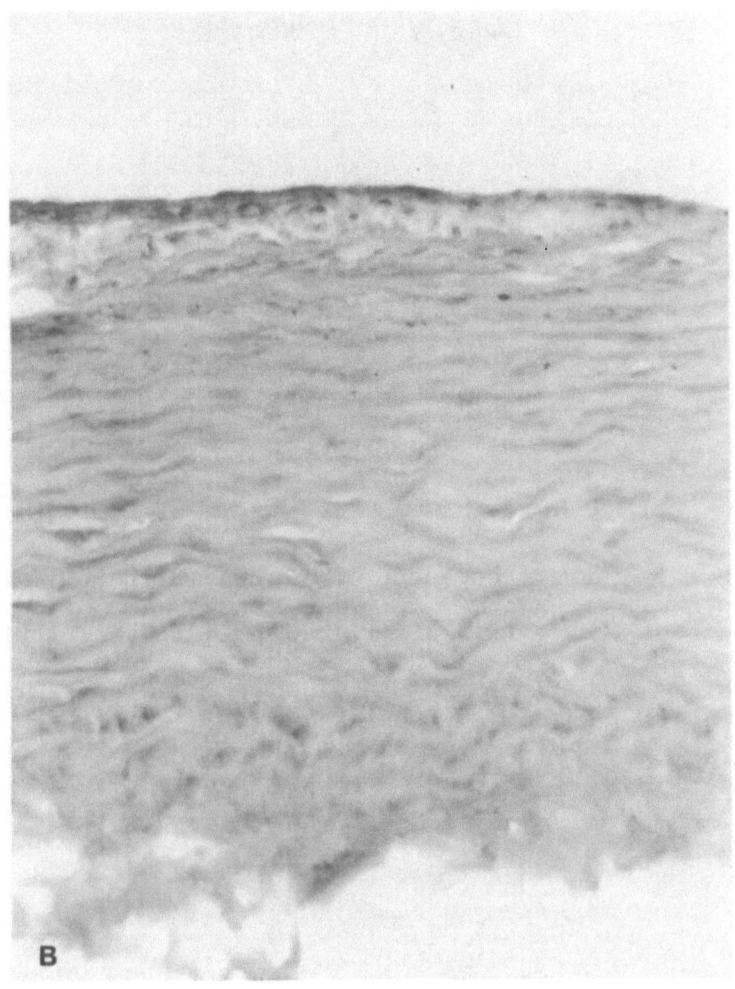

tion of calcium on the deranged elastica. Accumulations of GAGs (not shown) also were present in the lesions, mainly surrounding the damaged elastica and in areas of collagen accumulations. By contrast, treatment of rabbits with lanthanum (Fig. 9A) resulted in almost complete suppression of atherosclerosis, with the small lesions present consisting mainly of a thin layer of intimal foam cells over an otherwise normal aorta and no calcification or abnormal glycosaminoglycan depositions demonstrable (Fig. 9B). Similar lesion suppression was observed in rabbits treated with

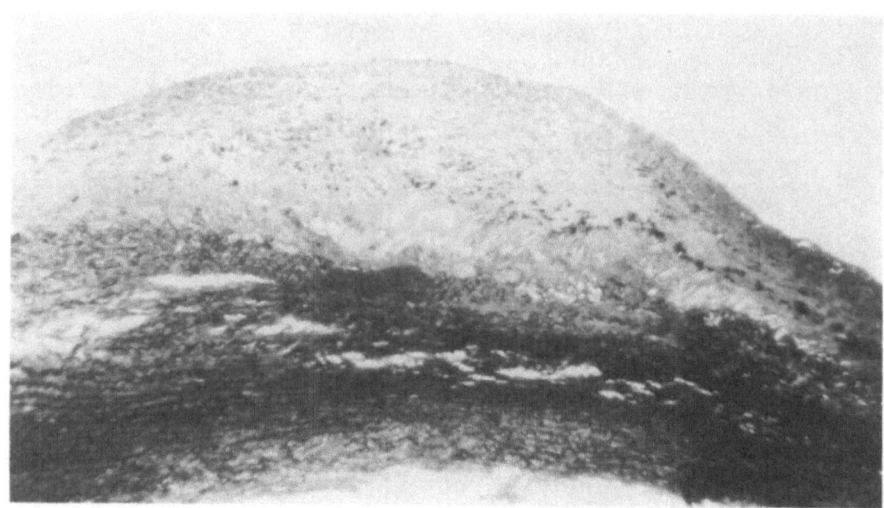

FIG. 10. Sections through one of the characteristic fibrous lesions of thoracic aorta in a sedentary monkey on the atherogenic
diet without drugs for 18 months. Note collagen containing
plaque capsule (grey) surrounding a core of necrotic foam cells;
the intimo-medial elastica (black) is fragmented and deranged.
Verhoeff's - Van Gieson, X 70

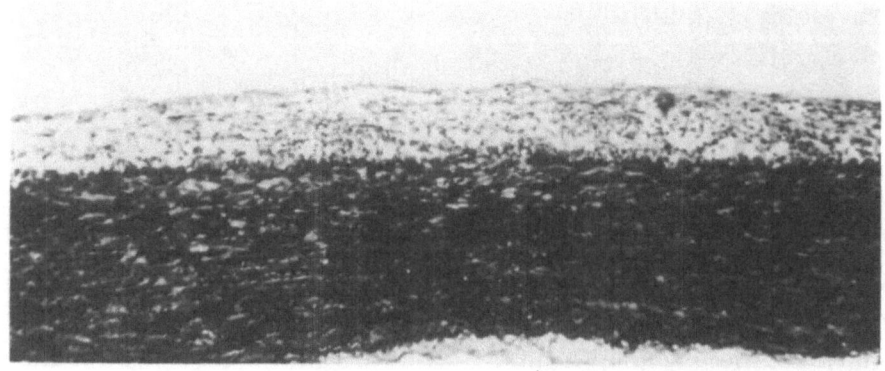

FIG. 11. Lesion of thoracic aorta in a sedentary monkey on the
atherogenic diet and treated with lanthanum for 18 months. The
lesion consists only of a few layers of (lipid-filled) foam cells in
the intima. No connective tissue changes (or calcifications) were
detectable in this lesion. Verhoeff's - Van Gieson, X 70

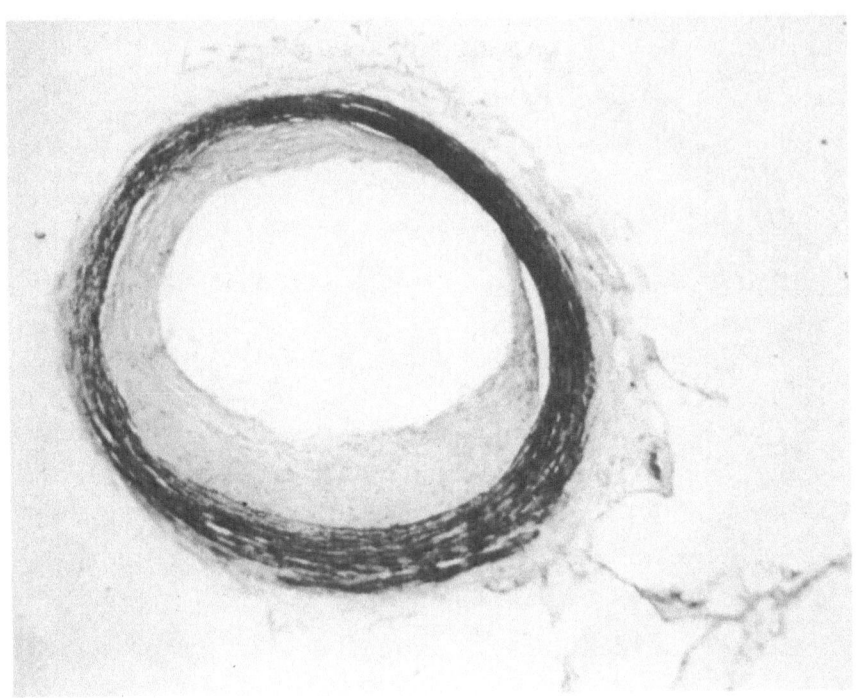

FIG. 12   Cross section of a fibrous plaque of proximal left anterior descending coronary artery in a sedentary monkey on the
atherogenic diet for 18 months without drugs.   The coronary
arteries were perfusion-fixed under the diastolic pressure of the
animal determined in vivo: 70 mm Hg.   The plaque is comprised
mainly of collagen accumulations in the intima (dark grey) ste-
nosing the arterial lumen by over 60%.   Verhoeff's - Van Gieson,
X 70

AHDP or Colcemid and EHDP in combination, in which small residual lesions were observed that were morphologically similar to
those in $LaCl_3$ treated animals.

Comparable morphologic results were observed in the nonhuman primates.   Figure 10 shows a section through one of the
more fibrous plaques of thoracic aorta in a nonexercising (sedentary) monkey on the atherogenic diet for 18 months without drug
treatment.   The lesion was more akin to a human fibrous plaque,
showing a dense fibrous (collagenous) cap overlying a partially

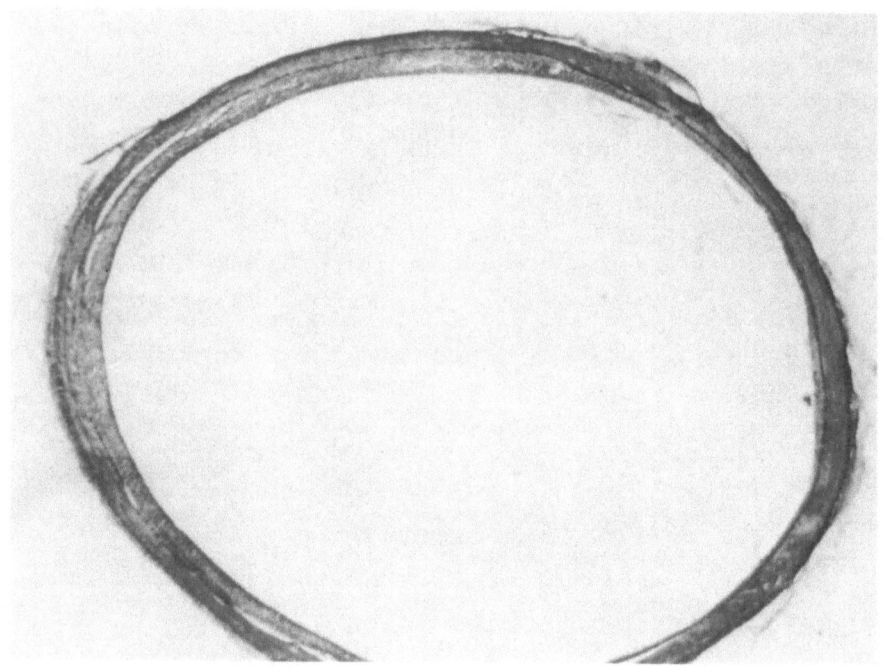

FIG. 13. Cross section through a lesion of proximal left anterior
coronary artery in an exercising monkey on the atherogenic diet
for 18 months. The coronary arteries were perfusion-fixed under the diastolic pressure of the animal determined in vivo: 70
mm Hg. The lesion is compromised of a thin layer of predominantly foam cells overlying an otherwise normal artery. The
normal arterial media appears to be thinner than in nonexercised
(sedentary) animals and the luminal diameter (determined by the
intact internal elastica - black) also is greater than normal. The
small lesion does not compromise the lumen. Verhoeff's - Van
Gieson, X 65

necrotic, lipid-filled core, and severely deranged elastica deep
into the media. Calcification (not shown) was present on the
deranged elastica as well as in the necrotic core, and massive
depositions of GAGs (not shown) were seen predominantly in the
fibrous cap. As in rabbits, treatment of these sedentary atherogenic monkeys with lanthanum resulted in much fewer and smaller
lesions characterized by a few layers of foam cells overlying an
essentially normal arterial wall (Fig. 11). A similar suppression

of atherogenesis, especially of the connective tissue and calcium abnormalities, was revealed by histology in EHDP or exercise treated monkeys.

Of special interest in monkeys were the extramural coronary arteries that in untreated sedentary atherogenic animals revealed large fibrous plaques (Fig. 12), causing considerable stenoses of the lumina. These coronary fibrous plaques were not seen in any of the treated animals except those treated with Colcemid. The coronary arteries of atherogenic monkeys treated with $LaCl_3$, EHDP, or exericse revealed only thin intimal foam cell lesions overlying an essentially normal arterial wall, which in the exercised monkeys, also appeared to be thinner than normal resulting in wider coronary artery lumina (Fig. 13).

Conclusion

While it is important to develop techniques of lowering serum lipids and lipoproteins in order to control vascular disease, one should not overlook alternative methods which may have a direct effect on the vascular wall regardless of serum cholesterol or lipoprotein levels. Of foremost importance for this purpose appear to be agents which influence the metabolism of vascular connective tissue and calcium.

Calcium homeostasis at the tissue level appears to be an important factor in the inhibition of atherogenesis. Recent studies by Robert et al. (1978) revealed that in rats with a certain experimental immunogenic injury, the formation of arterial lesions as well as elastolysis, calcification of arterial elastin, and the binding of secondary proteins to elastin were suppressed by daily injections of the hormone thyrocalcitonin, which provides calcium homeostasis independent of parathyroid mechanisms. As in the arterial lesion formation following the immunogenic injury produced by these workers, atherogenesis may be dependent on the availability of Ca^{++}. This would not be surprising in the present studies where the marked increases in total arterial calcium of untreated cholesterol-fed animals may have included increases in ionized arterial calcium. Presence of excessive amounts of Ca^{++} could have provided the increased availability of energy from Ca^{++} dependent ATP and GTP necessary for many atherogenic processes, such as increased cell migration and mitosis, endocytosis of lipids and lipoproteins, as well as of excessive synthesis and secretion of connective tissue elements and their degradation.

In vascular smooth muscle cells, as in any cell containing contractile proteins, the relaxation - contraction cycle is dependent on the myoplasmic concentration of Ca^{++} (Anderson 1973), with increasing amounts of Ca^{++} leading to increasing contractability. Moreover, a gradient of extracellular Ca^{++} appears to be instrumental in the directional movement of cells such as in chemotaxis (Boucek 1976). These cellular responses to focal increases in Ca^{++} content may account for the migration of cells into the atherosclerotic intima. The contraction of vascular endothelial cells also appears to be influenced by Ca^{++} (Numano et al. 1976), with increasing contraction presumably resulting in increased permeability of the endothelial barrier to blood-born elements such as lipoproteins as well as platelets and leucocytes. Calcium ions also have been implicated as intracellular messengers in the regulation of other important cellular functions such as the secretion of proteins (Hellman et al. 1976), including that of collagen and perhaps elastin from cultured arterial smooth muscle cells (Kramsch and Allam, unpublished work), as well as in mitosis (Berridge 1975; D'Amore and Shepro 1977). In addition, as discussed above, Ca^{++} appears to play a direct role in many important extracellular events in atherosclerosis such as the complexing of lipoproteins to arterial GAGs, the alterations of arterial elastin, and focal calcium mineralizations of arterial components.

Further evidence of the importance of ionic calcium in the formation of fibrous plaques is the increased inhibition of all atherogenic processes by increased doses of the specific calcium ion antagonist lanthanum. As reviewed by Weiss (1974) and Weiss and Goodman (1976), lanthanum is a potent competitor for Ca^{++} binding sites to which it adheres in a less reversible manner than does calcium. La^{3+} has been shown to displace and replace Ca^{++} on certain selected cell membrane loci, thereby blocking some, but not all, cellular influx and efflux of Ca^{++}, including that in arterial smooth muscle cells. Although confined to the extracellular space and adjacent membrane surfaces, larger amounts of La^{3+} profoundly inhibit in vitro the excitation - contraction coupling of muscle (skeletal, cardiac, smooth muscle), the stimulation - secretion coupling of many secretory processes, and the stimulus - division coupling of cell mitosis (D'Amore and Shepro 1977). The other inhibitors of calcium depositions into arteries employed in the present studies such as the diphosphonates and Methyl-ThCA may have produced suppression of atherogenesis in a similar manner as lanthanum, at least in part. The diphosphonate EHDP has been shown to inhibit calcium transport through cellular membranes (Guilland et al. 1974).

The beneficial effect of Colcemid and Vinblastine may be explained in part by their ability to disrupt microtubules. According to Marx (1976) these cellular organelles are involved in cell mitosis and cell motility; they also direct endocytosis and secretion of intracellular products. As discussed by Yin et al. (1972) Colcemid and Vinblastine, like Colchicine, bind specificially to the tubulin subunits and thereby disrupt microtubular assembly. This in turn appears to suppress, at least in part, excessive proliferation and motility of cells as well as to inhibit enhanced endocytosis and secretion of connective tissue elements. In the present studies, however, these microtubular disruptive agents appeared to have exerted their effect more in the inhibition of cell proliferation and migration than in the inhibition of endocytosis and secretion of connective tissue elements. This was particularly apparent in the treatment of atherogenic monkeys with Colcemid.

The beneficial effect of the comparatively moderate exercise may in part be explained by a small but significant increase in HDL-cholesterol content of exercising monkeys on the atherogenic diet (Kramsch et al. 1979). In addition, Wolinsky et al. (1979) recently have shown in normal rats that even mild exercise appears to increase several arterial enzymes involved in the catabolism of cholesterol, most notably acid cholesteryl hydrolase. However, as evidenced by the decreased arterial content of collagen, elastin, cholesterol, calcium, and phosphorus in exercising control-diet monkeys (compared to sedentary normal controls), exercise appears to have a direct effect on these arterial components. This effect may be due to a remodeling of the arterial wall in adaptation to altered hemodynamics, i.e., a decreased pulse rate in exercise conditioned animals. An increased production of connective tissue, especially of collagen, by arterial smooth muscle cells in culture exposed to rhythmical stretch compared to unstretched cultured cells has been observed by Glagov and co-workers (personal communication).

Taken together, the results of the studies presented indicate that agents capable of regulating functional calcium levels in arteries or influencing microtubular assembly may offer alternative methods in the treatment of atherosclerosis, even when elevated serum cholesterol levels and hyperlipoproteinemia cannot be effectively controlled. Equally beneficial appear to be adaptive changes in arteries brought about by moderate regular exercise.

Acknowledgment

The work was supported by U.S. Public Health Service Research Grants HL 15512, HL 13262, HL 18060 and the Henkel Co., Dusseldorf, Germany.

REFERENCES

Adams CWM, Tuqan NA (1961) Elastic degradation as a source of lipids in the early lesions of atherosclerosis. J Pathol Bacteriol 82: 131–139

Anderson R (1973) Rise of cyclic AMP and Ca^{++} in mechanical and metabolic events in isometrically contracting vascular smooth muscle cells. Acta Physiol Scand 87: 84–95

Anderson JC (1976) Glycoprotein of the connective tissue matrix. In: Hall, DA, Jackson DS (eds) International Review of Connective Tissue Research. Academic Press, New York, Vol 7, pp. 251–322

Armstrong ML (1976) Regression of atherosclerosis. In: Paoletti R, Grotto AM (eds) Atherosclerosis Reviews, Raven Press, New York, Vol 1, pp. 137–182

Armstrong ML, Megan MB (1975) Arterial fibrous proteins in cynomolgus monkeys after atherogenic and regression diets. Circ Res 36: 256–261

Ashe BM, Zimmerman M (1977) Specific inhibition of human granulocyte elastase by unsaturated fatty acids. Fed Proc 36: 678

Barnes MJ, Gordon JL, MacIntyre DE (1976) Platelet – aggregating activity of type I and type III collagens from human aorta and chicken skin. Biochem J 160: 647–651

Baumstark JS (1967) Studies on elastase-serum protein interaction. I. Molecular identity of the inhibitors in human serum and direct demonstration of inhibitor-elastase complexes by zone and immunoelectrophoresis. Arch Biochem Biophys 118: 619–630

Berridge M (1975) The interaction of cyclic nucleotides and calcium in the control of cellular activity. In: Greengaard P, Robinson GA (eds) Advances in Cyclic Nucleotide Research. Raven Press, New York, Vol 6, pp. 1–98

Bjorkerud S (1969) Reaction of the aortic wall of the rabbit after superficial, longitudinal, mechanical trauma. Virchows Arch Abt A, Pathol Anat 347: 197–210

Bladen HA, Martin GR (1962) Preferential mineralization of elastin in a matrix containing collagen. In: Fifth International Congress on Electron Microscopy. Academic Press, New York, pp. QQ-5

Blankenhorn DH (1977) Studies of regression/progression of atherosclerosis in man. In: Manning GW, Haust MD (eds) Atherosclerosis. Metabolic, Morphologic and Clinical Aspects. Adv Exp Med Biol Vol 82, pp. 453-458

Boucek M (1976) Calcium influx requirements for human neutrophil chemotaxis: inhibition by lanthanum chloride. Science 193: 905-907

Buchwald H, Moore RB, Varco RL (1974) Partial ileal by-pass operation in treatment of the hyperlipidemias. In: Kritchevsky D, Paoletti R, Holmes WL (eds) Drugs, Lipid Metabolism and Atherosclerosis. Adv Exp Med Biol Vol 63, pp. 221-230

Calatroni A, Donnelly PV, DiFerrante N (1969) Glycosaminoglycans of human plasma. J Clin Invest 48: 332-343

Clark JM, Glagov S (1977) The smooth muscle fascicle: arterial medial structure and function. Fed Proc 36: 393

D'Amore P, Shepro D (1977) Stimulation of growth and calcium influx in cultured bovine aortic endothelial cells by platelets and vasoactive substances. J Cell Physiol 92: 177-184

Ehrlich HP, Ross R, Bornstein P (1974) Effects of antimicrotubular agents on the secretion of collagen. A biochemical and morphological study. J Cell Biol 62: 390-405

Faris B, Salcedo LL, Cook V, Johnson L, Foster JA, Franzblau C (1976) The synthesis of connective tissue protein in smooth muscle cells. Biochem Biophys Acta 418: 93-103

Fleisch H, Russell RGG, Bisaz S, Muehlbauer RC, Williams DA (1970) The inhibitory effect of phosphonates on the formation of calcium phosphate crystals in vitro and on aortic and kidney calcification in vivo. Europ J Clin Invest 1: 12-18

Franzblau C (1971) Elastin. In: Florkin M, Stotz EH (eds) Comprehensive Biochemistry, Vol 26C, Elsevier, Amsterdam, pp. 659-712

Friedman M (1963) Pathogenesis of the spontaneous atherosclerotic plaque. Arch Pathol 76: 318-329

Fuller GC, Langner RO (1970) Evaluation of aortic proline hydroxylase: a biochemical defect in experimental arteriosclerosis. Science 168: 987-309

Gay S, Balleisen L (1977) Interaction of collagen types with platelets and transformation of collagen type synthesis in human atherosclerosis. In: Schettler G, Goto Y, Hata Y, Klose G (eds) Atherosclerosis IV. Springer, New York, pp. 366-367

Geerdink RA, Breel PM, Sander PC, Schillhorn-Van Veen JH (1973) Comparison of serum cholesterol values in Amerindians from Surinam with those of Dutch controls. Atherosclerosis 18: 173-178.

Gertler A (1971) The non-specific nature of the absorption of elastase and other basic proteins on elastin. Europ J Biochem 20: 541-546

Gotte L, Menegheli V, Castellani A (1965) Electron microscope observations and chemical analyses of human elastin. In: Fitton-Jackson S, Harkness RD, Tristram GR (eds) Structure and Function of Connective and Skeletal Tissue. Butterworth, London, pp. 93-101

Glagov S (1977) Presented at the annual Hugh Lofland Conference on Arterial Wall Metabolism

Grant ME, Prockop DJ (1972) The biosynthesis of collagen. Part III. N Engl J Med 286: 291-300

Guilland DF, Salis JD, Fleisch H (1974) The effect of two diphosphonates on the handling of calcium by rat kidney mitochondria in vitro. Calcif Tissue Res 15: 303-314

Harris ED Jr, Krane SM (1971) Effects of colchicine on collagenase and cultures of rheumatoid synovium. Arthritis Rheum 14: 669-684

Haust MD, Geer JC (1970) Mechanism of calcification in spontaneous arteriosclerotic lesions of the rabbit. Amer J Pathol 60: 329-338

Hellman B, Schlin S, Taljedahl I-B (1976) Calcium and secretion: distinction between two pools of glucose-sensitive calcium in pancreatic islets. Science 194: 1421-1423

Hoff HF, Glaubatz JW (1977) Ultrastructural localization of apolipoprotein B in human aortic and coronary atherosclerotic plaques. Exp Molec Pathol 26: 214-227

Hollander W, Colombo MA, Kramsch DM, Kirkpatrick B (1974a) Immunological aspects of atherosclerosis. Adv Cardiol 13: 192-207

Hollander W, Kramsch DM, Franzblau C, Padock J, Colombo MA (1974b) Suppression of atheromatous fibrous plaque formation by anti-imflammatory drugs. Circ Res 34 (suppl I): 131-141

Hornebeck W, Partridge SM (1975) Confirmational changes in fibrous elastin due to calcium ions. Europ J Clin Invest 51: 73-78

Jacotot B (1974) Intercellular macromolecules of the arterial wall and plasma lipids. In: Schettler G, Weizel A (eds) Atherosclerosis III. Springer, Berlin, pp. 207-218

Jacotot B, Monnier G, Beaumont JL (1971) In vivo incorporation of dietary 14C-cholesterol in rat serum lipoproteins and transfers into connective tissue. Clin Chim Acta 33: 95-100

Jacotot B, Beaumont JL, Monnier G, Szigeti M, Robert B, Robert L (1973) Role of elastic tissue in cholesterol deposition in the arterial wall. Nutr Metabol 15: 46-58

Janoff A, Scherer J (1968) Mediators of inflammation in leucocyte lysosomes. IX. Elastinolytic activity in granules of human polymorphonuclear leucocytes. J Exp Med 128: 1137-1151

John R, Thomas J (1972) Chemical composition of elastins isolated from aortas and pulmonary tissue of humans of different ages. Biochem J 127: 261-269

Jordon RE, Hewitt N, Lewis W, Kagan HM, Franzblau C (1974) Regulation of elastase-catalyzed hydrolysis of insoluble elastin by synthetic and naturally occurring hydrophobic ligands. Biochemistry 13: 3497-3503

Kagan HM, Lerch RM (1976) Amidated carboxyl groups in elastin. Biochim Biophys Acta 434: 223-232

Kagan HM, Hewitt NA, Salcedo LL, Franzblau C (1974) Catalytic activity of aortic lysyloxidase in an insoluble enzyme-substrate complex. Biochim Biophys Acta 365: 223-234

Kagan HM, Milbury P, Kramsch DM (1979) A possible role for elastin ligands in the proteolytic degradation of arterial elastic lamellae in the rabbit. Circ Res 44: 95-103

Keeley FW, Partridge SM (1974) Amino acid composition and calcification of human aortic elastin. Atherosclerosis 19: 287-296

Kramsch DM, Chan CT (1976) Increased in vivo synthesis of elastin and collagen in atherosclerotic arteries and its suppression by drugs. Fed Proc 35: 598

Kramsch DM, Hollander W (1968) Occlusive atherosclerotic disease of the coronary arteries in monkeys (Macaca irus) induced by diet. Exper Molec Pathol 9: 1-22

Kramsch DM, Hollander W (1973) The interaction of serum and arterial lipoproteins with elastin of the arterial intima and its role in the lipid accumulation in atherosclerotic plaques. J Clin Invest 52: 236-247

Kramsch DM, Franzblau C, Hollander W (1971) The protein and lipid composition of arterial elastin and its relationship to lipid accumulation in the atherosclerotic plaque. J Clin Invest 50: 1666-1677

Kramsch DM, Hollander W, Renaud S (1974a) Induction of fibrous plaques versus foam cell lesions in Macaca fascicularis by varying the composition of dietary fats. Circulation 48 (suppl IV): 41

Kramsch DM, Franzblau C, Hollander W (1974b) Components of the protein-lipid complex of arterial elastin. Their role in the retention of lipids in atherosclerotic lesions. Adv Exp Med Biol 43: 193-210

Kramsch DM, Aspen AJ, Abramowitz BM, Abell MA, Hood WB (1979) Cardiovascular effects of exercise in primate atherosclerosis. Circulation 60 (suppl. II): 167

Kramsch DM, Aspen AJ, Apstein CS (1980) Suppression of experimental atherosclerosis by the Ca^{++}-antagonist lanthanum. The possible role of calcium in atherogenesis. J Clin Invest 65: 967–981

Kritchevsky D, Tepper SA, Vesselinovitch D, Wissler RW (1971) Cholesterol vehicle in experimental atherosclerosis. Part II (peanut oil). Atherosclerosis 14: 53–64

Lansing AI, Alex M, Rosenthal TB (1950) Atheromatosis as a sequel to senescent changes in the arterial wall. J Gerontol 5: 314–318

Layman DL, Epstein EH, Dodson RF, Titus JL (1977) Biosynthesis of type I and III collagens by cultured smooth muscle cells from human aorta. Proc Natl Acad Sci USA 74: 671–675

Lee KT, Nam SC, Kwon OH, Kim SB, Goodale F (1963) Geographic pathology of arteriosclerosis: a study of the "critical level" of dietary fat as related to myocardial infarction in Koreans. Exp Molec Pathol 2: 1–13

Legrand Y, Caen J, Boyse FM, Raffelson EM, Robert B, Robert L (1973) Studies on human blood platelet proteases with elastolytic activity. Biochim Biophys Acta 309: 406–413

Levy RI (1980) Dietary prevention of coronary artery disease - a policy overview. In: Gotto AM, Smith LC, Allen B (eds). Atherosclerosis V, Springer, New York, pp. 199–218

Lian JB, Skinner M, Glimcher MJ, Gallop P (1976) The presence of gamma-glutamic acid in the proteins associated with ectopic calcification. Biochem Biophys Res Commun 73: 349–355

Lillie RD, Pizzolato P, Strong JP (1976) Elastin VII: Aging effects on vascular elastica staining by oil soluble nigrosin dyes. Virchows Arch A Pathol Anat Histol 371: 323–330

Lindner JP (1974) What is the morphological and (physico-) chemical evidence that connective tissue in lesions indeed is altered? In: Schettler G, Seizel A (eds) Atherosclerosis III. Springer, Berlin, pp. 218–228

Lloyd W, Fang VS, Wells H, Tashjian AH (1969) 2-Thiophene carboxylic acid: a hypocalcemic, antilipolytic agent with hypocalcemic and hypophosphatemic effects in rats. Endocrinology 85: 763-768

Loewen WA (1969) Elastolytic enzymes in the vessel wall. J Atheroscler Res 9: 35-46

Macarak EJ, Howard BV, Kefalides NA (1976) Biosynthesis of collagen and metabolism of lipids by endothelial cells in culture. Annals NY Acad Sci 275: 104-113

Marx JL (1976) Cell biology: cell surfaces and the regulation of mitosis. Science 192: 455-457

McCullagh KG, Page IH (1974) Increased collagen synthesis in early rabbit atherosclerosis and its inhibition by cis-hydroxyproline. In: Schettler G, Weizel A (eds) Atherosclerosis III. Springer, Berlin, pp. 239-241

McCullagh KA, Balian G (1975) Collagen characteristics and cell transformation in human atherosclerosis. Nature 258: 73-75

Minkin C, Rabadjija L, Goldhaber P (1974) Bone remodeling in vitro: the effects of diphosphonates on osteoid synthesis. Calcif Tissue Res 14: 161-168

Moczar M, Robert L (1970) Extraction and fractionation of the media of the thoracic aorta. Atherosclerosis 11: 7-25

Moon HD, Rinehart JF (1952) Histogenesis of coronary atherosclerosis. Circulation 6: 481-488

Mustard JF, Packham MA (1970) Factors influencing platelet functions: adhesion, release and aggregation. Pharmacol Rev 22: 97-187

Mustard JF, Packham MA, Moore S, Kinlough-Rathbone RL (1974) Thrombosis and atherosclerosis. In: Schettler G, Weizel A (eds) Atherosclerosis III. Springer, Berlin, pp. 253-267

Nikkari T, Heikkinnen O (1968) The lipids of collagen preparations. Acta Chem Scand 22: 3047-3049

Noma A, Takahashi T, Yamada K, Wada T (1979) Elastin-lipid interaction in the arterial wall, Part 1 (extraction of elastin from human aortic intima.) Atherosclerosis 33: 29-39

Numano F, Watanabe Y, Takeno K, Takano T, Arita M, Numano F, Maezawa H, Shimamoto T, Adachi K (1976) Microassay of

cyclic nucleotides in vessel wall. I. Cyclic AMP. Exp Molec
Pathol 25: 172-181

Osborn GR (1963) The Incubation Period of Coronary Thrombosis. Butterworth, London.

Ouzilou J, Robert AM, Robert L, Bouisson H, Pieraggi MT (1973)
Pario Arterielle 1: 105-116

Packham MA, Cazenave JP, Kinlough-Rathbone RL, Mustard JF
(1978) Drug effects on platelet adherence to collagen and
damaged vessel walls. Adv Exp Med Biol 109: 253-276

Parakkal PF (1969) Involvement of macrophages in collagen resorption. J Cell Biol 41: 345-354

Parker F (1960) An electron microscopic study of experimental
atherosclerosis. Amer J Pathol 36: 19-53

Partridge SM, Keeley FW (1974) Age related and atherosclerotic
changes in aortic elastin. Adv Exp Med Biol 43: 173-191

Potokar M, Schmidt-Dunker M (1978) The effect of new diphos-
phonic acids on aortic and kidney calcification in vivo. Atherosclerosis 30: 313-320

Radhakrishnamurthy B, Ruiz HA, Berenson GS (1977) Isolation
and characterization of proteoglycans from bovine aorta. J
Biol Chem 252: 4831-4841

Robert AM, Grosgogeat Y, Reverdy V, Robert B, Robert L
(1971) Lesion arterielle produites chez le lapin par immunisa-
tion avec l'elastine et les glycoproteines de structure de
l'aorte. Etudes biochimiques et morphologiques. Atherosclerosis 13: 427-449

Robert AM, Moczar M, Brechemier D, Godeau G, Miskulin M,
Robert L ((1978) Biosynthesis and degradation of matrix mole-
cules of the arterial wall. Regulation by drug action. In:
International Symposium. State of Prevention and Therapy in
Human Arterioclerosis and in Animal Models. Hauss WH,
Wissler RW, Lehmann R (eds) Abh Rhein - Westf Akad Wiss
Vol 3, Westdeutscher Verlag, Opladen, Germany, pp. 301-312

Robert L, Robert B (1973) Immunology and aging. Gerontologia
19: 330-350

Robert L, Robert B (1974) In: Fricke R, Hartman F (eds) Connective Tissue, Biochemistry and Pathophysiology. Springer, New York, p. 240

Robert L, Robert B, Robert AM (1972) Interactions entre lipides, lipoproteines et macromolecules fibreuses du tissu conjonctif. Exp Ann Biochim Med 31: 110-144

Rosenblum IY, Flora L, Eisenstein R (1975) The effect of sodium ethane-1-hydroxy-1,1-diphosphonate (EHDP) on a rabbit model of arterio-atherosclerosis. Atherosclerosis 22: 411-424

Ross R, Bornstein P (1969) The elastic fiber. I. Separation and partial characterization of its macromolecular components. J Cell Biol 40: 366-381

Ross R, Glomset JA (1973) Atherosclerosis and the arterial smooth muscle cell. Science 180: 1332-1339

Ross R, Glomset JA (1976a) The pathogenesis of atherosclerosis. Part I. N Engl J Med 295: 369-377

Ross R, Glomset JA (1976b) The pathogenesis of atherosclerosis. Part II. N Engl J Med 295: 420-425

Schaffner T, Elner V, Wissler RW (1977) Histochemical localization of acid lipase with alpha-naphthyl fatty acid esters. Fed Proc 36: 400

Schwarz W, Guldner FH (1967) Elektronenmikroskopische Untersuchungen des Kollagenabbaus im Uterus der Ratte nach der Schwangerschaft. Z Zellforsch Mikrosk Anat 83: 416-426

Schwartz CJ (1977) Presented at the annual Hugh Lofland Conference on Arterial Metabolism

Seligman M, Eilberg RG, Fishman L (1975) Mineralization of elastin extracted from human aortic tissue. Calc Tissue Res 17: 229-234

Serafini-Fracassini A (1963) Electron microscope and x-ray crystal analysis of calcified elastic tissue. J Atheroscler Res 3: 178-188

Slack HGB (1954) Metabolism of elastin in the adult rat. Nature 174: 512-513

Smith EB (1974) Acid glycosaminoglycans, collagen and elastin content of normal artery, fatty streaks and plaques. Adv Exp Med Biol 43: 125-139

Smith EB, Smith RH (1976) Early changes in aortic intima. In: Atherosclerosis Reviews, Paoletti R, Gotto AM (eds) Raven Press, New York, Vol 1, pp. 119-136

Smith EB, Evans PH, Downham MD (1967) Lipid in the aortic intima: the correlation of chemical and morphological characteristics. J Atheroscler Res 7: 171-186

Srinivasan SR, Lopez S, Radakrishnamurthy B, Berenson GS (1970) Complexing of serum pre-beta-and beta-lipoproteins and acid mucopolysaccharides. Atherosclerosis 12: 321-334

Stemerman MB, Ross R (1972) Experimental atherosclerosis. I. Fibrous plaque formation in primates, an electron microscope study. J Exp Med 136: 769-789

Stevens RL, Colombo M, Gonzales JJ, Hollander W, Schmid K (1976) Glycosaminoglycans of the human artery and their changes in atherosclerosis. J Clin Invest 58: 470-481

Szigeti M, Monnier G, Jacotot B, Navarro N, Robert L (1972) Distribution of ingested ^{14}C-cholesterol in the macromolecular fraction of rat connective tissue. Connect Tissue Res 1: 145-152

Trelstad RL (1974) Human aorta collagens. Evidence for three distinct species. Biochem Biophys Res Commun 57: 717-725

Urry DW, Cunningham WD, Ohnishi T (1973) A neutral polypeptide-calcium ion complex. Biochim Biophys Acta 292: 853-857

Vogel JJ, Boylan-Salyers BD (1976) Acidic lipids associated with the local mechanism of calcification. Clin Orthopaed 118: 230-241

Wagner WD, Clarkson TB (1973) Slowly miscible cholesterol pools in progressing and regressing atherosclerotic aortas. Proc Soc Exp Biol Med 143: 804-809

Wagner WD, Clarkson TB, Foster J (1977) Contrasting effects of ethane-1-hydroxy-1,1-diphosphonate (EHDP) on the regression of two types of dietary-induced atherogenesis. Atherosclerosis 27: 419–435

Wahl LM, Wahl SM, Martin GR, Mergenhagen SE (1974) Production of collagenase by macrophages exposed to lymphocyte products Fed Proc 33: 618

Walker WJ (1977) Changing United States life-style and declining vascular mortality: cause or coincidence? N Engl J Med 297: 163–165

Walton KW, Williamson N (1968) Histochemical and immunofluorescent studies on the evolution of the human atheromatous plaque. J Atheroscler Res 8: 599–624

Wartman A, Lampe TL, McCann DS, Boyle AJ (1967) Plaque reversal with MgEDTA in experimental atherosclerosis: Elastin and collagen metabolism. J Atheroscler Res 7: 331–341

Weiss GB (1974) Cellular pharmacology of lanthanum. In: Elliot HW, Okun R, George R (eds) Annual Review of Pharmacology. Annual Reviews, Palo Alto, Vol 14, pp. 343–354

Weiss GB, Goodman FR (1976) Distribution of lanthanide ([147]Pm) in vascular smooth muscle. J Pharmacol Ther 198: 366–374

Weissman G, Weissman S (1960) X-ray diffraction studies of human aortic elastin residues. J Clin Invest 39: 1657–1666

Werb Z, Gordon S (1975) Elastase secreted by stimulated macrophages. J Exp Med 142: 361–377

Wight TN, Ross R (1973) Ultrastructural and biochemical evidence for the production of glycosaminoglycans by primate arterial smooth muscle cells. J Cell Biol 59 (2): 371a

Wissler RW, Vesselinovitch D (1976) Studies of regression of advanced atherosclerosis in experimental animals and man. Ann NY Acad Sci 275: 363–378

Wolinsky H, Goldfischer S, Daly M, Kasak LE, Coltoff-Schiller B (1975) Arterial lysosomes and connective tissue in primate atherosclerosis and hypertension. Circ Res 36: 553–561

Wolinsky H, Goldfischer S, Katz D, Markle R (1979) Effects of regular physical activity on hydrolase activities of the rat aorta. Circulation 60 (Suppl. II): 167

Yin HH, Ukena TE, Berlin RD (1972) Effect of colchicine, col-
    cemid and vinblastine on the agglutination, by concanavalin
    A, of transformed cells. Science 178: 867-868
Yu SY (1971) Cross-linking of elastin in human atherosclerotic
    aorta. Lab Invest 25: 121-125
Yu SY, Blumenthal HT (1963) The calcification of elastic fibers.
    I. Biochemical studies. J Gerontol 18: 119-126
Yu SY, Yoshida A (1977) The fate of ^{14}C-elastin in the perito-
    neal cavity of rats. I. Biochemical studies. Lab Invest 37:
    143-149
Zamosciank H, Veis A (1966) The isolation and chemical charac-
    terization of a phosphate-containing sialoglycoprotein from
    developing bovine teeth. Fed Proc 25: 409
Zugibe FT, Brown KD (1960) Histochemical studies in atherogen-
    esis: human aortas. Circ Res 8: 287-295

Discussion

Rosenquist. Please give us a bit more information about the exercise: the frequency, duration and intensity that was effective.

Kramsch. The monkeys were run at a speed of three kilometers per hour in a drum - shaped treadmill. The monkeys weighed about 5 - 10 kilograms. This is a reasonable jogging speed for animals of this size. It certainly is not marathon running, since they were run for only about one hour every other day. That is moderate exercise. But the heart rates of exercised monkeys at rest and at exercise were 50% - 75% lower than in monkeys that were never exercised, indicating conditioning.

Turino. You clearly put the emphasis for the pathogenic mechanism on the interaction between calcium and some of the connective tissue components such as elastin and collagen in the wall of the blood vessel. Are you excluding a role for the proteolytic enzyme action in these mechanisms? Don't you think we have to include that as a part of the process? How do you see proteolysis interacting in the formation of plaque?

Kramsch. Of course, proteolysis is very important. However, some enzymes involved in elastolysis, for instance, macrophage elastase, require calcium for their action, and Kagan (unpublished work) has shown, in vitro, that pancreatic elastase activity also enhanced by increased concentrations of calcium ions. If it is true that pancreatic elastase circulates in the blood stream, then it could attack the arterial wall. I do not claim that calcium - dependent mechanisms are the only mechanisms involved in atherogenesis -- far from that, but I want to point out that there are quite a number of these mechanisms that require calcium. For instance, proteolysis can also be carried out by platelets, and the adherence of platelets to collagen, their aggregation, and their enzyme release reaction -- all of these mechanisms require calcium.

Snider. You mentioned the atherogenic stimulus and that not too much is known about it. Is the connective tissue altered primarily or secondarily?

Kramsch. That is a very good question which I cannot answer with certainty. We still are not at the point where we can say for sure whether fatty streaks, which usually have very little alteration, can develop into fibrous plaques as a secondary phenomenon. Some of them may, and some of them may have no relation to fibrous plaques which may develop as a primary phenomenon. There is great uncertainty as to what causes the specific responses of the arterial wall, that is, on the one hand, what causes the cells in the wall to take up lipids and lipoproteins and produce a fatty streak, and, on the other hand, what turns on the synthesis and degradation of connective tissue to form a fibrous plaque in which both the synthesis and degradation occur simultaneously. There are speculations that some diets may cause a more fibrogenic response than others. For instance, feeding monkeys cholesterol along with a variety of polyunsaturated fats, for example, cholesterol with corn oil or

cotton seed oil, doesn't produce much of a fibrogenic response;
however, feeding of butter with cholesterol does. And, for some
strange reason, diets rich in peanut oil also are fibrogenic in
rabbits and monkeys. Wissler et al. (Wissler RS, Vesselinovitch
D, Borensztajn J, Shaffner T, Hughes R [1976] Effects of various diets on progression of atherosclerosis in Rhesus monkeys.
Fed Proc 35: 294) have shown that peanut oil alone can produce
fibrous lesions in nonhuman primates. I am not sure whether it
is safe to say this in Georgia, but it is a fact. And this is how
I produce routinely a fibrogenic response in rabbits, by using
peanut oil and cholesterol as components of their diet.

McDonald. You spoke of preventing the plaque formation. Is
there much of a possibility of causing it to regress after it is
formed?

Kramsch. Our experiments after cessation of atherogenic
diets so far have shown that the cells of lesions may either lose
their lipid accumulations, or disappear entirely. Stary (Stary
HC [1974] Cell proliferation and ultrastructural changes in regressing atherosclerotic lesions after reduction of serum cholesterol. In: Schettler G, Weizel A [eds] Atherosclerosis, Third
International Symposium. Springer-Verlag, Berlin, pp 187-190)
has shown that in very early lesions, produced by feeding an
atherogenic diet to nonhuman primates for a short period of time,
so-called foam cells appear and then disappear after cessation of
that diet. However, fibrous plaques and even most foam cell
lesions in experimental animals do not regress, not even if you
do what you can never do in a human, that is, completely stop
all cholesterol and fats in the diet for prolonged periods of time.
In rabbits, even after cessation of an atherogenic diet for two
years, there is no regression. On the contrary, in rabbits such
a "regression" diet may increase the severity of the lesions;
they all become fibrous and calcified. Armstrong and Megan
(Armstrong ML, Megan BM [1974] Responses of two macaque species to atherogenic diet and its withdrawal. In: Schettler G,
Weizel A [eds] Atherosclerosis, Third International Symposium.

Springer-Verlag, Berlin, pp 336-338) showed some regression of accumulated arterial collagen in monkeys after withdrawal of atherogenic diets; however, no one has really shown any regression of a calcified plaque. Whether a massively calcified plaque can go away is highly doubtful, at least with the present methods.

Biochemistry of Collagen
with Special Reference to the Arterial Wall

R. KENT RHODES

Investigations of the last decade have produced major advances in collagen biochemistry (for reviews see Bornstein and Sage 1980; Bornstein and Traub 1979; Eyre 1980; Prockop et al. 1979; Miller and Gay, in press). Among the most significant has been the discovery of the genetically distinct collagens that spawned numerous studies concerning the characterization and distribution of the various collagen types. Such studies have also begun to elucidate some of the roles collagen can play in both normal and pathologic conditions (Gay and Miller 1978).

Genetically Distinct Collagens

Presently, three groups of collagens are recognized based on their anatomical distribution and compositional features (Miller and Gay, in press) namely, the interstitial, basement membrane, and pericellular collagens (Table 1). In addition, a fourth group of collagenous peptides have been characterized compositionally, but have not been localized within any given tissues (Furuto and Miller 1980). The nomenclature used in this report conforms to that proposed by Bornstein and Sage (1980).

The interstitial collagens are deposited as fibers or reticular matrices in the intercellular spaces and constitute the bulk of the

TABLE 1. The Genetically Distinct Types of Collagen

Collagens	Molecular Form	Tissue Form
Interstitial collagens		
Type I	$[\alpha1(I)]_2\alpha2(I)$	Large striated fibers of dense connective tissue
Type I-trimer	$[\alpha1(I)]_3$	Fibrillar form unknown
Type II	$[\alpha1(II)]_3$	Fibrils of hyaline cartilage
Type III	$[\alpha1(III)]_3$	Fine reticular networks
Basement membrane collagens		
Type IV	$[\alpha1(IV)]_3$ $[\alpha2(IV)]_3$	Structural elements of the morphologically-distinct basement membranes
Pericellular collagens		
Type V	$[\alpha1(V)]_2\alpha2(V)$ $[\alpha1(V)]_3$ $[\alpha2(V)]_3(?)$	Supporting elements of basement membrane-like exocytoskeletons
Collagenous polypeptides	40K–A $\Big\}$ 40K–B $\Big\{$ Disulfide bonded high-molecular-weight aggregates	Unknown

organic connective tissue matrix. Compositionally, these collagens are distinguishable from other groups by their high alanine
content and the lack of substantial quantities of hydroxylated
and glycosylated lysyl residues (Table 2). Type I, the most
abundant and best characterized collagen molecule, is composed
of two identical α1(I) chains and a third α2(I) chain. In situ,
these molecules form well ordered fibers ranging from 450 Å to
1800 Å in diameter and display a characteristic periodicity of
680 Å when stained with heavy metals and visualized in the electron microscope. The most ubiquitous of the collagens, type I,
is found in virtually every tissue and is the predominant collagen
in tissues which resist deformation, such as bone and tendon.

Akin to the type I molecule is the type I trimer, which contains three α1(I) chains. The fiber form and functional role of
this species is presently unknown. It has been found as a minor
component in skin (Uitto 1979) and dentine (Wohllebe and Carmichael 1978) and as a product of various cell types in culture
(Mayne et al. 1975; Crouch and Bornstein 1978; Munksgaard et
al. 1978; Narayanan et al. 1978).

The predominent collagen of hyaline cartilage is type II,
which is comprised of three α1(II) chains (Miller 1971; Trelstad
et al. 1970). More recent investigations have reported the occurrence of type II in certain structures of the embryonic eye as
well (Smith et al. 1976). Compositionally, type II contains more
hydroxylysine and hydroxylysine glycosides than the other interstitial species (Table 2). It is generally deposited in thin fibrils
that do not display a discernible cross-striation pattern.

Type III collagen is composed of three identical α1(III) chains
that are unique among the interstitial chains due to the presence
of cysteine in the helical portion of the molecule (Table 2)
(Chung and Miller 1974; Chung et al. 1974). Type III has a
widespread distribution throughout the organism and appears to
be more abundant in distensible tissues, such as the elastic
arteries, skin, and uterus. Fibers of type III are somewhat
smaller than those of type I, ranging from 50 Å to 400 Å in dia-

meter. In addition, much of the type III collagen retains the amino-terminal extension peptides of procollagen. These molecules do not align into striated fibrils, but participate in the formation of a reticular matrix which may associate with the larger fibers.

The basement membrane collagens are found distributed throughout the epithelial and endothelial basal laminae of various tissues. At present there are two relatively well-characterized chains, the α1(IV) and α2(IV) chains, which are distinguished by their low quantities of alanine, high levels of hydrophobic residues, and increased levels of hydroxylysine and hydroxylysine glycosides (Table 2) (Kresina and Miller 1979; Glanville et al. 1979; Gay and Miller 1979; Dixit 1979; Sate et al. 1979b). Extraction of amniotic fluid cells that synthesize basement membrane collagen (Crouch et al. 1980) and bovine lens capsules (Gay and Miller, unpublished data) yields primarily two chains of approximately 145,000 - 160,000 daltons, indicating that unlike other collagens the chains undergo little if any immediate post-translational cleavage. This material, however, when solubilized using limited pepsin digestion produces chains similar in size to the interstitial α chains, i.e., 95,000 daltons. The molecular configurations of the basement membrane chains is currently not known, but the proportions found in various tissues indicated that they probably exist separately as $[\alpha1(IV)]_3$ and $[\alpha2(IV)]_3$ collagen molecules.

The designation "type V" represents a group of collagens that includes three approximately α-size chains, the α1(V), α2(V), and α3(V) (Burgeson et al. 1976; Chung et al. 1976; Brown et al. 1978; Sage and Bornstein 1979). Compositionally, these chains have characteristic values for alanine, hydroxylysine, and hydrophobic residues which are intermediate between those of the interstitial and basement membrane collagens (Table 2). The molecular forms that these chains may participate in are not fully defined; however, two species have been identified, the $[\alpha1(V)]_2$-α2(V) and $[\alpha1(V)]_3$ (Table 1) (Bentz et al. 1978; Rhodes and

TABLE 2. Compositional Features of the Various Collagen Chains

	α1(I)[a]	α2(I)[a]	α1(II)[a]	α1(III)[b]	α1(IV)[c]	α2(IV)[c]	α1(V)[d]	α2(V)[d]	α3(V)[e]	40KA[f]	40KB[f]
Hydroxyproline	109	94	99	125	123	111	115	109	100	86	69
Proline	124	113	120	107	85	73	130	107	99	100	107
Glycine	333	333	333	350	334	324	332	331	332	293	304
Alanine	115	102	103	96	30	47	39	54	49	48	36
Cysteine	0	0	0	2	0	2	0	0	1	31	36
Hydrophobics[g]	65	96	76	65	159	171	91	101	122	92	84
Hydroxylysine	9	12	20	5	50	36	36	23	43	28	39
Lysine	26	18	15	30	6	7	14	13	15	11	18
Arginine	50	50	50	46	22	42	40	48	42	53	69
Gal-Hyl	1	1	4	0	2	2	5	3	7	5	5
Glc-Gal-Hyl	1	2	12	1	44	29	29	5	17	23	34
Glucosamine	0	0	0	0	0	0	0	0	0	24	10

[a]Miller and Gay, in press
[b]Chung and Miller (1974)
[c]Kresina and Miller (1979)
[d]Rhodes and Miller (1978)
[e]Sage and Bornstein (1979)
[f]Furuto and Miller (1980)
[g]Hydrophobic residues: sum of values for valine, methionine, isoleucine, leucine, and phenylalanine

Miller 1978; Haralson et al. 1980). It is obvious, considering
the existence of the α3(V) chain, that other molecular species
are present. Though these chains have been isolated from a
number of sources, they seem to be most abundant in vascular
tissue.

Another group of collagenous molecules that has recently been
identified are isolated initially as high molecular weight aggregates resulting from interchain disulfide bonding between polypeptides of approximately 40,000 daltons (Furuto and Miller 1980).
These components contain large quantities of cysteine, arginine,
and hydroxylysine and less than the usual one-third glycine content, suggesting the presence of short noncollagenous sequences.
The distribution of these polypeptides is uncertain; however,
they are abundant in highly vascularized tissues such as placenta and have been isolated from bovine aortas (Furuto and
Miller 1980; Chung et al. 1976).

Arterial Collagen

The elucidation of the various collagen types has led to the
investigation of numerous tissues with regards to their collagenous components. Studies of the vascular system have revealed
that in addition to containing the majority of the described collagen species, there exists a distinct distribution pattern within
the layers of the vessel wall.

The endothelial cells that rest on a basement membrane and
the subendothelial space constitute the intimal layer of the major
vessels. Studies using indirect immunofluorescence have been
used to show that the basement membrane contains type IV collagen (Gay et al. 1979; Timpl et al. 1978) and that the subendothelium contains small amounts of collagen types I, III and V
(Gay et al. 1975; Gay and Miller 1978). The presence of type
IV in vascular basement membrane has also been demonstrated
biochemically with the isolation of α1(IV) and α2(IV) chains from
purified glomerular basement membrane (Dixit 1979).

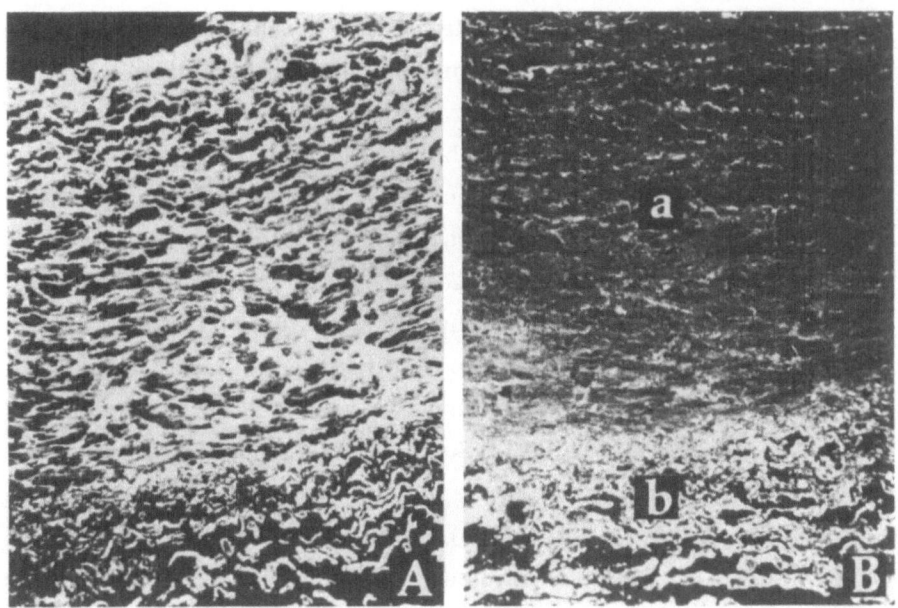

FIG. 1. Section from a carotid artery stained with antibodies to type III and type I collagen. In A, type III antibodies intensely stain the medial layers. In B, little staining for type I appears in the media (a), but it is very evident in the adventitia (b). (Gay and Miller 1978).

The collagens found in the intima are probably synthesized at least in part by the endothelial cells lining the lumen of the vessel. Studies on cultured vascular endothelial cells have shown that these cells synthesize collagen types III, IV, and V (Howard et al. 1976; Jaffe et al. 1976). Interestingly, Sage et al. (1979a) found that type III was secreted into the medium whereas types IV and V remained associated with the cell layer, indicating that certain factors operate to partition these secreted products.

The medial layer is composed almost entirely of smooth muscle cells in a matrix of collagen, elastin, and proteoglycan. Biochemical studies revealed that the media of normal aortas contains approximately 70% type III and 30% type I collagen (McCullagh and Balian 1975). Further investigation also demonstrated the presence of type V and the collagenous 40,000 dalton polypep-

tides (Chung et al. 1976; Furuto and Miller 1980). Immunohistochemical studies have also confirmed the presence of these collagen types and illustrate their proportionate distribution (Fig. 1)
(Gay and Miller 1978; Gay et al. 1975).

The ability of medial smooth muscle cells to synthesize the
various collagen types has been investigated using cell culture
techniques. Several laboratories have reported the synthesis of
types I and III by smooth muscle cells in culture with varying
ratios of type I to type III being observed as a result of differences in isolation procedure and culture conditions (Barnes et
al. 1976; Burke et al. 1977; Layman et al. 1977; Mayne et al.
1977; Rauterberg et al. 1977; Scott et al. 1977). However, proportions approximating those found in intact medial tissue were
reported by Burke et al. (1977), Mayne et al. (1977), and Scott
et al. (1977). Further studies by Mayne et al. (1978) using
monkey aortic smooth muscle cells also demonstrated the biosynthesis of type V collagen and a low molecular weight collagenous
peptide of 45,000 daltons (CP 45). CP 45 has not been isolated
from intact tissue. Thus, its possible significance as a functional protein in vivo is still uncertain.

The adventitial layer of the vasculature is a loosely arranged
connective tissue layer forming the outermost portion of the
vessel. Its cellular components are primarily fibroblasts which
secrete a matrix rich in type I collagen with small amounts of
types III and V also present.

Collagen in Artherosclerosis

Considerable attention has been given in recent years to
changes in collagen metabolism in atherosclerosis. Several proposed models (see Ross and Glomset 1976; Benditt 1977; Martin
and Sprague 1973) offer varied explanations for the initiation of
the now well recognized lesions of the artery, namely, the fibrous plaque and the complicated lesion. Fibrous plaques are
the hallmark of progressing atherosclerosis, appearing as gray-

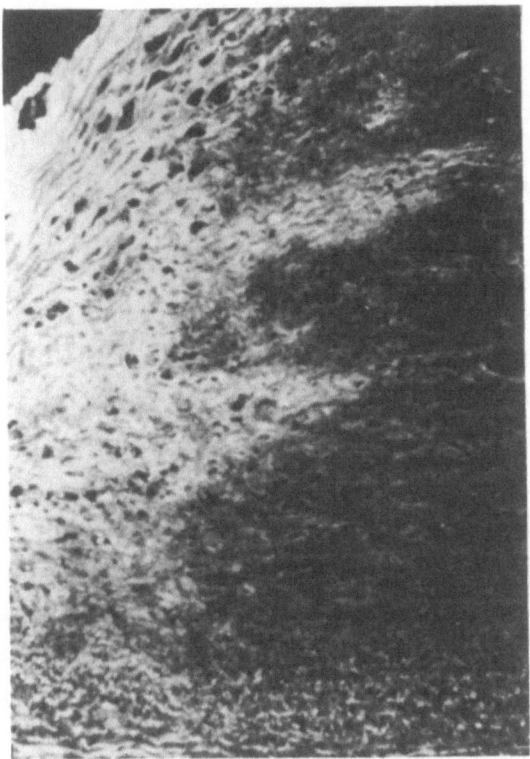

FIG. 2. Section from the margin of an early atherosclerotic lesion showing intense staining with antibodies for αI(V) collagen chains. (Gay and Miller 1978).

ish white thickenings on the arterial intima. They contain lipid-filled smooth muscle cells within a matrix rich in collagen, elastin, and proteoglycan that overlays deeper areas of extracellular lipid, cell debris, and invading macrophages. The fibrous plaque may progress to the complicated lesion, which is the most advanced stage of the disease. Mural thrombosis, cellular necrosis and calcification characterize this stage. In some instances the lesion itself may occlude the arterial lumen, but more importantly it can result in conditions which produce secondary thrombi that stop the flow of blood.

Results from biochemical and immunohistochemical studies reflect the changes in the collagenous matrix associated with the atheromatous lesions. McCullagh and Balian (1975), using normal and atherosclerotic tissues from human aortas, made comparisons of the type I to type III ratios. Atherosclerotic tissue was found to contain 65% type I and 35% type III which was nearly the reverse of the 70% to 30% ratio of type III to type I in normal tissue. By using type-specific antibodies to the various collagens, it has been possible to extend these studies to show that a progressive change in collagen type occurs. Smooth muscle cells of fibrous plaques in the early stages of development stain intensely when treated with antibodies to type V collagen (Fig. 2) (Gay and Miller 1978). In addition, type IV has been found to be present not only in the basal lamina but distributed throughout the plaque matrix (Gay and Gay, personal communication). Tissue sections taken from advanced lesions confirm the biochemical results, showing a matrix rich in type I with little staining for type III evident. These findings indicate that the atheromatous lesion follows the pattern of many fibrotic processes where newly synthesized collagen types appear in a predictable procession with the eventual replacement of the normal matrix by large amounts of type I collagen (Gay and Miller 1978). The resultant matrix in the case of the vascular wall is not a suitable replacement and leads to a loss of normal function.

Acknowledgment

The work done in the author's laboratory was supported by Grant DE-02670 and HL-11310 from the United States Public Health Service.

REFERENCES

Barnes MJ, Morton LF, Levene CI (1976) Synthesis of collagen types I and III by pig medial smooth muscle cells in culture. Biochem Biophys Res Commun 70: 339

Benditt EP (1977) The origin of atherosclerosis. Sci Am 236: 74

Bentz H, Bachinger HP, Glanville R, Kuhn K (1978) Physical evidence for the assembly of A and B chains of human placental collagen in a single triple helix. Europ Biochem 92: 563

Bornstein P, Sage H (1980) Structurally distinct collagen types. An Rev Biochem 49: 957

Bornstein P, Traub W (1979) The chemistry and biology of collagen. In: Neurath H, Hill RL (eds) The Proteins, Vol IV. Academic Press, New York

Brown RA, Shuttleworth CA, Weiss JB (1978) Three new α-chains of collagen from a non-basement membrane source. Biochem Biophys Res Commun 80: 866

Burgeson RE, El Adli FA, Kaitila II, Hollister DW (1976) Fetal membrane collagens: Identification of two new collagen alpha chains. Proc Natl Aca Sci USA 73: 2579

Burke JM, Bailan G, Ross R, Bornstein P (1977) Synthesis of types I and III procollagen by monkey aortic smooth muscle cells in vitro. Biochemistry 16: 3243

Chung E, Miller EJ (1974) Collagen polymorphism: Characterization of molecules with the chain composition $[α1(III)]_3$ in human tissues. Science 183: 1200

Chung E, Keele EM, Miller EJ (1974) Isolation and characterization of the cyanogen bromide peptides from the α1(III) chain of human collagen. Biochemistry 13: 3459

Chung E, Rhodes RK, Miller EJ (1976) Isolation of three collagenous components of probable basement membrane origin from several tissues. Biochem Biophys Res Commun 71: 1167

Crouch E, Bornstein P (1978) Collagen synthesized by human amniotic fluid cells in culture: Characterization of a procollagen with three identical pro α1(I) chains. Biochemistry 17: 5499.

Crouch E, Sage H, Bornstein P (1980) Structural basis for apparent heterogeneity of collagens in human basement membranes: Type IV procollagen contains two distinct chains. Proc Natl Aca Sci USA 77: 745

Dixit SN (1979) Isolation and characterization of two α-chain size collagenous polypeptide chains C and D from glomerular basement membrane. FEBS Letters 106: 379

Eyre DR (1980) Collagen: Molecular diversity in the body's protein scaffold. Science 207: 1315

Furuto DK, Miller EJ (1980) Isolation of a unique collagenous fraction from limited pepsin digests of human placental tissue. Biol Chem 255: 290

Gay S, Miller EJ (1978) Collagen in the Physiology and Pathology of Connective Tissue. Gustav Fischer, Stuttgart-New York

Gay S, Miller EJ (1979) Characterization of lens capsule collagen: evidence for the presence of two unique chains in molecules derived from major basement membrane structures. Archiv Biochem Biophys 198: 370

Gay S, Balleisen L, Remberger K, Fietzek PP, Adelmann BC, Kuhn K (1975) Immunohistochemical evidence for the presence of collagen type III in human arterial walls, arterial thrombi, and in leucocytes, incubated with collagen in vitro. Klin Worchensch 53: 899

Gay S, Kresina TF, Gay R, Miller EJ, Montes LF (1979) Immunohistochemical demonstration of basement membrane collagen in normal human skin and in psoriasis. Cutaneous Pathol 6: 91

Glanville RW, Rauter A, Fietzek PP (1979) Isolation and characterization of a native placental basement-membrane collagen and its component chains. Europ Biochem 95: 383

Haralson MA, Mitchell WM, Rhodes RK, Kresina TF, Gay R, Miller
    EJ (1980) Chinese hamster lung cells synthesize and confine
    to the cellular domain a collagen comprised soley of B chains.
    Proc Natl Aca Sci USA in press

Howard BV, Macarak EJ, Gunson D, Kefalides NA (1976) Char-
    acterization of the collagen synthesized by endothelial cells in
    culture. Proc Natl Aca Sci USA 73: 2361

Jaffe EA, Minick CR, Adelman B, Becker CG, Nachman R (1976)
    Synthesis of basement membrane collagen by cultured human
    endothelial cells. Exper Med 144: 209

Kresina TF, Miller EJ (1979) Isolation and characterization of
    basement membrane collagen from human placental tissue.
    Evidence for the presence of two genetically-distinct collagen
    chains. Biochemistry 18: 3089

Layman DL, Epstein EJ, Dodson RF, Titus JL (1977) Biothe-
    sis of type I and III collagens by cultured smooth muscle
    cells from human aorta. Proc Natl Aca Sci USA 74: 671

Martin GM, Sprague CA (1973) Symposium on in vitro studies
    related to atherogenesis: Life histories of hyperplastoid cell
    lines from aorta and skin. Exper Mole Pathol 18: 125

Mayne R, Vail MS, Miller EJ (1975) Analysis of changes in col-
    lagen biosynthesis that occur when chick chondrocytes are
    grown in 5-bromo-2'-deoxyuridine. Proc Natl Aca Sci USA
    72: 4511

Mayne R, Vail MS, Miller EJ, Blose SH, Chacko S (1977) Colla-
    gen polymorphisms in cell cultures derived from guinea pig
    aortic smooth muscle: Comparison with three populations of
    fibroblasts. Archiv Biochem Biophys 181: 462

Mayne R, Vail MS, Miller EJ (1978) Characterization of the col-
    lagen chains synthesized by cultured smooth muscle cells de-
    rived from rhesus monkey thoracic aorta. Biochemistry 17:
    446

McCullagh KA, Balian G (1975) Collagen characterization and cell
    transformation in human atherosclerosis. Nature 258: 73

Miller EJ (1971)   Isolation and characterization of a collagen from chick cartilage containing three identical α chains.   Biochemistry 10: 1652

Miller EJ (1976)   Biochemical characteristics and biological significance of the genetically-distinct collagens.   Molec Cell Biochem 13: 165

Miller EJ, Gay S (in press) The multiple types and forms of collagen - an overview.   In: Cunningham LW, Fredericksen DW (eds) Methods in Enzymology.   Academic Press, New York

Munksgaard EC, Rhodes M, Mayne R, Butler WT (1978) Collagen synthesis and secretion by rat incisor odontoblasts in organ culture.   Europ Biochem 82: 609

Narayanan AS, Page RC, Kuzan F (1978) Collagens synthesized in vitro by diploid fibroblasts obtained from chronically inflamed human connective tissue.   Lab Inves 39: 61

Prockop DJ, Kivirikko KI, Tuderman L, Guzman NA (1979) The biosynthesis of collagen and its disorders.   N Eng J Med 301: 77

Rauterberg J, Allam S, Brehmer U, Wirth W, Hauss WH (1977) Characterization of the collagen synthesized by cultured human smooth muscle cells from fetal and adult aorta.   Hoppe-Seyler's Zeitshr Physio Chem 358: 401

Rhodes RK, Miller EJ (1978) Physico-chemical characterization and molecular organization of the collagen A and B chains.   Biochemistry 17: 3442

Ross R, Glomset JA (1976) The pathogenesis of atherosclerosis.   N Eng J Med 295: 420

Sage H, Bornstein P (1979) Characterization of a novel collagen chain in human placenta and its relation to AB collagen.   Biochemistry 18: 3815

Sage H, Crouch E, Bornstein P (1979a) Collagen synthesis by bovine aortic endothelial cells in culture.   Biochemistry 18: 5433

Sage H, Wordbury RG, Bornstein P (1979b) Structural studies on human type IV collagen.   J Biol Chem 254: 9893

Scott DM, Harwood R, Grant ME, Jackson DS (1977) Characterization of the major collagen species present in procine aortae and the synthesis of their precursors by smooth muscle cells in culture. Connective Tissue Res 5: 7

Smith GN Jr, Linsenmayer TF, Newsome DA (1976) Synthesis of type II collagen in vitro by embryonic chick neural retina tissue. Proc Natl Aca Sci USA 73: 4420

Timpl R, Martin GR, Bruckner P, Wick G, Wiedemann H (1978) Nature of the collagenous protein in a tumor basement membrane. Europ J Biochem 84: 43

Trelstad RL, Kang AH, Igarashi S, Gross J (1970) Isolation of two distinct collagens from chick cartilage. Biochemistry 9: 4993

Uitto J (1979) Collagen polymorphism: isolation and partial characterization of α1(I)-trimer molecules in normal human skin. Archiv Biochem Biophys 192: 371

Wohllebe M, Carmichael DJ (1978) Type-I-trimer and type-I collagen in neutral-salt-soluble lathyritic-rat dentine. Europ J Biochem 92: 183

Discussion

Bustos. I have two questions. Both pertain to the biochemistry of collagen. First, is there any relationship between the hydrophobic amino acid residue distribution and the presence of cross striations in the collagen fibril?

Rhodes. The broad banding pattern normally seen in electron micrographs results from the staggered arrangements, or D spacing, of collagen molecules within the fibers. There are also cross striation patterns present in reconstituted fibers and segment - long - spacing (SLS) crystallites, which are a result of the clustering of polar and nonpolar amino acid residues along the molecule's sequence. These staining patterns have been correlated with the structure of the collagen chains (Bruns RR, Gross J [1973] Band patterns of the segment - long - spacing form of collagen. Its use in the analysis of primary structure. Biochemistry 12: 808–815; Meek KM, Chapman JA, Hardcastle RA [1979] The staining patterns of collagen fibrils. Improved correlation with sequence data. J Biol Chem 254: 10710–10714).

Bustos. Also, you showed us an electrophoretic pattern of the so - called linkage collagen, and then you showed a postulated model of how this was organized. Maybe the resolution you get in the first dimension is not representative; perhaps instead of having one polypeptide chain that is a homogeneous band, you may find that you have more if you use two - dimensional electrophoresis.

Rhodes. The band that you are referring to, the acidic component, is homogeneous. Dr. Don Furuto in our laboratory has characterized the cyanogen bromide peptides of the acidic 40,000 - dalton component. The sum of the molecular weights and amino acid compositions of the CNBr peptides are equivalent to the 40,000 - dalton polypeptide (Furuto DK, Miller EJ [1980] Isolation of a unique collagenous fraction from limited pepsin digests of human placental tissue. J Biol Chem 255: 290).

Foster. Have you tried to localize any of the Type of VI collagens in any organs?

Rhodes. There has been some preliminary work using immunofluorescent techniques which indicates that the Type VI material is located in the subendothelial layer of the vascular intima. It is close to the basement membrane but not a part of it.

Glagov. We recently advanced our concepts of the organization of the aortic media by fracturing frozen, distended arteries, examining the fracture surfaces by scanning electron microscopy and comparing these findings with transmission electron micrographs of the same material. We found that collagen occurred in two distinct organizational forms. Thick undulating bundles of collagen were found between the elastin plates of the fibrous layers, and a finer interlacing basket work was found around groups of cells in the cell layers. Steffen Gay of your group pointed out to us that these morphologic forms corresponded to the immunofluorescent localization of Type I and Type III collagens, respectively. We believe that the thick bundles contribute mainly to the tensile strength of the wall as a whole, while the pericellular sheaths encompass and help to coordinate functional muscle groups. In addition, we were able to find an orderly, uniformly spaced array of very fine fibrils on cell surfaces of normally distended vessels. These seem to correspond closely in both size and location to those you have called Type V. This correlation between distinct morphologic forms and collagen types would seem to suggest that each of the collagen types corresponds to a particular functional role.

Rhodes. We, of course, are interested in this concept and in evidence other than just immunofluorescent data. We would like to have morphological data and are also pursuing means of confirming the Type V as an exocytoskeleton.

Chandler. Before the smooth muscle cells were found to be the cells producing most of the collagen in atherosclerotic lesions, a lot of investigators thought that fibroblasts as well as endothelial cells were involved in this process. I would be very interested in your comments about the possibility that the endothelium may indeed be producing some type of collagen other than basement membrane collagen.

Rhodes. There is an increasing amount of evidence now that the endothelial cells, in addition to making the basement membrane collagens, do, at least in culture, synthesize Type III and Type V (Sage H, Crouch E, Bronstein P [1979a] Collagen synthesis by bovine aortic endothelial cells in culture. Biochemistry 18: 5433–5441). This is not surprising because the subendothelium contains all three of these types, that is, Type IV localized in the basement membrane, and beneath the basement membrane one finds Types I, III and V, with Type III being the most abundant. Thus endothelial cells have the potential to synthesize more than just the basement membrane types. Let me also add in support of the theory that Type V is a pericellular type of collagen and that cultured endothelial cells sequester Type V in the cell layer; it is not found secreted into the culture medium. Again, this is some evidence, though indirect, that it remains closely associated with the cell.

Oegema. Would you give us an idea of the 40,000 - dalton molecules distribution in tissues?

Rhodes. I wish I could give you some information concerning tissue distribution. The only definite thing I can say at this point is that we find it in vascular tissue. Others have reported finding the 40,000 - dalton components in other tissues. Rojkind (Rojkind M, Giambrone MA, Biempica L [1979] Collagen types in normal and cirrhotic liver. Gastroenterology 76: 710-719) has isolated it from cirrhotic liver, but in that case one doesn't know if it is from the liver vasculature or not. Without monospecific antibodies, I cannot give any definite answers. I have also heard of one report where it has been isolated from skin. In terms of concentration I can only relate it to the placenta. It constitutes on the order of 2% - 3% of the total collagen that we can extract using limited pepsin digestion, so it is a rather small proportion of the total tissue collagen. However, the features of the molecule are unique; it could be very reactive and thus important even in such small quantities.

Caulfield. In our work we see banded collagen inserting into basement membrane in a variety of areas, especially in heart, into the membrane that surrounds the myocyte. Do you have any notion of how these banded fibers are attached to the basement membrane, because actually quite a bit of force goes through them? They must be well stuck!

Rhodes. No, I do not. I cannot give any definitive answers based on the biochemical information available. The proposal of a linkage type of collagenous moiety is very attractive for building models of how collagen fibers could insert into an amorphous basement membrane. One of the things that has not been investigated thoroughly is the possibility that noncollagenous sequences at the ends of the procollagen molecules may play a role in matrix interaction. Particularly with Type III and IV collagens, there seems to be limited or no extracellular processing of the procollagen molecule. Thus the nonhelical sequences which contain sulfhydryl groups may be more reactive with other tissue components. Another possibility is that some of the more recently described matrix components such as fibronectin and, now, in the case of basement membranes, laminin, may be interacting. Fibronectin does not bind Type V very efficiently, but does bind strongly the 40,000 - dalton components (Furuto DK [personal communication]).

Part II
Connective Tissues in Pulmonary Disease

THOMAS H. ROSENQUIST, *Chairman*

Introduction

THOMAS H. ROSENQUIST

There are no other systems in the body wherein the fibers of the connective tissues have more immediate and vital significance than in the respiratory system, especially the lung. In many ways the organization and distribution of the collagen and elastin of the lung have more impact on the physiologic behavior of the organ than does the absolute quantity of these scleroproteins. In the first paper of this part of the symposium, Dr. Gordon L. Snider presents some powerful arguments in support of the significance of the relationship between connective tissue organization and the mechanical behavior of the lung. Collagen and elastin work together, with collagen limiting pulmonary distensibility at high lung volumes and elastin providing the basic compliant character of the lung.

The unique contribution of elastin to the elastic functions of tissues, especially the lung and the large vessels, is reinforced by the presentation of Dr. Judith Foster. Dr. Foster's discussion of elastin biochemistry is highlighted by the interesting recent discovery of two distinct forms of tropoelastin or soluble elastin, called the "a" and "b" forms, whose proportions are unique to specific tissues and whose functional significance surely will be the object of intensive investigation in the future.

Dr. Gerald M. Turino defines the anatomy and biochemistry of the most common disease that interrupts these tissues, and thus interferes with normal function -- emphysema. Dr. Turino presents an excellent hypothesis for the etiology of emphysema, where the basic balance between α-1 antiprotease on the one hand and neutrophil or macrophage protease on the other hand is interrupted, e.g., with tobacco smoke, with resulting connective tissue disruption.

Dr. Holde Puchtler, whom we have honored, gives the final presentation of the symposium. As is usual with Dr. Puchtler, her presentation begins with a comprehensive historical digest; continues through the state of the art; and concludes with an enlightening prospective. Those readers who are willing to plunge into the massive literature written by Dr. Puchtler over the years may not always be able to keep pace with her intellect upon first reading, but a persistent reader will be amply rewarded by her brilliant applications of basic chemistry and physics to stain - substrate interactions, which hold the promise of placing histochemistry on a more scientific basis.

Her work in histochemistry in the past has often presaged advances in biochemistry; the paper presented here indicates that she may have done so once more, for her discussions of the histochemistry of elastin indicate a heterogeneity that may be related to the heterogeneous forms of elastin defined biochemically by Dr. Judith Foster.

Connective Tissues
and the Mechanical Behavior of Lungs

GORDON L. SNIDER

It has been known for more than 150 years (1) that the lungs have elastic behavior; beginning with Orsos' 1907 (2) classic description of normal and emphysematous lungs, there has been an ever increasing body of knowledge on the anatomic distribution of the connective tissues in the lungs. Histologic, ultrastructural, biochemical, and physiologic studies in the past 20 years on human lung disease and experimental models of lung disease have provided important new insights. Although much has been learned of the relation between the static mechanical properties of the lungs and the nature and disposition of their framework, there are still many unanswered questions regarding the role of some of the components of the connective tissues and the matrix in which they reside.

In this presentation, I briefly review our current understanding of the relation between the connective tissues of the normal lung and its mechanical behavior. This is followed by a discussion of these interrelations in two pathologic processes that appear to have a major impact on the connective tissues of the lungs: pulmonary emphysema and interstitial pulmonary fibrosis.

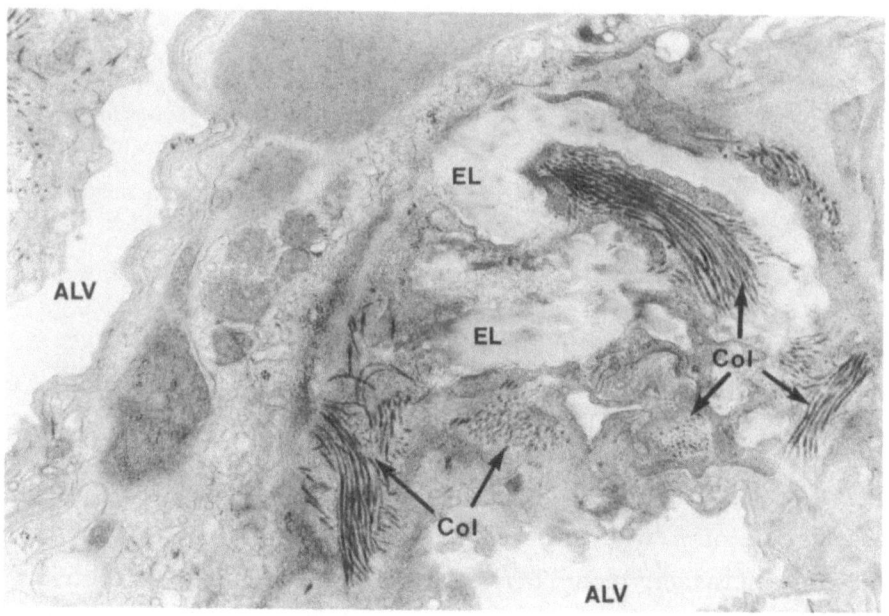

FIG. 1. Transmission electron micrograph of normal hamster lung showing connective tissue in the parenchymal interstitium. ALV, alveolar space; COL, collagen fiber bundles; EL, elastic fibers. Note the amorphous appearance of the elastic fibers. The collagen fiber bundles take a serpiginous course so that some are cut longitudinally, some obliquely, and some in cross section. X 12,200 (Courtesy of Drs. Shirley Morris and John Albright)

Connective Tissue Framework of the Lung

For many years anatomists and pathologists, basing their classification on differential staining properties in histologic sections (3), have described two main types of connective tissue fibers in the lungs: collagen fibers, which stain deeply with aniline dyes, and elastic fibers, which stain bluish-black to black with resorcinol - iron - fuchsin and purplish-red with orcein - iron hematoxylin. The connective tissue fibers are embedded in amorphous, acellular material that fills the extracellular space and is known as "ground substance."

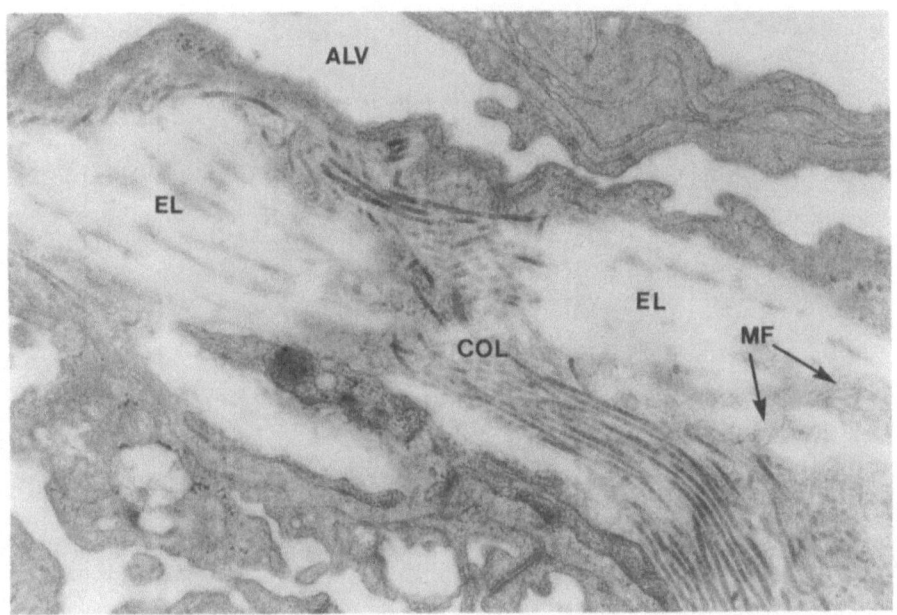

FIG. 2. Transmission electron micrograph of normal hamster lung showing connective tissues in the parenchymal interstitium. ALV, alveolar space; COL, collagen fibers; EL, elastic fibers. The cross banding of the collagen fibers can be faintly seen; the fibers are cut longitudinally, obliquely, and in cross section. Microfibrils (MF) are seen at the periphery of one of the amorphous elastic fibers. Note the granular appearance of the ground substance in which the fibers lie. X 22,800 (Courtesy of Drs. Shirley Morris and John Albright)

Transmission electron microscopy (4) resolves additional structural differences between collagen and elastin. Collagen fibers (5) appear as bundles of densely packed fibrils with a regular periodicity of 640 Å when stained with uranyl acetate and lead citrate (Figs. 1 and 2). Major bands result from the staggered packing of tropocollagen elements during laying down of the fibrils. Each major band is equivalent to the space left between the N-terminal end of one tropocollagen molecule and the C-terminal end of the adjacent molecule. Minor cross striations result from the alignment of polar amino acids from adjacent tropocollagen moieties that overlap in the fibril. These fiber bundles al-

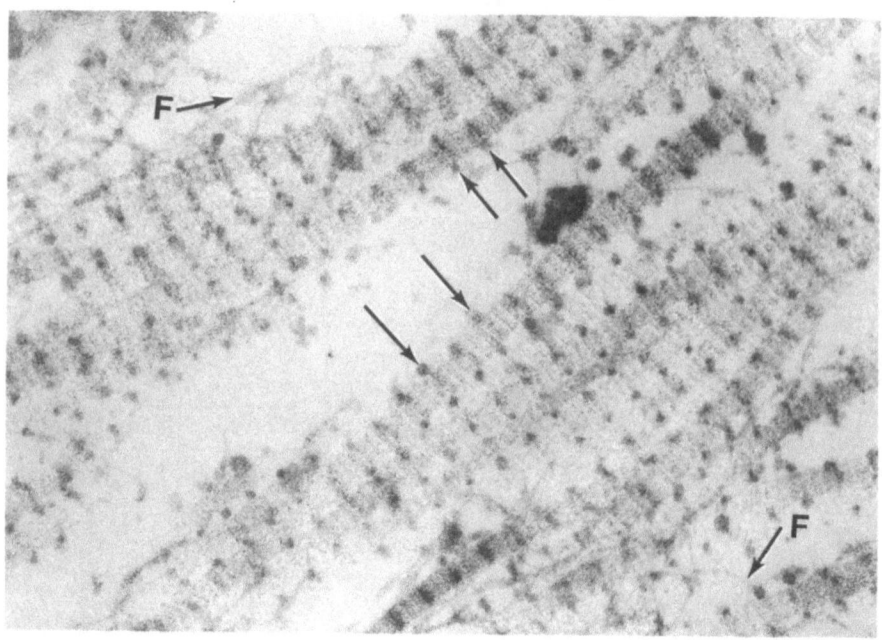

FIG. 3. Transmission electron micrograph of cross-banded collagen in rat lung. Numerous 10 - 40 nm granules are seen attached to the major collagen doublet band (arrows). Filaments (F) 3 - 10 nm in diameter are seen in some instance interconnecting granules and collagen fibrils. After digestion with chondroitinase ABC or papain the granules disappear, indicating that they represented proteoglycans containing chondroitin or dermatan sulfate. Tissues were treated with triton X-100 to improve stain penetration and were stained with ruthenium red. X 86,800 (From Vaccaro CA, Brody JS (1979) Am Rev Resp Dis 120: 901)

ways appear to take a serpiginous course in the lung. Basement membrane collagen is different in that it occurs as relatively homogeneous layers in which many small (10 nm) unbanded fibrils seem to merge with fibrils in the interstitial space.

Elastic fibers (6) are composed of predominant amorphous and less evident fibrillar components (Figs. 1 and 2); the latter are known as microfibrils (Fig. 2). The amorphous component, which is positively charged, stains poorly with cationic stains (uranyl acetate, lead citrate), but can be clearly identified with anionic stains such as phosphotungstic acid and palladium (7). Microfibrils are negatively charged and stain best with cationic stains. They are fibrillar structures, 10 - 12 nm thick, with a denser periphery than center, a property which gives them a tubular appearance. They are usually best observed at the periphery of the amorphous component of the elastic fibers.

Vaccaro and Brody (10) have recently shown the ultrastructural features of proteoglycans in lung by using ruthenium red staining and enzymatic digestion. Granules attached to the major doublet band of collagen were thought to represent proteoglycan aggregates containing chondroitin or dermatan sulfate (Fig. 3). Collagen fibers were enmeshed in an intrafibrillar matrix of 3 - 10 nm filaments, which was thought to comprise a protein of glycoprotein not containing glycosaminoglycans (Fig. 4).

Krahl (8) and more recently Weibel (9) have emphasized the concept that the connective tissues in the lung are composed of pleural, interstitial, and bronchovascular networks that merge to form a fibrous continuum. In the pleura, a dense layer of fibrous tissue lies immediately beneath the mesothelium, melding with a deeper spongy layer in which a network of small vessels run in a comparatively loose connective tissue network. This spongy layer, in turn, is in immediate contact with the fibrous limiting membranes of the subpleural pulmonary alveoli. Connective tissue fibers from the pleura are interlaced with fibers which pass into the interlobular and interalveolar lung septae, thus firmly binding the pleura to the underlying lung. Collagen and elastic fibers are found running together in the subpleural and septal connective tissues. Within the alveolar walls, collagen and elastic fibers weave in and out through the capillary rete. The fibers are seen between the capillary and alveolar epithelial basement membranes in the interstitial space and account for the thick portion of the alveolar septum. The alveolar fiber network communicates in turn with the fibers in the adventitia of the membranous bronchioles and the small pulmonary vessels; the latter are continuous with the rich connective tissue elements of the

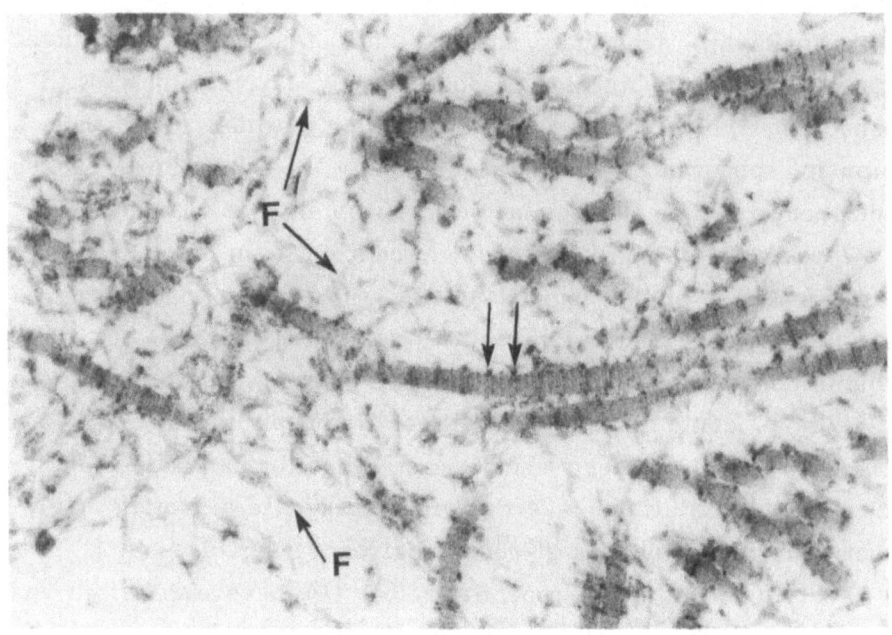

FIG. 4. Transmission electron micrograph of rat lung after mor-
danting tissue blocks with tannic acid. Collagen fibrils with
electron-dense granules at the major doublet band (arrows) are
clearly seen. Filaments (F) form a net-like matrix intertwined
with collagen and granules. This network was resistant to collagenase and glycosidase digestion but was removed by papain
treatment, suggesting that it was a protein or glycoprotein that
did not contain glycosaminoglycans. Triton X-100 followed by
ruthenium red stain. X 70,700 (From Vaccaro CA, Brody JS
(1979) Am Rev Resp Dis 120: 901)

larger vessels and bronchi. The continuity of the connective
tissues throughout the lungs is the basis for the interdependence
of the various elastic elements of its connective tissue framework;
forces are distributed relatively uniformly throughout the organ.

Measuring the Elastic Properties of Lung Tissues

Opening the thoracic cavity in a mammal promptly results in
collapse of the lungs toward the hilum. This tendency of the

lungs to recoil explains the subatmospheric pressure within the pleural space. The static elastic behavior of the lungs can be measured by studying the relation between the volume of the lungs (V_L) and the pressure difference between the airway opening (Pao) and the pressure on the pleural surface of the lungs, the transpulmonary pressure (Ppl). Thus, the static transpulmonary pressure [Pst(L)] is readily calculated from the equation: Pst(L) = Pao - Ppl. In practice, in both humans and animals, it is less invasive and more convenient to use intraesophageal pressure as a measure of pleural pressure. Although esophageal pressure is not precisely equivalent to pleural pressure, changes in esophageal pressure generally mirror changes in pleural pressure. Since pressure over the surface of the lung varies as a result of the effects of gravity, a measurement of pleural pressure at a single point over the lung would also not give an exact measure of mean pleural pressure.

Using a constant-volume, variable-pressure plethysmograph and a water-filled esophageal catheter, we have measured transpulmonary pressures and lung volumes in anesthetized hamsters (11). Such measurements reflect a combination of the elastic properties of lung tissues and of the elastic properties of the alveolar air - fluid interfaces. Using the plethysmographic system, transpulmonary pressure was measured as the difference between intraesophageal pressure and airway opening pressure, and lung volume was determined. A representative quasi-static inflation - deflation, volume - pressure (VP) curve from a normal anesthetized hamster is shown in Figure 5.

Ideally, volume - pressure relations of the lungs should be studied by making static measurements of volume and pressure at a number of different points. The term "static" implies that a given lung volume has been maintained long enough to allow development of equilibrium among all of the stresses within the lungs. That is to say, all forces due to the viscoplastoelastic properties of the tissues involved have had time to reach equilibrium. It is not usually convenient, under experimental condi-

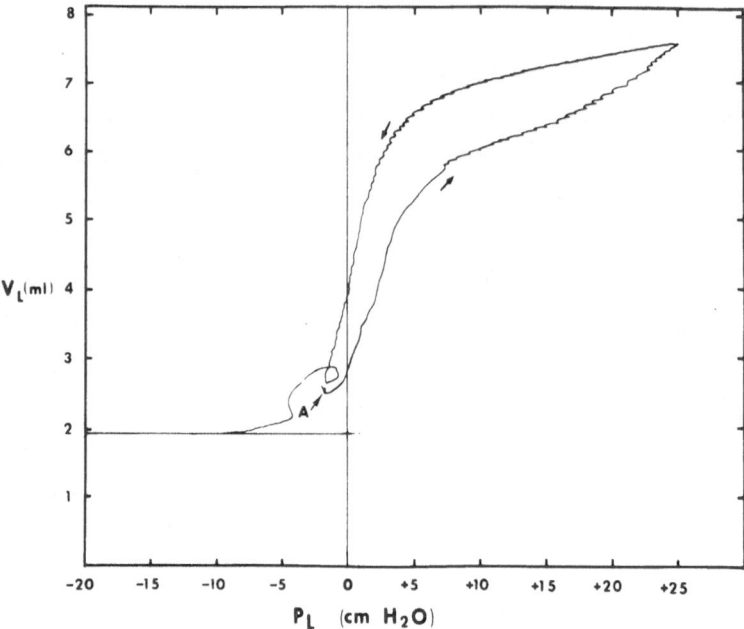

FIG. 5.   Tracing of a representative quasi-static, inflation - deflation, volume - pressure curve obtained from a normal anesthetized hamster.   Lung volume (V_L) is plotted against transpulmonary pressure (P_L). V_L at P_L = 25 cm H_2O is designated
total lung capacity (TLC_{25}) and measures 7.6 ml.   Lung volume
at P_L = -20 cm H_2O is designated residual volume (RV_{-20}) and
measures 1.9 ml.   Point A represents the functional residual
capacity (FRC) and measures 2.5 ml.   The vital capacity (VC)
measures 5.7 ml.   (From Snider GL, Karlinsky JB (1977) In:
Ioachim HL (ed) Pathobiology Annual.   Appleton-Century-Crofts,
New York, Vol 7, pp 115-142)

tions, to provide enough time for truly static properties to
develop, and the term "quasi-static" is therefore used to indicate
that static conditions may not have been completely met.

The anesthetized animal is rendered apneic by hyperventila-
tion, and the lungs are inflated to a transpulmonary pressure of
25 cm H_2O by applying positive pressure at the airway opening.
Decreases in volume and pressure are then allowed to occur
slowly but continuously during deflation.   The volume of air in
the lungs at a transpulmonary pressure of 25 cm H_2O is designated the total lung capacity or TLC_{25}, the subscript denoting

the transpulmonary pressure at which this volume is measured. This volume is analogous to the total lung capacity in man or the volume of air in the lungs at maximal inspiration. As maximal passive emptying is reached, a transpulmonary pressure of -20 cm H_2O is applied to empty the lungs completely. The volume of air in the lungs at this point is designated the residual volume, or RV_{-20}. This volume is meant to be analogous to the residual volume in man or the volume of air in the lungs at full expiration. The volume of air exhaled between TLC_{25} and RV_{-20} is the vital capacity (VC). The volume of air in the lungs at the resting-end expiratory position is known as the functional residual capacity (FRC) and is measured by the principle of Boyle's law. The volume of air between FRC and RV_{-20} is designated the expiratory reserve volume (ERV) and subtraction of ERV from FRC gives the RV_{-20}.

The quasi-static compliance of the lungs [Cst(L)] is defined as the slope of a straight line fitted to the deflation curve just above FRC. This ratio is a measure of the steepest part of the curve in the mid-lung volume range. Chord compliance is defined as the slope of a line joining any two designated points on the deflation VP curve. For example, chord compliance between 15 and 25 cm H_2O, designated $C_{st}L_{15-25}$, is a measure of compliance of the lungs at high lung volume. The VP curve may also be analyzed by fitting it to an exponential curve (15).

It is important to note that variations in lung volume will have an important influence on the VP curve and the indices used to describe it. For example, consider a hamster lung in which the compliance, $\Delta V_L / \Delta Pst(L)$, equals 5 ml/5 cm H_2O or 1.0 ml/cm H_2O. If one were then to halve V_L without changing Pst(L) by occluding a main bronchus, compliance would fall to 2.5 ml/5 cm H_2O or 0.5 ml/cm H_2O even though the elastic behavior of the inflated lung tissue had not changed (see also Table 3). It is apparent that caution must be exercised in drawing the conclusion that an alteration in compliance necessarily reflects a change in the modulus of elasticity of lung tissue. Variations in VP data in individuals of different size can be volume-corrected for differences in lung volumes among subjects by expressing V_L as percent of predicted VC or TLC using regressions of lung volume on some index of body size such as nose-to-tail length or body weight (or body height and age in the case of man). Methods of dealing with this problem in disease states are discussed later.

The Viscoplastoelastic Properties of Lung Tissue

The inflation and deflation limbs of the VP curve follow different courses, that is, they display hysteresis (Fig. 5). The inflation limb lies to the right of the deflation limb because higher pressures are developed during inflation than during deflation. Some of the higher pressure required during inflation is necessary to open alveoli, a phenomenon which occurs mostly in the lower third of the VP curve. Forces arising from the gas - tissue interface and as a result of time-dependent properties of tissues, such as creep and stress - relaxation, also contribute to hysteresis. For all of these reasons, the deflation limb of the VP curve above the FRC is thought to better reflect the combination of tissue and surface forces than the inflation limb (16).

Surface forces can be eliminated by studying the VP curve of the saline-filled, excised, gas-free lung (12). The lung is gas freed by asphyxiating the anesthetized animal after ten minutes of 100% oxygen breathing; during asphyxiation all of the oxygen is absorbed from the lungs. In the saline-filled lung, Pst(L) is diminished one-third to one-half of the value required to produce the same volume in air-filled lungs. However, pressures comparable to those in air-filled lungs are readily attained without reaching the yield or rupturing point of the lungs. Hysteresis is less in saline-filled than in air-filled lungs since it is due almost entirely to the viscoplastoelastic properties of the tissues.

The question may reasonably be asked whether tissue forces are due entirely to the connective tissue framework of the lung or whether contractile and noncontractile cells and vascular engorgement play any role. The VP curves of lungs stored for several days remain quite constant (13). Since storage might be presumed to have markedly altered cells, this phenomenon suggests that noncontractile cells contribute little to the viscoplasto-elastic behavior of lungs. Smooth muscle and other contractile elements may contribute in an important way to the viscoplasto-elastic properties of lung tissue. Changes in smooth muscle tone induced by drugs have great effects on the static VP curves of animals; in humans, differences in resting airway tone appear to have much less effect (14). Vascular engorgement of saline-filled lungs increases resting lung volume and the V_L reached at high Pst(L) is slightly reduced. Compliance of the lung is slightly decreased (14). Thus it appears reasonable to consider that the connective tissue framework of the lung is the major determinant of the quasi-static deflation saline-filled VP curve.

Evaluation of the VP Curve

Ideally, if no information is to be lost, VP curves describing different lungs should be compared throughout their volume range. This may be done by visual inspection after plotting them on the same coordinates, or some statistical method may be used to compare the volume measured at designated values of Pst(L) throughout the VP curve. The use of quasi-static compliance and of chord compliance at various designated regions of the VP curve was referred to earlier. Note also that in animal studies, where TLC is defined by an arbitrarily chosen Pst(L), say 25 cm H_2O, the TLC_{25} is also a statement of the chord compliance of the lung between 0 and 25 cm H_2O.

The VP Curve and the Elements of the Connective Tissue Framework of the Lung

Single collagen fibers from human tendon have a high modulus of elasticity and can be lengthened to only about 2% of their resting length before reaching their yield point (17). Elastic fibers from bovine neck ligament exhibit rubberlike elasticity with high extensibility. Both single elastic fibers and strips of neck ligament can be readily extended to 100% of their resting length without yielding, although tensions developed in the strip are much lower than those developed in the single fiber (18).

Assuming that collagen and elastic fibers in the lungs have similar mechanical properties, how do they contribute to the sigmoid shape of the pulmonary VP curve? As noted earlier, ultrastructural studies always show pulmonary collagen fibers to be arranged in serpentine fashion. The significance of this is that nonyielding fibers arranged in an interweaving or coiled fashion may contribute to the elastic behavior of a structure even though the individual fibers have little extensibility. A useful analogy is the inextensibility of the nylon monofilament as compared with the highly elastic, leg-conforming properties of the nylon stocking. Setnikar (19) developed and Mead (20) extended a model describing the mechanical behavior of the lungs based on the deformation of the collagen and elastic fibers of the connective tissue network. At low lung volumes the steep slope of the VP curve was attributed to the stretching of the readily extensible elastic fibers combined with the nylon stocking-like elasticity displayed by the coiled and interwoven collagen fibers. As lung volume increased, the wavy collagen fibers straightened, and as stress was applied to these inextensible fibers, the result was falling compliance of the combined networks and greatly increased stiffness of the lungs at maximal lung volumes. These two networks were considered to be acting in parallel with the collagen network functioning at high lung volumes to limit pulmonary distensibility.

Virtually nothing is known of the relative elastic contributions of the microfibrillar or amorphous components of the elastic fiber, and the contribution of the ground substance to elastic behavior is largely speculative. It seems likely that the ground substance contributes little to static elastic properties but may play an important role in the viscoplastoelastic or time-dependent properties of the connective tissue network.

Biochemical Measurements of Lung Collagen and Elastin

Biochemical measurements of lung collagen and elastin may also be used to evaluate the integrity of the connective tissue framework of the lung. Total lung collagen is relatively easily estimated, using the amino acid hydroxyproline as a marker. Hydroxyproline is found in only three proteins present in the lungs: collagen, elastin, and the C1q component of complement. Hydroxyproline comprises about 10% of the amino acid residues of collagen but only about 1% of the amino acid residues of elastin. Collagen is the most abundant protein in the lung, making up about 10% of its dry weight. Since elastin comprises only about 2.5% and the C1q component of complement is under 1% of dry lung weight, a measure of total lung hydroxyproline is a reasonable estimate of lung collagen. Subtraction of hydroxyproline attributable to elastin refines the measurement.

Measurement of whole lung elastin is not so simple because of technical problems in using the marker amino acids of elastin, desmosine and isodesmosine, to identify elastin. It is not feasible to measure desmosine and isodesmosine in whole lung hydrolysates without first carrying out some purification procedure. The use of harsh treatment, such as alkali denaturation of all other proteins at high temperature, the so-called Lansing procedure, has been widely used but results in loss of some of the soluble moieties of elastin. The most gentle procedures which have been developed may not yield all of the elastin of the lung for measurement.

In any event, it is important to recognize that biochemical measurements are most useful for providing a statement of the total quantity of the protein of interest and for evaluating the chemical properties of the protein. However, these measurements give little or no information about the location of the proteins unless some procedure has first been applied to separate the lung into fractions rich in one or another of the components

of the lung such as pleura, bronchi, blood vessels, or lung
parenchyma.

Alterations of the Connective Tissue Network and the VP Curve

The validity of the Setnikar-Mead theory of the role of the
collagen and elastic fiber networks has been studied by enzymatic alteration of the connective tissues of excised lungs and by
studying disease states, occurring spontaneously in man and induced in experimental animals, in which connective tissue alterations play a key role.

In Vitro Alterations

Johanson and Pierce (21) treated excised rat lungs with elastase, collagenase and papain solution. In their air-filled system
they could demonstrate no abnormality in the VP curves of lungs
treated with collagenase, but lungs treated with elastase and
papain (the latter has elastolytic activity) demonstrated increased
compliance at low and mid-transpulmonary pressures. Senior and
co-workers (22) incubated lung slices and Martin and Sugihara
(23) incubated alveolar walls with collagenase and elastase and
found changes consistent with the Setnikar-Mead hypothesis.
Turino and colleagues (24) demonstrated that elastase treatment
of excised rat tracheal segments increased compliance at low and
mid-distending volumes. On the other hand, collagenase treatment increased compliance only at very high distending pressures.

Karlinsky et al. (12) studied saline-filled VP curves made in
excised hamster lungs after incubation with endotracheally instilled clostridial collagenase or porcine pancreatic elastase solutions. Ultrastructural studies of lung tissue treated in vitro
with these enzyme solutions showed only disruption of collagen
fibers in lungs treated with collagenase and disruption of elastic
fibers in lungs treated with elastase. Mean deflation curves
from these studies are shown in Figure 6. Chord compliance in

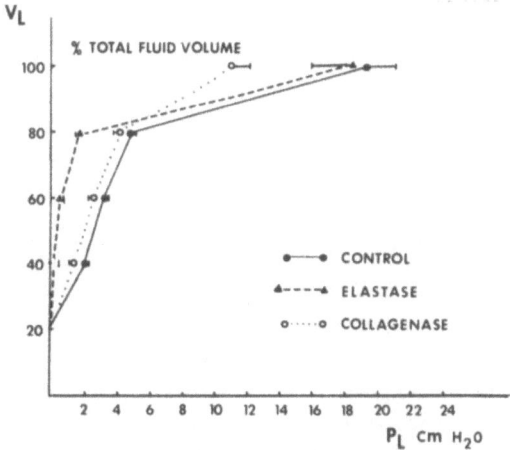

FIG. 6. Mean deflation saline-filled volume - pressure curves of excised lungs treated with pancreatic elastase or clostridial collagenase for 30 min at 37°C; control lungs were similarly treated with saline. Bars show SE of mean; V_L = lung volume; P_L = transpulmonary pressure. Note that at mid-volume range (40% - 60% total fluid volume) the elastase-treated lungs are more compliant than the control or collagenase groups; at high volume range (80% - 100% total fluid volume) the collagenase lungs are more compliant than the control or elastase groups. (From Karlinsky JB, Snider GL, Franzblau C, Stone PJ, Hoppin FG Jr. (1976) Am Rev Resp Dis 113: 769)

lungs treated with collagenase was significantly greater at high lung volumes than in elastase-treated or control lungs. Chord compliance in lungs treated with elastase was significantly higher at mid-volume range than collagenase-treated or control lungs. Thus, all of the available in vitro studies support the Setnikar-Mead theory of parallel functioning of elastic and collagen fibers.

In Vivo Alterations

Interesting observations regarding the relation between the connective tissue framework of the lung and its mechanical behavior have emerged from studies of experimental emphysema (25). Within a few hours after a single endotracheal injection of

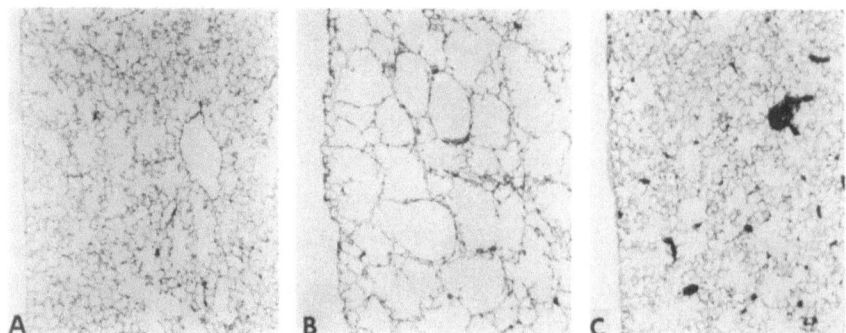

FIG. 7. Photomicrographs of hamster lungs. (A) Untreated normal lung; (B) 20 days following endotracheal porcine pancreatic elastase treatment; note diffuse and extensive dilatation and disruption of alveoli; (C) 16 days after treatment with endotracheal clostridial collagenase. There is no abnormality except for a plaque of pleural fibrosis. Hematoxylin and eosin stain. X 28 (From Snider GL, Sherter CB, Koo KW, Karlinsky JB, Hayes JA, Franzblau C (1977) J Appl Physiol Resp, Env Exercise Physiol 42: 206)

crystalline porcine pancreatic elastase or bacterial collagenase is administered to an anesthetized hamster, extensive pulmonary hemorrhage is noted. Twenty-one days later, the hemorrhage has cleared except for a few residual siderophages. The lungs of the elastase-treated hamster show remarkable distortion of the architecture with uniform dilatation of the alveoli characteristic of human panlobular emphysema; the collagenase-treated lungs are normal (Fig. 7).

Measurements of lung volumes and VP curves in anesthetized elastase-treated hamsters at 21 days (Fig. 8) show that the TLC_{25}, FRC, and RV_{-20} are increased and the VP curves are shifted upward and to the left. $C_{st}(L)$ is increased (1.119 ± 0.045 for elastase vs 0.669 ± 0.019 ml/cm H_2O ± SE for control, p = 0.05), but $C_{st}(L)_{15 - 25}$ remains unchanged from control. In collagenase-treated animals, the only change from control is an increase in VC and TLC_{25}, and inspection of the VP curve

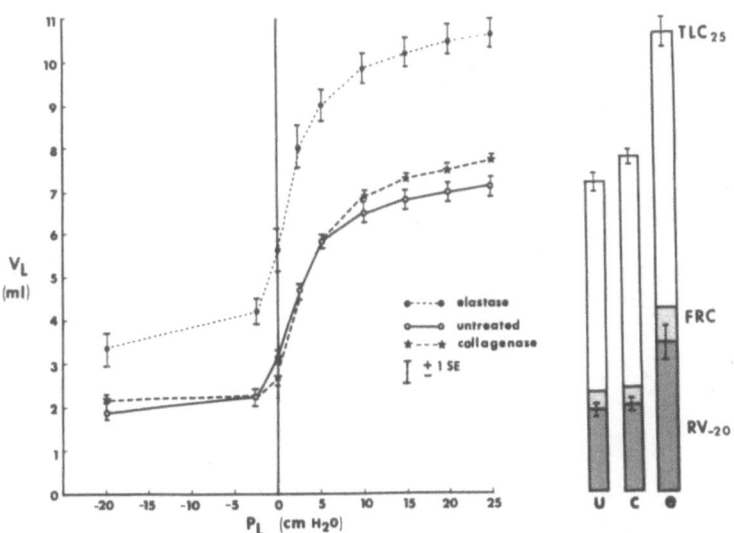

FIG. 8.   Mean ± SE lung volume (V_L) is plotted against selected values of transpulmonary pressure (P_L), measured from quasi-static deflation volume - pressure curves of groups of anesthetized hamsters.   The bar diagram to the right summarizes the lung volumes, showing the volume of air in the lungs at P_L 25 cm H_2O (TLC_{25}) and -20 cm H_2O (RV_{-20}) and functional residual capacity (FRC).   Groups comprised 15 untreated hamsters (U), 12 hamsters instilled endotracheally with clostridial collagenase (C) and 8 hamsters instilled endotracheally with pancreatic elastase (E) 18-21 days before study.   (From Snider GL, Karlinsky JB (1977) In: Ioachim HL (ed) Pathobiology Annual. Appleton-Century-Crofts, New York, Vol 7, pp 115-142)

shows that this is due to an increase in the slope of the VP curve in the higher reaches of lung volume. The $C_{st}L_{15 - 25}$ is significantly increased in the collagenase-treated animals as compared with controls (0.046 ± 0.01 for collagenase vs 0.033 ± 0.01 ml/cm H_2O ± SE for controls, p = 0.05); $C_{st}L$ is unchanged from controls in the collagenase-treated animals.   Similar changes were observed in VP curves of saline-filled lungs made in hamsters treated approximately 21 days previously with these enzymes (Fig. 9), thus confirming that the changes observed in air-filled lungs reflect alterations in the lung connective tissue networks and are not due to alterations in surface forces.

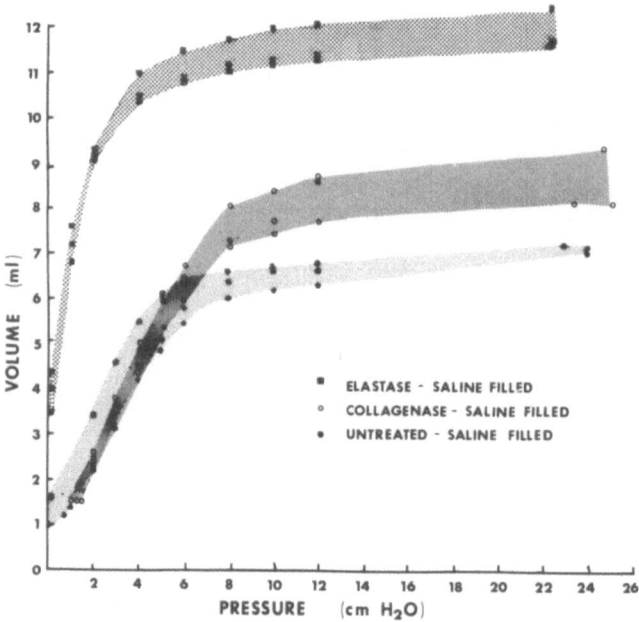

FIG. 9. Saline-filled deflation pulmonary volume - pressure curves for groups of 3 hamsters untreated or instilled endotracheally approximately 21 days earlier with pancreatic elastase or clostridial collagenase. Data points represent lung volume at selected values of transpulmonary pressure of saline for individual animals. Note that the volume of saline that could not be withdrawn from the lungs is greater for the elastase-treated animals than the other two groups. Compliance in mid-volume range and the maximum volume instilled into the lungs is greatest in the elastase group. Compliance in mid-volume range is the same in the collagenase-treated hamsters as in the untreated hamsters. However, compliance is higher at high lung volume (between 5 and 7 ml) in the collagenase group than in the untreated hamsters. These findings confirm that the changes described in Figure 8 are due to altered tissue forces. (From Snider GL, Sherter CB, Koo KW, Karlinsky JB, Hayes JA, Franzblau C (1977) J Appl Physiol Resp, Env Exercise Physiol 42: 206)

The alterations in $C_{st}L$ and $C_{st}L_{15-25}$ after elastase and collagenase treatment are in agreement with the Setnikar-Mead hypothesis. However, this hypothesis does not provide a rational explanation for the increase in TLC_{25} that is observed after elastase treatment. Since elastase does not attack native collagen, the collagen fiber network should have been unaffected and

thus the distensibility of the lung should have remained unchanged.   However, it is known that elastase will attack the
ground substance of the connective tissues and collagen may
have been altered by endogenous proteolytic hydrolases released
from inflammatory cells during the course of the response to the
elastase injury in the hamster lung.   It is known that collagen
synthesis is increased dramatically after elastase injury, suggesting that the structural forms of these proteins present at 21
days may be quite different than in the normal lung.   The repair
process itself may account for the increase in observed TLC_{25}.

Emphysema

In this discussion, the literature relating biochemical, physiologic and structural data in experimental and human emphysema
is briefly summarized.   The importance of disruption of the elastic fiber network in the production of experimental emphysema
by means of treatment with enzymes has now been clearly established.   The effectiveness of papain, a proteolytic enzyme of
plant origin, relates to its elastolytic and not to its esterolytic
properties (26).   The potency of several proteolytic enzymes of
bacterial and fungal origin has also been shown to be related to
their potency as enzymes capable of solubilizing elastin (27).   As
already noted, endotracheal treatment with clostridial collagenase
fails to produce emphysema; the same is true of trypsin and
chymotrypsin.   A genetic model of impaired cross-linking has
been described in blotchy mice which have an x-linked blotchy
allele causing defective cross-linking of both elastin and collagen
(28).   The lungs of these animals show air-space dilatation, and
saline-filled VP curves show increased compliance between 30%
and 70% of TLC.

Hoffman and associates administered DM-penicillamine (29) and
Stanley et al. gave β-amino-proprionitrile (30) to weanling rats
to inhibit the cross-linking of elastin and produced a physiologic
pattern of increased compliance most apparent in the low to mid-

volume range. Kuhn and Starcher (31) gave β-amino-proprionitrile and penicillamine to hamsters treated with elastase and demonstrated a more severe lesion than in animals given elastase
alone; Fedullo et al. (32) administered penicillamine to adult hamsters and demonstrated an increase in the soluble collagen and
an increase in compliance at high lung volumes. There was no
disruption of lung architecture in any of the adult animals
treated with lathyrogens alone. However, Kida and Thurlbeck
(33) found that administering β-amino-proprionitrile to rats in
the first four weeks of life resulted in changes compatible with
emphysema -- the lungs were large, had too few and too large
alveoli, and had diminished elastic recoil. Recovery did not occur four weeks after cessation of feeding of the lathyrogen (34).
Copper is an essential co-factor for lysyloxidase, a key enzyme
in the cross-linking of elastin. When pregnant rats are made
copper deficient and the copper deficiency is maintained in the
offspring, the pups demonstrate structural changes resembling
emphysema (35).

It has been known for more than 70 years that disruption of
the elastic tissue framework occurs in human emphysema (2),
and contemporary pathologists have confirmed this observation
(36). Physiologic studies in humans have shown a normal or
increased TLC, an increase in $C_{st}L$, and a decrease in transpulmonary pressure at TLC. Interestingly, biochemical studies
have failed to reveal any change in quantity of elastin in human
emphysema when elastin is expressed as total lung elastin or
percent dry weight (37-39). In elastase-induced emphysema in
hamsters total quantity of elastin per lung is normal or even
slightly increased (40). Amino acid analysis of elastin from
human emphysematous lung has yielded conflicting results. Some
studies have shown no difference when compared with normal
tissues (40, 41); others have revealed that elastin from emphysematous lung has a higher ratio of polar to nonpolar amino acids
(42-44).

Although ultrastructural studies show no abnormality of elastic fibers in human or experimental emphysema, light microscopic studies show irregularity and beading of the elastic fibers, especially in the pleura, and fraying of fibers in the alveolar walls is also seen (36, 37, 40). Thus, although the quantity of elastin within the lung may be normal or even increased, its disposition within the lung parenchyma may be grossly abnormal so that its structural competence is compromised.

Interstitial Pulmonary Fibrosis

Interstitial pulmonary fibrosis (IPF) may be the end result of many different injuries to the lungs. Drugs used in cancer chemotherapy, such as bleomycin and cyclophosphamide, ionizing radiation, viral infections, and chronic exposure to inorganic dusts are known to result in fibrosis. Pulmonary fibrosis is also a part of the multisystem disorders known as the collagen - vascular diseases: rheumatoid disease, systemic lupus erythematosis, progressive systemic sclerosis, and dermatomyositis. Many of these diseases have overtones of disordered immunologic processes.

Regardless of etiology, the pathologic process in the lungs tends to be similar. The abnormalities tend to be patchy or inhomogeneous even though the process is widespread. Early in the course, edema, perhaps with hyaline membranes, mild hemorrhage, and cellular infiltration predominate. Polymorphonuclear leukocytes are the major inflammatory cells seen early, with subsequent predominance of lymphocytes and macrophages. Within a few days, fibrotic thickening of alveolar walls occur with organization of alveolar exudate and incorporation of alveoli into the interstitium. Persons with interstitial pulmonary fibrosis tend to have similar alterations in lung mechanics with diminished lung volumes and quasi-static compliance.

Earlier histochemical studies and more recent biochemical studies (32, 45, 46) indicate that the increased connective tissue

elements are made up of collagen, elastin, and glycosaminoglycans. In normal lungs, type III collagen constitutes about 33%
of the total collagen with the remainder being type I; in idiopathic interstitial pulmonary fibrosis, the relative content of type
III collagen is markedly diminished, ranging from 12% to 24% in
different patients (47).

Naturally enough, given the noncompliant nature of collagen
fibers investigators have attempted to correlate the severity of
fibrosis with the alterations in lung mechanics. There are many
problems in attempting to carry out such correlations. As noted
above, biochemical measurements indicate the quantity of a protein, while giving no information as to its anatomic disposition
within the lung. Furthermore, there are important problems of
sampling and of the units to be used in expressing lung connective tissue components.

Fulmer et al. (48) in a recent publication reported collagen
concentration as collagen per dry weight of lung. There were
no significant differences in the collagen content among nine patients with interstitial pulmonary fibrosis as compared with six
control subjects. There was also no correlation between collagen
concentration and the morphologic assessment of the degree of
fibrosis. Examination of data from several studies of experimental interstitial pulmonary fibrosis and one carefully done
human study provides an explanation for this seeming paradox.
McCullough et al. (49) studied the lobes and lungs of baboons
receiving bleomycin, 45 - 95 units/kg body weight. There was
an approximately 1.5 times increase in collagen per lung and a
doubling to tripling of elastin per lung. However, collagen per
unit dry weight was either unchanged or was actually decreased
as compared to control. There were slight increases in elastin
concentration per unit dry weight. Relations between elastin
and collagen and total protein or DNA were similar. Starcher et
al. (45) showed an approximate doubling of collagen and elastin
per lung in hamsters treated with endotracheal bleomycin.

TABLE 1. Relation Between Lung Collagen Content and Ratios of Collagen Content to Dry Weight, Deoxyribonucleic Acid (DNA) and Total Protein[a]

Group	Time (days)	Collagen/ lung	Collagen/ dry lung wt.	Collagen/ DNA	Collagen/ total protein
Normal	--	100	100	100	100
Bleomycin	8	104	81	82	91
Bleomycin	30	143	96	118	109
Bleomycin	60	195	152	154	163
Bleomycin	90	179	143	178	156

[a]All data are expressed as percent normal. Calculated from the data in Tables 2 and 3 of Goldstein et al. (46).

Goldstein et al. (46), studying the evolution of bleomycin-induced pulmonary fibrosis in hamsters, showed that ratios of collagen to dry lung weight, DNA, and total protein were decreased at 8 days, a time when total lung collagen was unchanged (Table 1). At 30 days, when lung collagen was increased to 143% of control, the ratios of collagen to dry lung weight, DNA, and total protein were either unchanged or were only slightly increased. It was not until 60 days, when the collagen per lung was almost doubled, that the ratios of collagen to dry lung weight, DNA, and total protein were increased by about 150%. The responses of elastin were similar to those of collagen.

Zapol et al. (50) measured collagen, dry lung weight, and dry lung weight after extraction of hemoglobin in 12 patients who died at various times after severe, acute respiratory failure and in 9 normal lungs. Approximately 50 samples of each lobe of lung were analyzed. Collagen concentration of the lungs was expressed as micrograms per milligram of lyophilized dry weight; total collagen, expressed in grams per square meter of body surface area, was calculated from the total dry weight of the lung and the individual's calculated body surface area. After

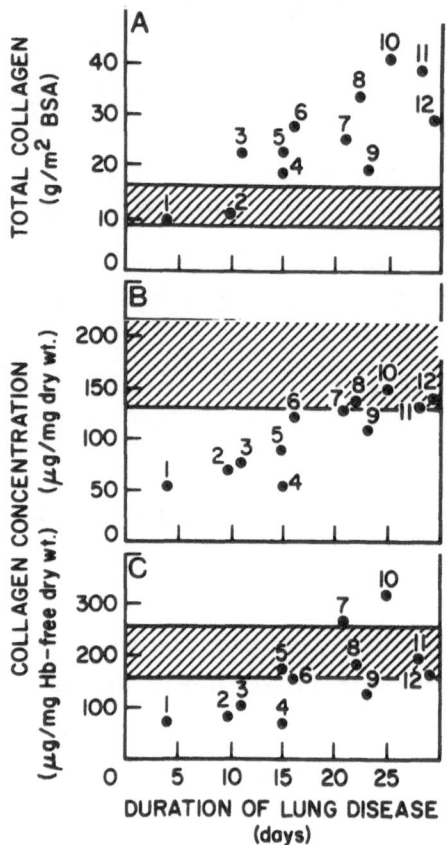

FIG. 10. Total collagen [g/m² body surface area (BSA)] and collagen concentration in the lungs of patients at various times after the onset of acute respiratory failure. Each point is the mean of a large number of postmortem lung samples (see Fig. 11); the patient numbers are given above each point. The shaded areas represent the range for normal lungs. Note that total lung collagen increased with increasing duration of disease; all but two lungs were above the range of normal. On the other hand, the collagen concentration of all lungs was within or below the range of normal, although the values also increased with increasing duration of lung disease. Expressing concentration as µg/mg hemoglobin-free dry lung weight shifted the values upward but only two lungs were above the range of normal. (From Zapol WM, Trelstad RL, Coffey JW, Tsai I, Salvador RA (1979) Am Rev Resp Dis 119: 517)

three to four weeks of severe, acute respiratory failure, the lungs of all patients had severe and diffuse interstitial fibrosis as seen by histologic assessment. Total collagen content of these lungs was increased two- and three-fold (Fig. 10). Within the first 10 days of the disease several lungs remained in the range of normal. Mean collagen concentration was within or below the range of normal for all lungs. The concentrations increased significantly when collagen was expressed per unit hemoglobin-free dry weight, although only two lungs were above the range of normal. The findings are similar to those in the animal studies: large amounts of inflammatory proteins and cells increase the dry weight, protein, and DNA content of tissue samples and prevent accurate calculation of the collagen concentration. Determining the mean collagen concentration is further complicated by marked sample-to-sample variation in collagen concentration, which must be taken into consideration whenever measurements are made on human or large animal lungs (Fig. 11).

These studies clearly explain the contradictory findings of morphologic evidence of severe pulmonary fibrosis in lungs that have normal or low values of collagen concentration. Analysis of a small lung biopsy specimen for collagen cannot provide a reliable chemical assessment of fibrosis because one does not know the weight of the lung in an undiseased state. When the collagen is expressed as a ratio of DNA, total protein, dry lung weight, or virtually any other index, the ratio is meaningless since both the numerator and denominator may have changed as a result of the disease process.

Relation Between Pulmonary Function and Connective Tissue Composition in IPF

McCullough et al. (49) in their baboons found that pulmonary function tests revealed similar abnormalities in bleomycin-treated animals at all stages. Lung volumes and compliance were reduced, but these abnormalities of physiology were associated with highly variable histology, including nearly normal lung structure, intense inflammation, or marked fibrosis. Pulmonary

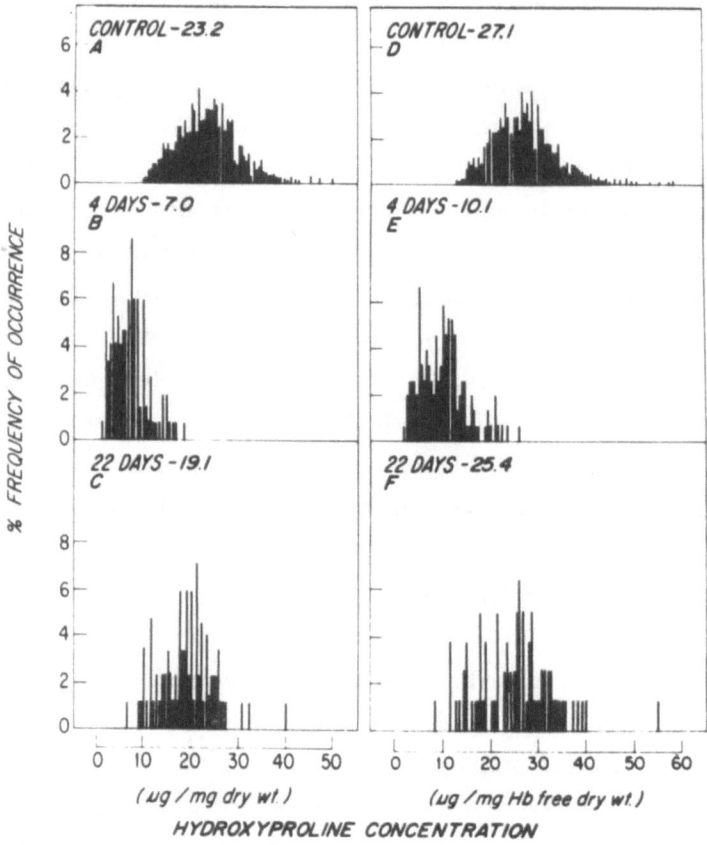

FIG. 11. Histograms of hydroxyproline concentration of 939 samples from 9 normal lungs (A) and (D); (B) and (E) are values from 150 samples from the lungs of a patient who died 4 days after severe thoracic trauma (patient 1 in Fig. 10); (C) and (F) are values from 84 samples from the lungs of a patient who died after 22 days of acute respiratory failure (patient 8 in Fig. 10). The concentrations in the left panels are calculated from dry lung weight; those on the right were calculated from hemoglobin-free dry lung weight. The mean concentration is given in the upper left corner of each panel. Note the increased concentration calculated from hemoglobin-free dry lung weight and the wide variation of concentrations in individual samples in both normal and diseased lungs. The confusion which could result from studying a single random sample is evident as is the need for dealing with the difficult sampling problem whenever lung connective tissue elements are to be measured. (From Zapol WM, Trelstad RL, Coffey JW, Tsai I, Salvador RA (1979) Am Rev Resp Dis 119: 517)

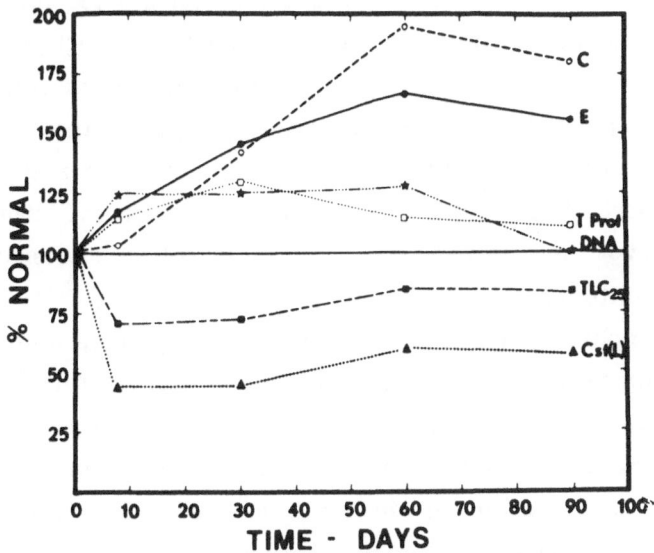

FIG. 12. Biochemical and physiologic alterations after endotracheal bleomycin treatment in hamsters expressed as percent of control and plotted against time. C, collagen; E, elastin; T Prot, total protein; DNA, deoxyribonucleic acid; TLC$_{25}$, volume of air in the lungs at a transpulmonary pressure of 25 cm H$_2$O; Cst(L), quasi-static compliance. Note the discordance, except for total protein values, between the physiologic and biochemical data. See text for further discussion. (From Goldstein RH, Lucey EC, Franzblau C, Snider GL (1979) Am Rev Resp Dis 120: 67)

function tests were not helpful in predicting either histologic or biochemical findings. The results of Goldstein et al. (46) summarized in Figure 12 show diminution in TLC$_{25}$, VC, C$_{st}$(L), and C$_{st}$L$_{15 - 25}$, which were striking by day 8 when there were no increases in lung collagen or elastin but DNA was increased by 25%. At 30 days, lung volumes and compliance were not changed, but collagen and elastin showed a definite increase. At 60 days, when collagen and elastin were maximally increased, compliance and lung volume were returning toward normal. Significant correlations of lung compliance and VC with collagen were not found. The lack of correlation persisted even when the 8-day data, when collagen was not yet increased, were excluded from analysis. On correction of compliance for lung volume, compliance remained significantly lower in bleomycin-induced IPF than in the control groups, and the correlation with collagen was not improved. These calculations suggest that the alterations in compliance is due to more than a diminution in lung volume. Correcting compliance for dry lung weight similarly did not improve the discrepancy between compliance alterations and collagen content.

It is apparent that the decreases in compliance and lung volume in bleomycin-induced IPF are not just a function of the amount of connective tissue present. Early in the process, alveoli are rendered airless by edema and cellular infiltration, giving rise to a diminution in lung volume and resulting in decreased compliance before connective tissue elements are increased. Altered surface forces may also play a role at this time. Later, focal areas of fibrosis contribute to the increased modulus of elasticity of the lung, but in some regions of the lung, focal scars may be so noncompliant that they contribute little to the alteration in lung mechanics except to decrease lung volume, yet they contribute in a major way to the increase in lung collagen. Finally, late in the course of the fibrotic process, compensatory lung growth of relatively uninvolved lung tissue may occur. This process, which has been clearly demonstrated in radiation-induced interstitial fibrosis in the baboon by Collins et al. (51), accounts for some restoration of net compliance toward normal at a time when connective tissue content of the lung remains high. Finally, as we have observed in both cadmium-induced and bleomycin-induced IPF in hamsters (52, 53), paracicatricial emphysema may develop late in the course of the disease and the algebraic sum of excessively compliant and excessively stiff areas of lung may cause compliance to return toward normal despite the persistence of high levels in the lungs of connective tissue elements.

While simple volume - pressure relations are generally a poor indicator of the connective composition of the lungs, a recent

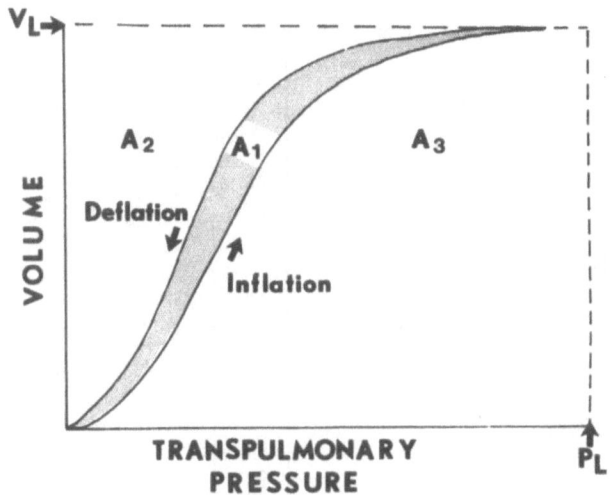

FIG. 13.   Definition of hysteresis and hysteresis ratio.   Hysteresis is the area enclosed by the inflation and deflation limbs of the saline-filled volume - pressure curve, area A_1.   Hysteresis ratio (HR) is the percentage of the rectangle enclosing the volume - pressure curve which is occupied by area A_1.   HR = A_1 (100)/V_L x P_L.   (From Fedullo AJ, Jung-Legg Y, Snider GL, Karlinsky JB (1980) Am Rev Resp Dis 122: 47)

experiment in our laboratory raises the question of whether this is always so.   Rinaldo et al. (54) confirmed that there was no relation between elastance (the reciprocal of compliance) and collagen content of the lungs in bleomycin-induced pulmonary fibrosis.   However, in combined injury with bleomycin and 0.6 atmospheres of oxygen, there was a high correlation between collagen content of the lungs and the change in elastance between the bleomycin-treated and the bleomycin/oxygen-treated animals.   Furthermore, the intercept of the line of regression with the Y axis fell at the level of collagen content of the bleomycin-treated lungs.   These observations suggested that the increased lung collagen in the animals with the combined injury might have been disposed more uniformly through the lung than the patchy deposition of collagen which is known to occur in bleomycin-induced pulmonary fibrosis.

TABLE 2. <u>Saline-filled Lung Statics and Hysteresis Data (Mean + SE) in Both Lungs and Right Lungs of Hamsters</u>[a]

Group	$TLC_{25}(S)$ (ml)	$C_{st} L(S)$ (ml/cm H_2O)	$\dfrac{C_{st} L(S)}{TLC_{25}(S)} \times 100$ (1/cm H_2O)	HA (in^2)	HR (%)
Both lungs	7.45 ± 0.31	1.1 ± 0.07	14.6 ± 0.56	4.98 ± 0.33	13.4 ± 0.62
Right lungs	4.65 ± 0.23*	0.5 ± 0.03*	11.8 ± 0.48*	3.42 ± 0.27	15.4 ± 0.90

[a]Abbreviations: $TLC_{25}(S)$, the volume of saline in the lungs at transpulmonary pressure 25 cm H_2O; $C_{st} L(S)$, the slope of the straight part of the deflation limb of the saline-filled volume – pressure curve; HA, the area of hysteresis, A_1 in Fig. 13; HR, the hysteresis ratio, in Fig. 13. (Data selected from Table 2 of Fedullo AJ, Jung-Legg Y, Snider GL, Karlinsky JB (1980) Am Rev Resp Dis 122: 47)

*Asterisk indicates p < 0.05

TABLE 3. Characterization of Hamsters with Bleomycin-Induced Pulmonary Fibrosis with Normal and Increased Hysteresis Ratio[a]

Group	n	HR (%)	TLC$_{25}$(S) (ml)	C$_{st}$L(S) (ml/cm H$_2$O)	HA (in.^{2})	LDI (%)
Normal HR	13	13.4 ± 0.52	5.58 ± 0.29	0.69 ± 0.05	4.02 ± 0.33	3.3 ± 0.56
Increased HR	9	27.6 ± 1.81*	5.01 ± 0.47	0.55 ± 0.08	7.19 ± 0.95*	7.0 ± 1.2*

[a]Abbreviations: LDI, lung disease index, a stereologically measured index of the proportion of total lung which is diseased; other abbreviations as in Table 2. (Data selected from Table 1 of Fedullo AJ, Jung-Legg Y, Snider GL, Karlinsky JB (1980) Am Rev Resp Dis 122: 47)

*Asterisk indicates $p < 0.05$.

Fedullo et al. (55) have evaluated the viscoplastoelastic properties of normal and diseased hamster lungs by determining the hysteresis ratio (HR). The HR is defined as the area enclosed within the inflation and deflation limbs of a saline-filled VP curve expressed as a percentage of the rectangle enclosing the curve (Fig. 13). In the right lung only, $C_{st}L(S)$ and $TLC_{25}(S)$ were diminished compared to both lungs, but HR was normal (Table 2). When bleomycin-treated animals were subdivided into groups with normal and elevated HR, compliance and lung volumes were similar for the two groups, but the lung disease index, an index of the amount of disease observed histologically, was greater in the animals with elevated HR (Table 3). Thus, HR might provide an additional indicator of the mechanical integrity of lung tissue.

Summary

The elastic recoil and viscoplastoelastic properties of the lungs are thought to be due primarily to the mechanical properties of the connective tissue fibers and the surface tension forces generated at the air - fluid interface in the alveoli. Tissue cells and vascular engorgement are believed to be of minor importance in health but the former particularly may assume a key role in disease. Deflation volume - pressure curves at volumes above 30% or 40% of VC are useful in assessing mechanical behavior of the lungs. Variations in volume contribute greatly to apparent variations in elastic behavior of the lungs as identified in static volume - pressure curves; there are no entirely satisfactory ways of analyzing data to separate changes due to alterations in lung volume from those due to changes in lung tissue properties. The hysteresis ratio, a measure of irrecoverable work done on the lungs, may prove to be a useful indicator of the viscoplastoelastic properties of the lungs.

Elastic fibers are mostly responsible for the great distensibility and recoil properties of the lungs. Collagen fibers are coiled at resting volume and, when extended, limit the distensibility of the lungs. Little is known of the mechanical roles played by the microfibrillar constituents of the elastic fiber or of the ground substance.

Disruption of the elastic fiber is the basis of experimental emphysema and is the likely basis of this lesion in man. Although collagen, elastin, and the glycosaminoglycans are increased in interstitial pulmonary fibrosis, there is a poor relation between the mechanical properties of the lungs and the content or concentrations of these proteins. In evaluating alterations in the connective tissue content of these lungs, it is essential that the connective tissues be expressed in absolute terms and not as ratios to some other measurement, such as total protein, dry lung weight, or DNA. In small animal lungs, this is best accomplished by measuring the protein content in the entire lung; in the lungs of larger animals and humans, the lungs must be extensively sampled and the concentration of the protein of interest must be related to the weight of the entire organ.

Acknowledgment
The work was supported by Program Project Grant HL-19717 from the National Heart, Lung and Blood Institute and the Veterans Administration Research Service.

REFERENCES

1. Carson J (1820) On the elasticity of the lungs. Philos Trans R Soc Lond (Biol) 110: 29

2. Orsos F (1907) Ueber das elastische Gerust der normalen und der emphysematosen Lungen. Beitr Pathol 41: 95

3. Luna LG (1968) Manual of histologic staining methods of the Armed Forces Institutes of Pathology. McGraw-Hill, New York

4. Schubert M, Hammerman D (1968) A primer on connective tissue biochemistry. Lea and Febiger, Philadelphia

5. Piez KA, Miller A (1974) The structure of collagen fibrils. J Supramol Struct 2: 121

6. Ross R (1973) The elastic fiber: a review. J Histochem Cytochem 21: 199

7. Morris SM, Stone PJ, Rosenkrans WA, Calore JD, Albright JT, Franzblau C (1978) Palladium chloride as a stain for elastin at the ultrastructural level. J Histochem Cytochem 26: 635

8. Krahl VE (1964) Anatomy of the mammalian lung. In: Fenn WO, Rahn H (eds) Handbook of physiology, respiration, Vol 1 Am Physiol Soc, Washington DC, p 213

9. Weibel ER, Gil J (1977) Structure-function relationships at the alveolar level. In: West JB (ed) Bioengineering aspects of the lung. Marcel-Dekker, Inc., New York, pp 1-81

10. Vaccaro CA, Brody JS (1979) Ultrastructural localization and characterization of proteoglycans in the pulmonary alveolus. Am Rev Resp Dis 120: 901

11. Koo KW, Leith DE, Sherter DB, Snider GL (1976) Respiratory mechanics in normal hamsters. J Appl Physiol 40: 936

12. Karlinsky JB, Snider GL, Franzblau C, Stone PJ, Hoppin FG Jr (1976) In vitro effects of elastase and collagenase on mechanical properties of hamster lungs. Am Rev Resp Dis 113: 769

13. Radford EP Jr (1964) Static mechanical properties of mammalian lungs. In: Fenn WO, Rahn H (eds) Handbook of physiology, respiration Vol 1. Am Physiol Soc, Washington DC, p 429

14. Gilson GJ, Pride NB (1976) Lung distensibility. The static pressure-volume curve of the lungs and its use in clinical assessment. Br J Dis Chest 70: 143

15. Salazar E, Knowles JH (1964) An analysis of pressure-volume characteristics of the lungs. J Appl Physiol 19: 97

16. Milic-Emili J (1974) Pulmonary statics. In: Guyton AC, Widdicombe JG (eds) MTP international review of science, physiology, Vol 2. University Park Press, College Park, Maryland, pp 105-137

17. Minns RJ, Soden PD, Jackson DS (1973) The role of the fibrous components and ground substance in the mechanical properties of biological tissues: a preliminary investigation. J Biomech 6: 153

18. Carton RW, Dainauskas J, Clark JW (1962) Elastic properties of single elastic fibers. J Appl Physiol 17: 547

19. Setnikar I (1955) Origine e significato delle proprieta meccaniche del polmone. Arch Fisiol 55: 349

20. Mead J (1961) Mechanical properties of lungs. Physiol Rev 41: 281

21. Johanson WG Jr, Pierce AK (1972) Effects of elastase, collagenase and papain on structure and function of rat lung in vitro. J Clin Invest 51: 288

22. Senior RM, Bielefeld DR, Abensohn MK (1975) The effects of proteolytic enzymes on the tensile strength of the human lung. Am Rev Resp Dis 111: 184

23. Martin CJ, Sugihara T (1973) Simulation of tissue properties in irreversible diffuse obstructive pulmonary syndrome: enzyme digestion. J Clin Invest 52: 1918

24. Turino GM, Lourenco RV, McCracken GH (1968) Role of connective tissues in large pulmonary airways. J Appl Physiol 25: 645

25. Snider GL, Sherter CB, Koo KW, Karlinsky JB, Hayes JA, Franzblau C (1977) Respiratory mechanics in hamsters following treatment with endotracheal elastase or collagenase. J Appl Physiol Resp 42: 206

26. Snider GL, Hayes JA, Franzblau C, Kagan HM, Stone PJ, Korthy AL (1974) Relationship between elastolytic activity

and experimental emphysema-inducing properties of papain preparations. Am Rev Resp Dis 110: 254

27. Blackwood CE, Hosannah Y, Perman E, Keller S, Mandl I (1973) Experimental emphysema in rats: elastolytic titer of inducing enzyme as determinant of the response. Proc Soc Exp Biol Med 144: 450

28. Fisk DE, Kuhn C (1976) Emphysema-like changes in the lungs of the blotchy mouse. Am Rev Resp Dis 113: 787

29. Hoffman L, Mondshine RB, Park SS (1971) Effect of DL-penicillamine on elastic properties of rat lung. J Appl Physiol 30: 508

30. Stanley NN, Cherniak NS, Altose MD, Saldana NM, Fishman AP (1972) Effects of beta-aminoproprionitrile on the mechanical properties of rat lung (Abstr) Am Rev Resp Dis 105: 999

31. Kuhn C, Starcher BC (1980) The effect of lathyrogens on the evolution of elastase-induced emphysema. Am Rev Resp Dis 122: 453

32. Fedullo AJ, Lucey EC, Karlinsky JB, Goldstein RH, Snider GL (to be published) Effect of penicillamine on bleomycin pulmonary fibrosis in hamsters. J Appl Physiol

33. Kida K, Thurlbeck WM (to be published) The effects of beta-amino-proprionitrile on the growing rat lung. Am J Pathol

34. Kida K, Thurlbeck WM (1980) Lack of recovery of lung structure and function after the administration of beta-amino-proprionitrile in the postnatal period. Am Rev Resp Dis 122: 467

35. O'Dell BL, Kilburn KH, McKenzie WN, Thurston RJ (1978) The lung of the copper-deficient rat. Am J Pathol 91: 413

36. Wright RR (1961) Elastic tissue of normal and emphysematous lungs: a tridimensional study. Am J Pathol 29: 355

37. Hayes JA, Korthy AL, Snider GL (1975) Pathology of elas-
    tase-induced panacinar emphysema in hamsters. J Pathol
    (London) 117: 1

38. Pierce JA, Hocott JB, Ebert RV (1961) The collagen and
    elastin content of the lung in emphysema. Ann Intern
    Med 55: 210

39. Bruce RM, Adamson JS, Pierce JA (1970) Collagen and elas-
    tin content of the lung in antitrypsin deficiency. Clin
    Res 18: 89A

40. Kuhn C, Yu S, Chraplyvy ML, Lindner HE, Senior RM
    (1976) The induction of emphysema with elastase. II.
    Changes in connective tissue. Lab Invest 34: 372

41. Fitzpatrick M, Hospelhorn VD (1962) Studies of human pul-
    monary connective tissue. I. Amino acid composition of
    elastins isolated by alkaline digestion. J Lab Clin Med
    60: 799

42. Fitzpatrick M (1967) Studies of human pulmonary connec-
    tive tissue. III. Chemical changes in structural pro-
    teins with emphysema. Am Rev Resp Dis 96: 254

43. Fitzpatrick M (1968) Studies of human pulmonary connective
    tissue. IV. Some differences in polypeptides derived
    from elastic protein. Am Rev Resp Dis 97: 248

44. Keller S, Mandl I (1972) Qualitative differences between
    normal and emphysematous human lung elastin. In:
    Mittman C (ed) Pulmonary emphysema and proteolysis.
    Academic Press, New York, p 251

45. Starcher BC, Kuhn C, Overton JE (1978) Increased elastin
    and collagen content of the lungs of hamsters receiving
    an intratracheal injection of bleomycin. Am Rev Resp
    Dis 117: 299

46. Goldstein RH, Lucey EC, Franzblau C, Snider GL (1979)
    Failure of mechanical properties to parallel changes in
    lung connective tissue composition in bleomycin-induced
    pulmonary fibrosis in hamsters. Am Rev Resp Dis 120:
    67

47. Seyer JM, Hutcheson ET, Kang AH (1976) Collagen polymorphism in idiopathic chronic pulmonary fibrosis. J Clin Invest 57: 1498

48. Fulmer JD, Bienkowski RS, Cowan MJ, Breul SD, Bradley KM, Ferrans VJ, Roberts WC, Crystal RG (1980) Collagen concentration and rates of synthesis in idiopathic pulmonary fibrosis. Am Rev Resp Dis 112: 289

49. McCullough B, Collins JF, Johanson WG Jr, Grover FL (1978) Bleomycin-induced diffuse interstitial pulmonary fibrosis in baboons. J Clin Invest 61: 79

50. Zapol WM, Trelstad RL, Coffey JW, Tsai I, Salvador A (1979) Pulmonary fibrosis in severe acute respiratory failure. Am Rev Resp Dis 119: 547

51. Collins JF, Johanson WG Jr, McCullough B, Jones MA, Waugh HJ Jr (1978) Effects of compensatory lung growth in irradiation-induced regional pulmonary fibrosis in the baboon. Am Rev Resp Dis 117: 1079

52. Snider GL, Karlinsky JB (1977) Relation between the elastic behavior and the connective tissues of the lungs. In: Ioachim HL (ed) Pathobiology annual, Vol 7, Appleton-Century-Crofts, New York, pp 115-142

53. Snider GL, Hayes JA, Korthy AL (1978) Chronic interstitial pulmonary fibrosis produced in hamsters by endotracheal bleomycin; pathology and stereology. Am Rev Resp Dis 117: 1099

54. Rinaldo JE, Goldstein RH, Snider GL (1980) The toxicity of oxygen in hamsters with bleomycin-induced interstitial pneumonia. Am Rev Resp Dis (Abstr) 122: 183

55. Fedullo AJ, Jung-Legg Y, Snider GL, Karlinsky JB (1980) Hysteresis ratio: a measure of the mechanical efficiency of fibrotic and emphysematous hamster lung tissue. Am Rev Resp Dis 122: 47

Discussion

Oegema. I have a question about the relation between lung collagen and the mechanical function of the lungs. Have you looked for histological evidence of collagen deposition in focal areas of the lungs and tried to relate this to function?

Snider. Although semiquanitative estimates of the degree of fibrosis have been done, I do not know of anyone who has been successful with morphometric studies. We tried and failed to develop a reproducible morphometric index of fibrosis. Large areas of collagen deposition were readily identified with a Masson trichrome stain, but it was very difficult to be certain that the fine, green fibrillar structures were collagen and even more difficult to develop a sufficiently cheap measurement technique. The sampling problems are just too great. For example, in studies on human lungs (Zapol WM, Trelstad RL, Coffey JW, Tsai I, Salvador A [1979] Pulmonary fibrosis in severe acute respiratory failure. Am Rev Respir Dis 119: 547) (50) of patients dying of acute respiratory failure, the mean of an average of 50 samples per lung was required to overcome the sampling problems. The reason for the sampling problem is that the disease is patchy despite its widespread distribution.

An additional response to your question is in order. One should remember that each measurement serves a useful purpose, but doesn't serve all purposes. I am not sure at the moment whether we should define pulmonary fibrosis by the appearance of fibrillar structures in dye-stained light microscopic preparations of the lungs, or whether we should define fibrosis in terms of a measured increase in total lung collagen. What is quite certain, however, is that a biochemical measurement of total lung collagen will never tell you how the protein is disposed; histological or ultrastructural study is essential for the latter. On the other hand, if you want to know whether you are looking at collapsed lung parenchyma or an excess of collagen, then you must go to biochemical measurements.

Caulfield. You mentioned that the collagen might be distributed something like nylon mesh and that would give it some viscoelastic properties. If you increase the diameter of the collagen fibers, you can increase the amount of collagen tremendously without affecting the elasticity much. If, however, you distort the weave without increasing the amount of collagen, it will affect the viscoelastic properties. Have you seen a weave of sorts in the lung or is this simply a proposition?

Snider. In disease states, the uniform bundles of collagen fibers that I showed you ultrastructurally in the normal lung are not observed. One sees a coarse feltwork of collagen fibers in areas of severe fibrosis. Whether these areas are capable of responding to stretch or whether they are quite silent, masquerading as areas of lost lung volume, is not known. I was thinking of the nylon mesh as an analogy to explain why you can have a very compliant lung at low lung volume despite the abundance of collagen fibers in the lung. Given these noncompliant fibers, one has to explain how the lung can have rubber-like recoil properties in its midvolume. Dr. Rosenquist, would you like to comment?

Rosenquist. I think that rather than a weave, the connective tissue in the lung is organized in helices of fibers. The paper of Orsos (Orsos F [1907] Über das elastische Gerüst der normalen und der emphusematösen Lunge. Beitr Path Anat Allg 41: 95-121) and others since indicate that as the way that the lung distributes the collagen to give it its elastic properties. We have found that the helical arrangement of collagen fibers continues all the way into the intervascular spaces in the alveolar septa.

Lathyrism and the Biochemistry of Elastin

JUDITH ANN FOSTER, CELESTE B. RICH
and ROGERS M. FRED III

Elastic recoil is of paramount importance in the structural integrity and function of large blood vessels and key connective tissue elements of pulmonary tissue. The elasticity of these tissues is due primarily to the presence of elastic fibers. These fibers can be shown both morphologically and chemically to be composed of at least two major proteins. One of the components, elastin, possesses an amorphous appearance in electron micrographs and has a unique amino acid composition consisting of approximately 95% nonpolar amino acids (Ross and Bornstein 1969; Partridge and David 1955). The other major component, the microfibril, displays a fibrillar structure in electron micrographs and possesses an amino acid composition characterized by a high content of polar amino acids and a significant amount of cysteine residues (Ross and Bornstein 1969). Although the microfibrillar component has not yet been chemically well defined, it is possible that this component may represent a single or a family of related glycoproteins (Serafini-Fracassini et al. 1975). The relationship between the two components of elastic fibers is not chemically well understood; however, ultrastructural studies have provided strong evidence that during development of the elastic fibers the microfibril appears first in the extracellular matrix. The insolubilized microfibril is thought to act as a framework

upon which soluble elastin is aligned and subsequently insolubilized (Ross 1971).

This paper will deal exclusively with the elastin component of
elastic fibers.

Physical and Chemical Properties

Elastin, as its name implies, behaves as a rubber–like elasto-
mer. It exhibits rapid extensibility of two or three times its
resting length under tension, with an equally rapid recovery to
the original size when the tension is relieved. This property
imparts to the elastin tissue its characteristic mechanical ability
to sustain repeated reversible deformability without loss of tissue
integrity. Consequently, elastin is distributed primarily in those
organs subjected to continual stress, with the actual distribution
being aorta (30% - 40%), lung (5% - 8%), skin (2% - 5%), and
ligament (78% - 80%) (Partridge 1962). Significantly, the highest
percentage of elastin within the circulatory system is located in
the walls of the aorta and other arteries of large diameter that
are subjected to the immediate effects of systolic stretch and
diastolic recoil.

Morphologically, elastin fibers exhibit significant fluorescence,
a high refactility, a distinct yellow color, a filament-like branching structure, and an easy compliance to stretching (Partridge
1962). Histologically, elastic fibers are stained selectively with
orcein and Weigert's resorcin-fuchsin (Hall et al. 1952). Since
elastin contains very few polar amino acids, dyes with predominantly acidic or basic functions exhibit a low fixation with elastin
while binding strongly with collagen. Thus, the two major protein components of connective tissue can be stained differentially
for histochemical investigations.

Wide-angle X-ray diffraction studies of elastin have thus far
not been able to demonstrate any significant molecular orientation
of the protein fibers (Partridge 1962). Electron micrographs of
the elastic fibers from arteries, tendons, and ligaments revealed

an amorphous appearance with little defined structure (Ross and
Bornstein 1969) and no periodicity such as the 640 Å spacing
exhibited by native collagen fibrils. The ligament fibers appear
to exist as a network of fine, interwoven fibrils about 10 mμ in
diameter (Partridge 1962) shaped into a poorly braided rope with
no free ends or specific orientation.

Isolation and Composition

The most frequently used tissue for the isolation of elastin is
bovine ligamentum nuchae of which the protein comprises up to
78% - 80%. Aortic tissue is also commonly employed, which, even
though it contains a lesser amount of elastin (20% - 30%), it remains an important source because of its significance in cardiovascular investigations.

Since elastin is an extremely insoluble protein, its isolation
and purification necessitate rather drastic conditions to solubilize
and remove all other connective tissue components. Thus, depending upon the tissue source and the information sought, many
different methods are reported that have as their end a homogeneous elastin preparation with a constant amino acid composition.
For example, isolation of elastin from aorta requires that the
tissue be heated with 0.01M NaOH at 98°C for 45 minutes to
remove a closely associated glycoprotein (Lansing et al. 1952).

Regardless of the method used, the resulting elastin preparations show a unique and constant amino acid composition. In
elastin, as in collagen, one-third of the amino acid residues are
glycine and one-ninth of the residues are proline. In contrast
to collagen, elastin contains a high content of the nonpolar amino
acids, valine, leucine, and isoleucine, an increase in the tyrosine
content, very little hydroxyproline (1%), and no hydroxylysine.
Elastin has only a small content of the polar amino acids aspar-
atic acid, glutamic acid, lysine, or arginine. Table 1 gives the
amino acid compositions of chick aortic elastin together with
chick aorta microfibrillar protein.

TABLE 1. Amino Acid Compositions of Elastic Fiber Components[a]

Amino acid	Elastin[b]	Microfibril[c]
Cysteic acid	1	12
Lysine	4	50
Histidine	1	22
Arginine	5	47
Aspartic acid	2	82
Threonine	3	38
Serine	5	72
Glutamic acid	12	119
Proline	128	72
Glycine	352	157
Alanine	176	108
Valine	175	70
Isoleucine	19	42
Leucine	47	70
Tyrosine	12	7
Phenylalanine	23	31
Allysine[d]	6	–
ACP[e]	12	–
Lysinonorleucine	1	–
Isodesmosine	3	–
Desmosine	3	–
Merodesmosine	2	–

[a]Compositions are expressed as residues per 1000 amino acid residues.

[b]From J.A. Foster, R. Shapiro, P. Voynow, G. Crombie, B. Faris and C. Franzblau Biochemistry, 14: 5343 (1975).

[c]Unpublished data.

[d]Allysine, determined as hydroxynorleucine, the reduced derivative.

[e]ACP is the aldol condensation product of two allysine residues determined as the reduced derivative. Crosslinks are expressed as lysine equivalents.

Elastin Crosslinks

Much of the early emphasis in elastin research was directed toward understanding the mechanisms of elastin insolubilization. Partridge et al. (1955), studying the elastin from ligamentum nuchae, showed that this protein could be solubilized by treatment with 0.25N oxalic acid at 100°C for 1-hour periods. Although this procedure is quite drastic, these investigators were able to separate elastin into two fractions designated α-elastin and β-elastin. Fluorodinitrobenzene treatment of these fractions revealed that the α-protein contained approximately 17 chains, while the β-protein possessed 2 chains. The conclusion from this data suggests that elastin contains a significant number of crosslinks.

Solubilization of elastin by enzymatic digestion has permitted some understanding of the nature of the crosslinks. The ultraviolet absorption spectrum of α-elastin exhibits a maximum at 275 mμ, which cannot be explained by the known amount of tyrosine and phenylalanine residues present in elastin. Isolation of the specific peptide responsible for the absorption maximum and subsequent analyses of the peptide led to the discovery of two polyfunctional amino acids containing a pyridine ring alkylated in four positions. Thomas et al. (1963) described these new compounds as desmosine and isodesmosine and suggested that these compounds were involved in elastin crosslinks.

Franzblau et al. (1969), while investigating desmosine- and isodesmosine-enriched peptides of elastin, observed another previously undescribed compound. This polyfunctional compound, characterized and designated lysinonorleucine, was also suggested to exist in a cross-linking capacity.

Reduction studies of ^{14}C-lysine-labeled elastin by Lent el al. (1969) were performed in order to elucidate the biosynthesis of lysinonorleucine. Using ^{14}C-lysine-labeled elastin, reduction was performed with sodium borotritide. Significantly, the alkaline hydrolysates of the reduced elastin revealed a new, prominent

radioactive compound. Mass spectrum, periodate and perman-
ganate oxidation, hydrogenation over palladium, and the calculated specific acitivity suggested that this compound is a reduced
derivative of an aldol condensation product of two residues of
α-aminoadipic acid-δ-semialdehyde. It was reported that there
are 4 to 5 aldol condensations products per thousand residues of
amino acids in elastin and that the aldol condensate may play a
cross-linking role in elastin.

In summary, there have been three unique amino acids isolated from elastin that are thought to function as crosslinks. On
the basis of reported data, elastin isolated from ligamentum
nuchae contains, per 1000 amino acid residues, 1.4, 1.0, 1.15,
and 4 - 5 of desmosine, isodesmosine, lysinonorleucine, and aldol
condensation residues, respectively (Franzblau and Lent 1969).

Biosynthesis of Elastin Crosslinks

The first clue to the origin and formation of the proposed
elastin crosslinks came from the work of Partridge et al. (1963).
These investigators subjected the isolated desmosine and isodesmosine molecules to mild oxidation with alkaline ferricyanide.
The oxidation products resulted in a significant formation of lysine residues, which suggested the involvement of this amino
acid in the eventual synthesis of the desmosine compounds.

Confirmation of this hypothesis was achieved by two independent laboratories working with ^{14}C-lysine-labeled aortae. Miller
et al. (1964) working with ^{14}C-lysine-labeled chick embryo as
well as young and adult chicken aortae showed that the amino
acid composition of elastin samples extracted at increasing time of
development exhibited a decrease in lysine residues with an
accompanying increase in the desmosines. Further, pulse experiments showed a decrease in the specific activity of the ^{14}C-ly-
sine fraction with a concomitant increase of radioactivity in the
desmosine fractions. These results further pointed to the formation of the desmosine compounds via lysine residues bound in
peptides bonds.

Partridge et al. (1966), working with aortae from rats injected with ^{14}C-lysine, showed that in the older specimens (25-day-old rats) the molar specific activity of the desmosine fraction was four times that of the lysine fraction.

The above data suggest that four lysine residues are involved in the formation of the desmosine compounds. Three of the lysine residues appear to be modified by removal of the ε-amino group in a way to permit their combination with an intact lysine residue to form the pyridinium ring.

Information on the common origin of elastin crosslinks was gained by the independent work of Franzblau et al. (1965), who investigated ^{14}C-lysine-labeled aortae of chick embryos. They found that in the maturing aortic tissue, the concentration of lysinonorleucine increased at the same rate as that of the desmosines and that by specific activity measurements, two lysine residues are incorporated into one lysinonorleucine residue. Their results also confirmed the previous data that four lysine residues are involved in the synthesis of the desmosine residues. These investigators (Franblau et al. 1969) also proposed that the biosynthesis of lysinonorleucine proceeds through: 1) oxidative deamination of the ε-amino group of a lysine residue, 2) reaction of this modified lysine residue with another intact lysine to form a Schiff base condensation product, and 3) reduction of the double bond to form the stable crosslink, lysinonorleucine.

Intrinsic to both of the proposed mechanisms for desmosine and lysinonorleucine synthesis is the deamination of one or more lysine residues to form α-aminoadipic acid-δ-semialdehyde (referred to as allysine). Both Miller and Fullmer (1966) and Lent et al. (1969) have independently demonstrated the existence of allysine in elastin.

The key step in elastin crosslink formation is the initial oxidation of lysyl residues catalyzed by the enzyme lysyl oxidase (Pinnell and Martin 1968; Harris et al. 1974). An overall scheme for the formation of elastin crosslinks is given in Figure I.

It should be pointed out at this time that several of the ly-

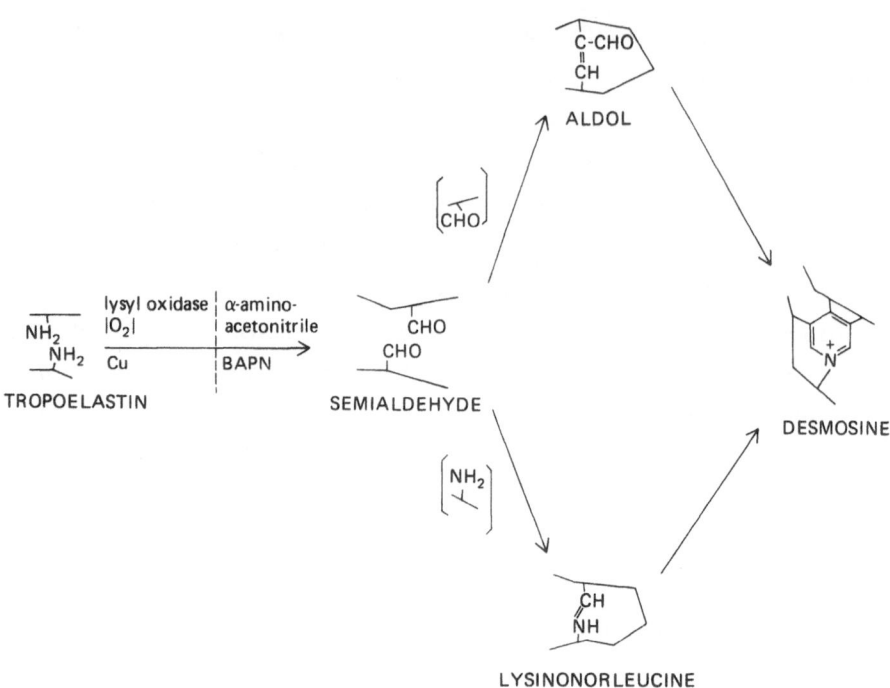

FIG. 1. Scheme for formation of elastin crosslinks.

sine-derived crosslinks described above are also found in another connective tissue protein, collagen. However, in the various genetically different types of collagen thus far described,
varying percentages of lysyl residues are hydroxylated. Consequently, collagen crosslinkage includes participation of modified
residues as well as unmodified residues such as are present in
elastin. Further, the desmosines are unique to elastin whereas
the involvement of histidine residues together with modified lysine residues is unique to collagen (Tanzer et al. 1973).

Several laboratories have been engaged in examining the area
surrounding elastin crosslinkages through the isolation and characterization of elastin crosslinked peptides. It should be pointed
out that this type of study is complicated by the fact that the
generation of elastin peptides must be accomplished by nonspeci-

fic agents. Elastin is not susceptible to specific enzymes such
as trypsin or chemical agents such as cyanogen bromide. Hence,
one is reduced to using general proteases such as elastase, sub-
tilisin, and thermolysin to solubilize elastin. The resulting peptide mixture is quite similar in size, contains little distinct
charge between individual peptides upon which to base ionic
separations, and contains great amounts of overlapping peptides.
For these reasons, primary sequence data on insoluble elastin
has progressed very slowly relative to information obtained on
soluble elastin.

Partridge (1962) and Franzblau et al. (1965) independently
demonstrated that the immediate environment of the desmosine
and lysinonorleucine crosslinks was greatly enriched in alanine.
Foster et al. (1973) found the same alanine clustering in the
area of the aldol condensate crosslink. Direct sequencing of
purified desmosine peptides by Gerber and Anwar (1975) and
Foster et al. (1974) have demonstrated polyalanine type sequences in the immediate vicinity of the desmosine crosslink.

Gerber and Anwar (1975) further reported that the desmosine
peptides fall into two broad categories based on the amino acid
residue C-terminal to the desmosine crosslink. One of these
groups possesses a hydrophobic group (phenylalanine, tyrosine,
or leucine) while the other possesses alanine as the NH_2-terminal.
Because of this distinction, it was proposed that the hydrophobic
amino acid residues prevent the oxidative deamination of the adjacent lysine ε-amino group, which contributes its nitrogen to
the pyridinium ring of the desmosine. Also of interest, these
investigators have suggested that tyrosine residues, which are
found in high concentration adjacent to lysyl residues in porcine
elastin, are substituted for by phenylalanine residues in bovine
elastin. At approximately the same time the above study was
reported, Foster et al. (1974) published data on the primary
sequence and conformation of desmosine cross-linked peptides
isolated from bovine ligamentum nuchae. The purified desmosine
peptides revealed several unique features in their amino acid

compositions. On a molar basis each of the peptides contained 1 serine, 1 glutamic acid, 1 tyrosine, and 2 - 3 residues of phenylalanine per peptide. The combined amount of the above-mentioned amino acid residues in the total ligament elastin is only 6% - 7%, which would suggest some clustering of these residues within the area of the desmosine crosslink. Evidence for the association of tyrosine, glutamic acid, and phenylalanine within the sites destined for elastin crosslinks is seen in the soluble elastin precursor.

The purified desmosine peptides were sequenced on an automated Beckman Sequencer directly. The actual interpretation of the sequencing data obtained was complicated by the fact that more than one peptide was sequenced simultaneously because the peptide is crosslinked. Results from this study indicated that the desmosines crosslink two chains based on: 1) micromoles of NH_2-terminal amino acids recovered per micromole of desmosine contained in the peptide; and 2) the finding of two peptide sequences comparable to those obtained from the soluble elastin precursor.

Lathyrism

Since the insolubilization of elastin is absolutely dependent upon crosslink formation, lysyl oxidase action is the key step in deposition of functional elastic fibers. Any loss or inhibition of lysyl oxidase may well have disasterous effects on the structure and functionality of elastin. There are two experimental conditions, copper deficiency and lathyrism, in which lysyl oxidase activity can be inhibited both in vivo and in vitro. Lysyl oxidase is a copper metallo-protein (Siegel et al. 1970) and hence requires copper for activity. By restricting copper from the diet of a young developing animal, a copper-deficient state can be maintained that results in significant inhibition of the crosslinking enzyme, lysyl oxidase. Primarily due to the efforts of Sandberg et al. (1969), a soluble, non-crosslinked elastin was isolated from the aortae of piglets maintained on a copper-deficient diet. Although not 100% effective, copper deficiency does allow for the accumulation of significant amounts of soluble elastin. The physiologic consequences of copper deficiency to the animal is fatal since major blood vessels are tremendously weakened and aneurysms are quite common.

Another situation in which the crosslinking of elastin is inhibited involves the state of lathyrism. The term lathyrism derives from a disease associated with the ingestion of certain types of sweet pea originating from the genus Lathyrus odoratus (Geiger et al. 1933). In brief, the active agent in the peas is β-aminopropionitrile (BAPN) (Bachhuber et al. 1955), which was found to be a competitive inhibitor of the enzyme lysyl oxidase (Narayanan et al. 1972). Lathyrism is now commonly referred to as a state in which an animal has been fed a lathyrogen (BAPN) to inhibit lysyl oxidase, therefore resulting in the accumulation of soluble forms of elastin as well as soluble forms of collagen.

Our laboratory has been especially interested in the use of lathyrogens for the isolation of the soluble, precursor forms of elastin. For this reason we have gained much experience in the use of lathyrogens and have thus been able to optimize conditions for lysyl oxidase inhibition and soluble elastin isolation (Foster et al. 1979, 1980a).

In order to isolate soluble elastin from chicks we normally maintain 1-day-old chicks on a diet supplemented with 0.1% BAPN (wt/wt). Recently, we have discovered that the extent of lathyrism produced and the yields of tropoelastin obtained varied depending on the quantity of fumarate present in the commercially bought BAPN preparations. The differences seen are not attributable purely to the actual amount of BAPN in the diet. If we use BAPN-fumarate purchased from Sigma wherein the ratio is 1:2 (BAPN to fumarate), the chicks become lathyritic; however, the fatality rate is greater than 10% and the recovery of tropoelastin is very poor (4 mg/100 g aortae). Increasing the BAPN to 0.2% results in a higher fatality rate but the same yield of tropoelastin. If we use BAPN-fumarate purchased from Aldrich (1:1 ratio) the recovery of tropoelastin increases (40 mg/100 g aortae) however the fatality rate remains approximately 10%. All of the reports concerning the use of BAPN-fumarate that we were able to find in the literature are based on weight rather than moles.

Because preparations of BAPN and fumarate are variable, depending upon which commercial source used, we decided to explore the possibility that either BAPN and/or fumarate may have biologically important actions distinct from crosslink inhibition. In light of the fact that soluble elastin is very susceptible to proteolytic degradation, we decided to test the effect of BAPN and fumarate on proteolytic enzymes. Since BAPN does resemble a lysine residue, trypsin and the enzyme associated with tropoelastin were examined. In summary, our results showed that at low concentrations of BAPN-fumarate and fumarate, tryptic activity was slightly stimulated. At concentrations above 0.01M, BAPN-fumarate was inhibitory.

In order to examine the tryptic inhibition by BAPN-fumarate, a Lineweaver Burke plot was constructed using 0.1M BAPN-fumarate and azo-casein as substrate. The results demonstrated that BAPN-fumarate acts as a competitive inhibitor. Similar results were obtained on the tropoelastin associated enzyme using (^{3}H) valine-labeled tropoelastin as a substrate. In order to examine each of the compounds separately, the tropoelastin enzyme was assayed in the presence of BAPN by itself, BAPN-fumarate, fumarate by itself, and ε-aminocaproic acid. BAPN, BAPN-fumarate, and ε-aminocaproic acid were inhibitory whereas fumarate maintained a slightly enhanced activity at concentration up to 0.1M. This latter effect was not due to a pH change since the stock solution of fumarate was adjusted to pH 8.0 prior to addition to the assay mixture.

The data obtained from these studies is interesting, especially as regards the inhibitory action of BAPN. How significant the stimulatory action of fumarate is in vivo or in vitro is not known.

As an extension of these studies, we have induced lathyrism in chicks on a diet of 0.1% α-aminoacetonitrile-HCl. This compound is one carbon less than BAPN and contains no fumarate. Within 5 days the chicks developed lathyrism; however, the fatality rate was less than 1%. The yield of purified tropoelastin from the aorta of these chicks was approximately 65 mg/100 g of tissue (wet weight). The yield of tropoelastin from lung tissue, however, was not improved. We have found further that if the chicks are maintained on a normal diet for 1 week prior to the administration of the lathyrogen, the yield of soluble elastin is even greater (Foster et al. 1980a).

Figures 2 - 5 illustrate the histologic and electron microscopic consequences of lathyrism on the thoracic aortae of chicks maintained on a diet of α-aminoacetonitrile-HCl.

Soluble Elastin

A major advance in elastin research came with the isolation of an elastin-like, soluble component from the aortae of copper-deficient swine (Sandberg et al. 1969). Further purification and characterization of this soluble protein have led to the proposal that it is indeed the precursor to insoluble elastin, and accordingly, it has been designated tropoelastin (Sandberg et al. 1969). Soluble elastin, as well as the mature insoluble elastin, is rich in glycine (33%) and the nonpolar amino acids alanine, valine, and proline. It differs from the insoluble protein in its high content of lysine residues and lack of any crosslinks (see Table 1).

Recently, Sandberg et al. (1971) have reported a strong clustering of alanine and lysine residues in the soluble protein, as evidenced by the structures of small tryptic peptides and of the carboxy-terminal fragments of the large tryptic peptides. This clustering of alanine near the lysine residues of the molecule is in agreement with the isolation of alanine-enriched, crosslinked peptides from mature elastin. Through the characterization of large tryptic peptides, Foster et al. (1973) have recently been

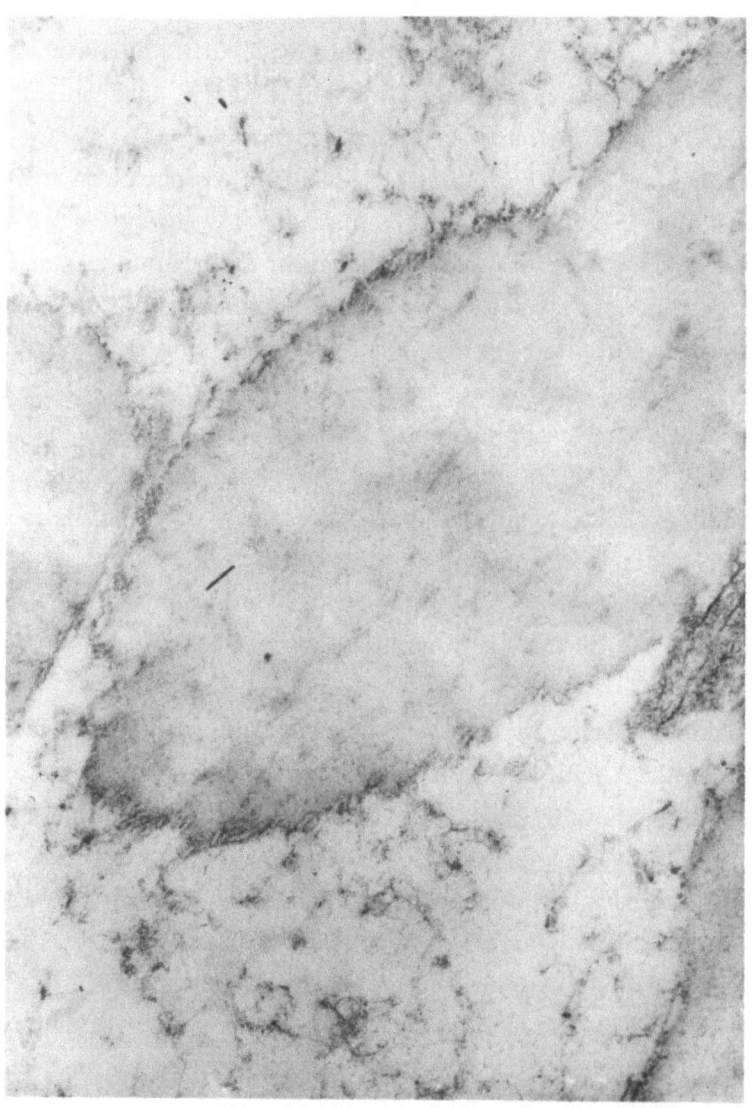

FIG. 2. Day-7 chick aorta, control. Elastic fiber composed of a peripheral layer of short, dense microfibrils investing an amorphous, relatively electron lucent material (elastin). Uranyl acetate - lead citrate stain. X 48,000

able to sequence over 400 residues that correspond to approximately half of the residues present in the tropoelastin molecule.

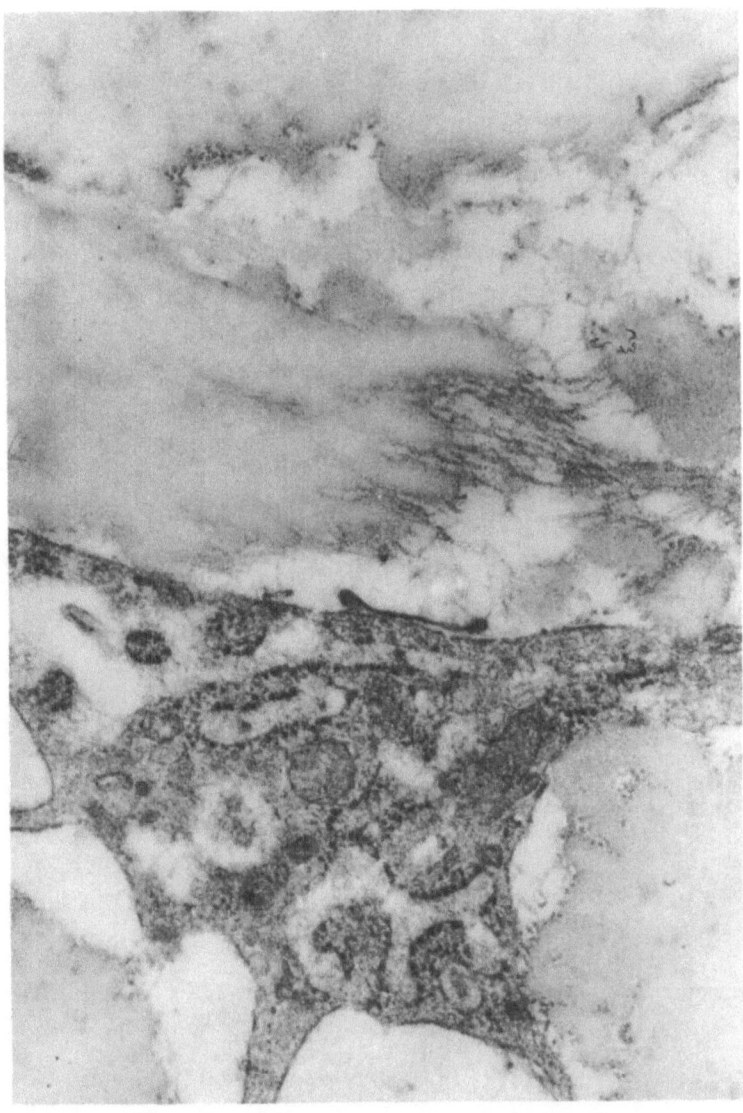

FIG. 3.   Day-8 chick aorta, lathyritic.   Elastic fiber with irregular, indented border at end and microfibrils protruding from indentations.   Note microfibrils sectioned transversely and cell process with dilated rough endoplasmic reticulum filled with amorphous material.   Uranyl acetate - lead citrate stain.   X 51,000

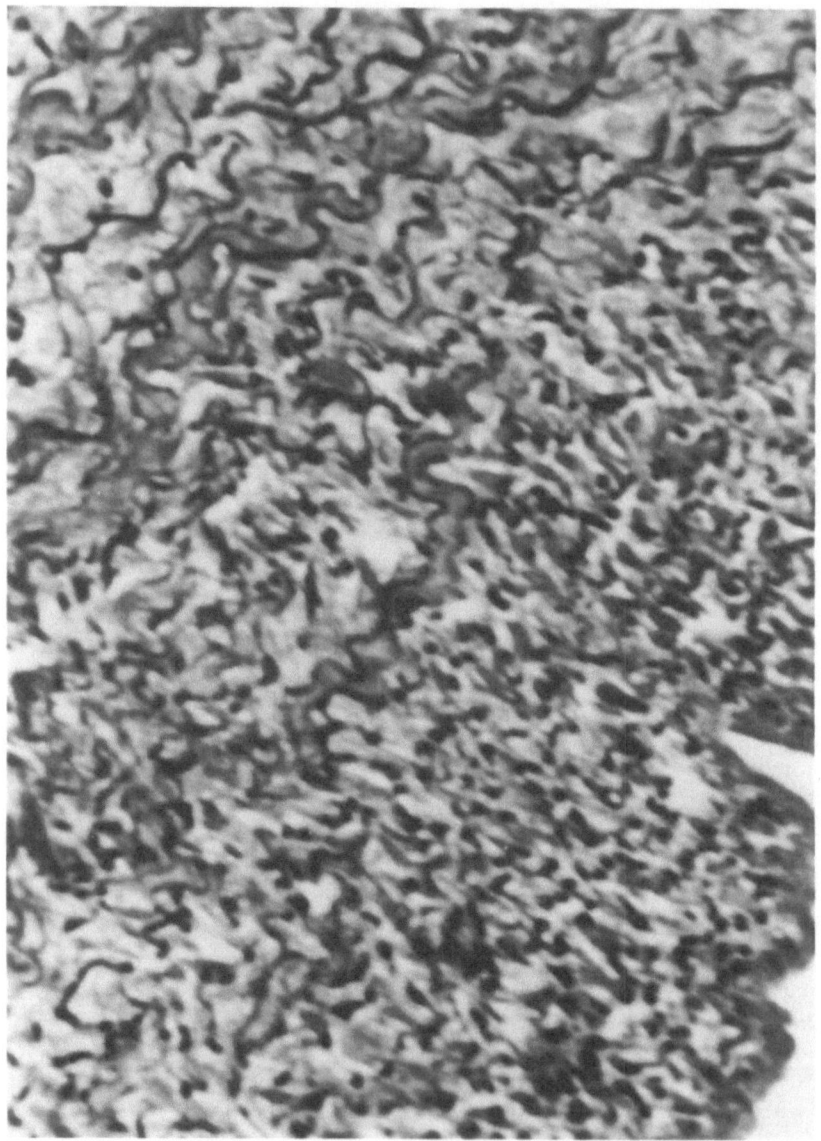

FIG. 4. Day-8 normal chick aorta, intima, and media. Flattened
endothelial cells with elastic fibers oriented obliquely to the plane
of section or parallel to long axis of the vessel comprise the intimal layer. Note appearance of longer, circumferentially arranged
elastic fibers bordering surface of smooth muscle cells in the in-
nermost third of the medial layer. Verhoeff stain. X 320

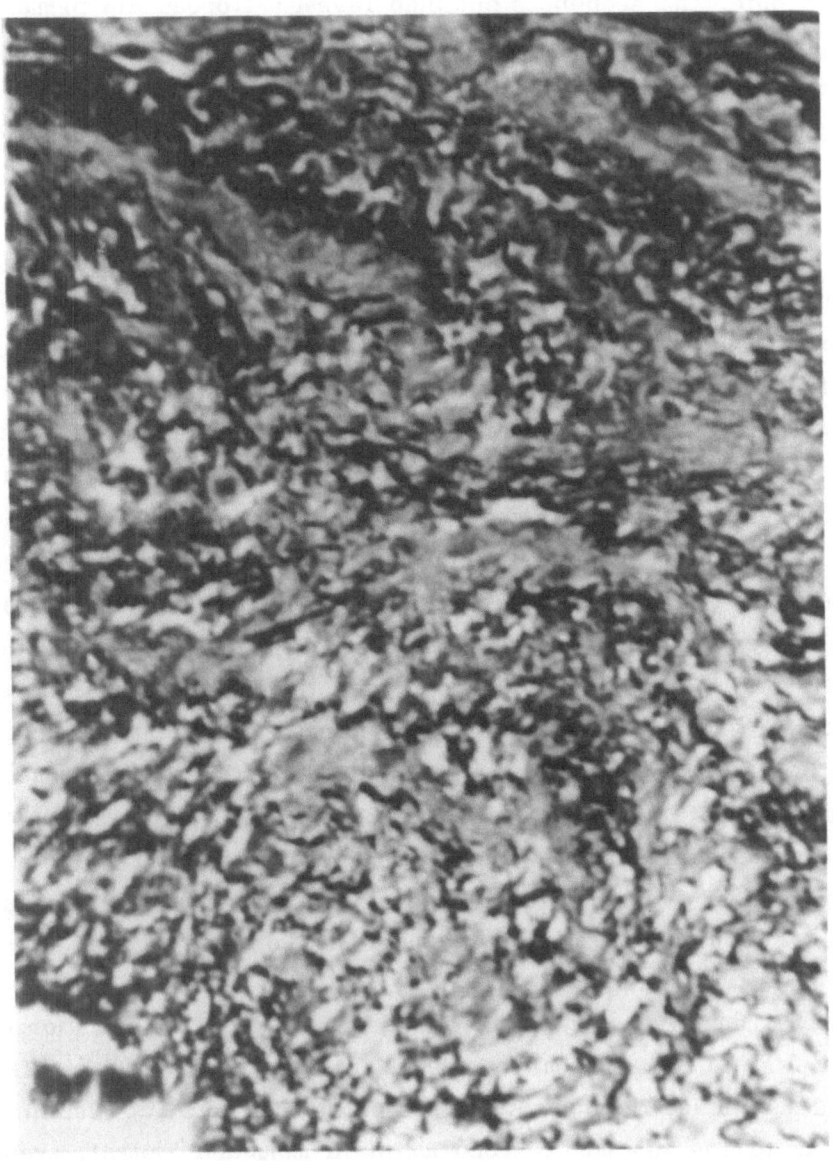

FIG. 5. Day-8 lathyritic chick aorta, intima, and media. Note swollen endothelial cells detached from subendothelial elastin fibers and generalized disorganization of vessel wall. Verhoeff stain. X 320

To date, the sequences obtained reveal a tropoelastin primary structure quite distinct from that of tropocollagen. Tropoelastin possesses repeated units of a tetrapeptide, Gly-Gly-Val-Pro, a pentapeptide, Pro-Gly-Val-Gly-Val, and a hexapeptide, Pro-Gly-Val-Gly-Val-Ala. In addition, alanine residues are close to the lysyl residues of elastin. Several of the peptides contain a partial substitution of hydroxyproline for proline, especially in the sequences Gly-Leu-Pro-Gly and Gly-Ile-Pro-Gly. Since the sequences of these peptides resemble those of other tropoelastin peptides and also lack glycine in every third position (contrary to collagen), we feel that this is definitive evidence for the existence of hydroxyproline in elastin. The combined data of the sequences from soluble elastin have led to a model of elastin which resembles a huge extension of coiled springs with the desmosines located in alanine-rich areas (Gray et al. 1973).

Sykes and Partridge (1974), Rucker et al. (1975), and Foster et al. (1975) have reported on the isolation of tropoelastin from chick aorta. The chick tropoelastin possesses the same molecular weight (70,000) as the pig aortic tropoelastin. The primary structure of the NH_2-terminal region of chick tropoelastin is homologous to that of the pig tropoelastin, with the exception of glycine inserted in residue 11 and several conservative substitutions attributable to one base change in the coding triplet (Foster et al. 1975; Rucker et al. 1975).

More recently our laboratory has reported on the isolation of tropoelastin from pig ear cartilage (Foster et al. 1980b). The results obtained demonstrate that the pig cartilage tropoelastin is similar to the pig aortic tropoelastin in molecular weight, amino acid composition, immunologic determinants, and primary structure as examined by limited trypsin proteolysis. The only differences which were found between the aortic and cartilage tropoelastins were the content of hydroxyproline and lysine residues. Both of these differences are associated with post-translational events and can not be ascribed to genetic differences.

Elastin Biosynthesis

Investigations into the biosynthesis of elastin have centered primarily on the identification of tropoelastin in aortic organ cultures (Murphy et al. 1972; Rucker et al. 1975), aortic cell suspensions (Uitto et al. 1976; Rosenbloom and Cywinski 1976), and smooth muscle cell cultures (Abraham et al. 1974; Narayanan et al. 1976). The majority of the data thus far accumulated suggest that elastin is synthesized first as a 68,000 - 75,000 dalton protein which is secreted into the extracellular matrix and rapidly incorporated into insoluble elastin fibers via lysine-derived crosslinks (Siegel et al. 1970). More recently, we have reported on the isolation of a high-molecular-weight protein from lathyritic chick aortae, which was shown to be both chemically and immunologically related to tropoelastin (Foster et al. 1976). The finding of a similar, large elastin-like protein was confirmed in cultures of rabbit aortic smooth muscle cells (Foster et al. 1978). These observations led us to hypothesize that the high-molecular-weight protein was the primary gene product and a precursor to tropoelastin. Since that time, Rucker et al. (1977) have confirmed the presence of high-molecular-weight elastin-like protein in chick embryonic aorta organ cultures and copper-deficient chick aortae. These authors further point out that the putative proelastin is very labile and its demonstration necessitates short-term pulse experiments and the presence of significant amounts of proteolytic inhibitors.

The main question concerning the synthesis of elastin has been the size of the primary elastin gene product. Ryhanen et al. (1978) identified tropoelastin as a 70,000 dalton protein synthesized in vitro by chick aortic polysomes. Burnett and Rosenbloom (1979), in the translation of chick aortic mRNA, also found a 70,000 dalton protein identified as tropoelastin by immunoprecipitation with antisera prepared against chick insoluble elastin. Foster et al. (1980b), examining cell-free translations of chick aortic mRNA and chick embryonic aortic organ cultures, have found two distinct proteins of molecular weight 70,000 and 73,000 shown to be elastin by isotope incorporation, immunoprecipitation, collagenase and cyanogen bromide sensitivity, and 2-dimensional gel electrophoresis. The 70,000 dalton protein, due to its behavior on sodium dodecyl sulfate gel electrophoresis and N-terminal sequence data, is believed to be authentic tropoelastin. The 73,000 dalton protein was seen in organ culture only if extracted with urea in the presence of reducing and alkylating agents. In addition to the molecular weight difference, the two have been shown to have different primary structure, cysteine content, and isoelectric points, indicating that they are products of separate genes. Recently, in the translation of sheep lung and nuchal ligament mRNA, Shibahara et al. (1980) have found a doublet 1×10^3 to 2×10^3 daltons larger than tropoelastin.

There is now general agreement that there are two forms of soluble elastin, the 73,000 dalton species (a) and the 70,000 dalton species (b). However, the ratios of the two and how they differ with development are unresolved questions. We have recently undertaken a study on the ratio of tropoelastin a to b during embryonic development of chick lungs and aortae. The most important outcome of this study has been the finding that the ratios of the two tropoelastin polypeptides differ with development as well as with tissue. Specifically, in embryonic lung tissue the ratio of the two tropoelastins remains essentially constant throughout development, showing 50% of each tropoelastin form. However in the aorta the ratio of tropoelastin b to a increases dramatically. In the 14-day embryo the total tropoelastin content is approximately 70% tropoelastin b. This ratio increases to 86% tropoelastin b in the 17-day embryo and maintains this proportion until hatching. It is especially important that the proportions of tropoelastin a and b are essentially identical both in the cell-free and organ culture systems. This suggests that regulation of gene expression of the two tropoelastins is due to transcriptional rather than translational control.

The fact that the ratios of the two elastin polypeptides are unique to specific tissues suggests a differential expression of the elastin genes, implying separate regulatory mechanisms. The differences in amount of the two species of elastin is not unique to the elastin system. A similar occurrence has been found in chick gizzard actin during development, wherein Saboria et al. (1979) have found conspicuous changes in the content of the iso forms of actin with development.

Elastin and Disease

The biologic distribution of elastin in the mammalian system is such that the highest concentration is found in those tissues which are subjected to continual physical deformation, tension, and high pressure differentials. Because of the intrinsic "elastic" nature of elastin, its presence in a tissue imparts a stretchability and subsequent recoil that is dependent only on the application of some physical force. Its elastic behavior is independent of extrinsic stimuli such as hormones or O_2 tension, rendering elastin devoid of any environmental controls, as is the case with muscle protein. Because of this unique physical property, elastin plays a major role in the structural integrity and function of large blood vessels and the pulmonary aveolar wall. The high concentration of elastin in these vital connective tissues makes this protein a likely candidate for some involvement in functional changes which accompany the process of aging and pulmonary and cardiovascular disease states. Evidence from the literature is strongly supportive of this involvement.

The large elastic arteries of the cardiovascular system are adapted to receive and transmit the pulsatile output of the left ventricle by virtue of possessing a relatively large amount of elastic tissue. In the media of large arteries, significant amounts of elastic tissue are arranged as thick, fenestrated concentric cylinders of elastin (Kadar 1979). The most prominent of these rings is the internal elastic lamella that marks the boundary between the intima and media of the vessel. A hallmark of the structural changes that occur in the normal aging process and the development of degenerative arteriopathies is reflected in the changes in the elastic fibers of the arteries. These changes include calcification and fragmentation of elastic fibers and often the concomitant deposition of lipid material. All of these events, whether occurring singularly or in unison, result in a loss of elasticity, a property essential for maintenance of normal intra-arterial pressure. Although it is not intended to suggest that elastin abnormalities are the causative factors in the pathogenesis of aging or disease, their involvement and contribution to the eventual malfunction of large arteries has been well established.

A number of investigations have been directed at studying the involvement of elastin in aging and the arterio- and athero-sclerotic processes. Partridge and Keeley (1974) have studied age- and atherosclerotic-related changes in human aortic elas-tin. They found that the amino acid composition of insoluble elastin contains a higher proportion of polar acids in the area of plaque formation of the diseased tissues. Kramsch et al. (1974) have also found this change in the composition of elastin when examining the aortic tissue of rabbits maintained on an athero-genic diet. John and Thomas (1972) in addition to examining the amino acid composition of elastin from aged aortic tissue also quantitated crosslinks. Their data demonstrate that elastin iso-lated from aged individuals contains less desmosine than elastin isolated from younger individuals. However, this type of data should be interpreted with some degree of caution since the elas-tin isolated from aged tissue contains polar contaminants. Hence what can be positively ascribed to loss of the desmosines versus dilution of the desmosine is not certain.

Other investigators have confirmed the changes in the elastin and have also reported on a high degree of calcification (Urry 1974) and fragmentation (Kadar 1979) of elastic fibers in diseased aortic tissue. It is interesting to note that the fragmentation of elastin in diseased tissue, identified both morphologically and chemically, has suggested the possible involvement of elastolytic enzymes in the degradation of elastic fibers. In this regard it has been demonstrated that both Ca^{++} (Hall 1970) and anionic fatty acids (Kagan et al. 1972) stimulate the digestion of insoluble elastin by pancreatic elastase. Hence, potentially, the factors found in arteriosclerosis (Ca^{++}) and atherosclerosis (lipid, Ca^{++}) do present a milieu for enhanced proteolytic attack of elastic fibers.

The studies described above regarding the chemical nature of elastin involvement in aging and arterial disease are very limited in their description of the actual events resulting in the loss of tissue elasticity. Techniques available to characterize insoluble elastin are insensitive to subtle molecular events that occur presumably over a long period of time prior to the drastic fragmentation and loss of elastic fibers. Data describing the change that occurs in elastin amino acid composition and the increase in NH_2-terminal amino acids found in diseased tissue offers no insight into the mechanism of such changes. Although it has been demonstrated by some investigators that elastin synthesis is increased in experimental animals fed atherogenic diets (Kramsch et al. 1971), little to nothing is known concerning the fate of the newly synthesized elastin except that "normal" functional elastin does not appear to be laid down in the diseased tissues. This appears to be a key factor in the loss of tissue elasticity since the inability to repair damaged elastin is a central event in the transition of an elastic, healthy artery to a hardened, diseased artery. If the mechanisms underlying this transition are to be elucidated, an understanding of the normal elastic structure and metabolism must be known.

Acknowledgment

The authors acknowledge the financial support of the National Institutes of Health Grant HL 22208 and Council for Tobacco Research 1179.

REFERENCES

Abraham PA, Smith DW, Carnes WH (1974) Synthesis of soluble elastin by aortic medial cells in culture. Biochem Biophys Res Commun 58: 597

Bachhuber TE, Lalich JJ, Angevine DM, Schilling ED, Strong FM (1955) Lathyrus factor activity of beta-aminopropionitrile and related compounds. Proc Soc Exp Biol Med 89: 294

Burnett W, Rosenbloom J (1979) Isolation and translation of elastin mRNA from chick aorta. Biochem Biophys Res Commun 86: 478

Foster JA, Bruenger E, Gray WR, Sandberg SB (1972) Isolation and amino acid sequences of tropoelastin peptides. J Biol Chem 248: 2876

Foster JA, Gray WR, Franzblau C (1973) Isolation and characterization of crosslinked peptides from elastin. Biochim Biophys Acta 303: 363-369

Foster JA, Mecham RP, Franzblau C (1976) A high molecular weight species of soluble elastin. Biochem Biophys Res Commun 72: 1399

Foster JA, Mecham RP, Rich CB, Cronin MF, Levine A, Imberman M, Salcedo LL (1978) Proelastin. J Biol Chem 253: 2797

Foster JA, Rich CB, Berglund N, Huber S, Mecham RP, Lange G (1979) The anti-proteolytic behavior or lathyrogens. Biochim Biophys Acta 587: 477

Foster JA, Rich CB, DeSa MD, Jackson AS, Fletcher S (1980a) Improved methodologies for the isolation and purification of tropoelastin. Anal Biochem (in press)

Foster JA, Rich CB, DeSa MD (1980b) Comparison of aortic and ear cartilage tropoelastins isolated from lathyritic pigs. Biochim Biophys Acta (in press)

Foster JA, Rubin L, Kagan H, Franzblau CB, Luenger E, Sandberg LB (1974) Isolation and characterization of elastin crosslinked peptides. J Biol Chem 249: 6191

Foster JA, Shapiro R, Voynow P, Faris B, Crombie G, Franzblau C (1975) Isolation of soluble elastin from lathyritic chicks. Comparison to tropoelastin from copper-deficient pigs. Biochemistry 14: 5343

Franzblau C, Faris B, Papaioannoy R (1969) Lysinonorleucine. A new amino acid from hydrolysates of elastin. Biochemistry 8: 2833-2837

Franzblau C, Lent RW (1969) Studies on the chemistry of elastin structure, function and evolution in proteins. Brookhaven Sympos Biol 21: 358-377

Franzblau C, Sinex FM, Faris B, Lampidis R (1965) Identification of a new crosslinking amino acid in elastin. Biochem Biophys Res Commun 21: 575-581

Geiger BJ, Steenback H, Persons H (1933) Lathyrism in the rat. J Nutr 6: 427

Gerber GE, Anwar RA (1975) Comparative studies of the crosslinked regions of elastin from bovine ligamentum nuchae and bovine, porcine and human aorta. Biochem J 149: 685-695

Gray WR, Sandberg SB, Foster JA (1973) Molecular model for elastin structure and function. Nature 246: 461

Hall DA (1970) Coordinately bound calcium as a crosslinking agent in elastin and as an activator of elastolysis. Gerontologia 16: 326

Hall DA, Reed R, Tunbridge RE (1952) Structure of elastic tissue. Nature 170: 264

Harris ED, Gonnerman WA, Savage JE, O'Dell BL (1974) Amine oxidases in aorta. II Purification and partial characterization of lysyl oxidase in chick aorta. Biochim Biophys Acta 341: 322-344

John R, Thomas J (1972) Chemical compositions of elastins isolated from aortas and pulmonary tissues of humans of different ages. Biochem J 127: 261

Kadar A (1979) The elastic fiber. Normal and pathological conditions in the arteries. In: Experimental Pathology Suppl 5. VEB Gustav Fischer Verlag

Kagan HM, Crombie GD, Jordan RE, Lewis W, Franzblau C (1972) Proteolysis of elastin-ligand complexes. Stimulation of elastase digestion of insoluble elastin by sodium dodecyl sulfate. Biochemistry 11: 3412

Kramsch DM, Franzblau C, Hollander W (1971) The protein and lipid composition of arterial elastin and its relationship to lipid accumulation in the atherosclerotic plaque. J Clin Invest 50: 1666

Kramsch DM, Franzblau C, Hollander W (1974) Components of the protein-lipid complex of arterial elastin: their role in the retention of lipid in atherosclerotic lesions. Adv Exp Med Biol 43: 193

Lansing AI, Rosenthal TB, Alex M, Dempsey EW (1952) The structure and chemical characterization of elastic fibers as revealed by elastase and by electron microscopy. Anat Rec 114: 555–575

Lent RW, Smith B, Salcedo LL, Faris B, Franzblau C (1969) Studies on the reduction of elastin. II Evidence for the presence of α-aminoadipic acid δ-semialdehyde and its aldol condensation product. Biochemistry 8: 2837–2845

Miller EJ, Fullmer HM (1966) Elastin: diminished reactivity with aldehyde reagents in copper deficiency and lathyrism. J Exp Med 123: 1097–1106

Miller EJ, Martin GR, Piez KA (1964) The utilization of lysine in the biosynthesis of elastin cross-links. Biochem Biophys Res Commun 17: 248–253

Murphy S, Harsch M, Mori T, Rosenbloom J (1972) Identification of a soluble intermediate during synthesis of elastin by embryonic chick aortae. FEBS Lett 21: 113

Narayanan AS, Sandberg SB, Ross R, Layman DL (1976) The smooth muscle cell. Elastin synthesis in arterial smooth muscle cell culture. J Cell Biol 68: 411

Narayanan AS, Siegel RC, Martin GR (1972) On the inhibition of lysyl oxidase by β-aminopropionitrile. Biochem Biophys Res Commun 46: 745

Partridge SM (1962) Elastin. Advanc Protein Chem 17: 227–302

Partridge SM, David HF, Adair GS (1955) The chemistry of connective tissues. Two soluble proteins derived from partial hydrolysis of elastin. Biochem J 61: 21

Partridge SM, Elsden DF, Thomas J (1963) Constitution of the cross-linkages in elastin. Nature 197: 1297–1298.

Partridge SM, Elsden DF, Thomas J, Dorfman A, Telser A, Ho PL (1966) Incorporation of labelled lysine into the desmosine cross-bridges in elastin. Nature 209: 399–400

Partridge SM, Keeley FM (1974) Age related and atherosclerotic changes in aortic elastin. Adv Exp Med Biol 43: 173

Pinnell SR, Martin GR (1968) The crosslinking of collagen and elastin: enzymatic conversion of lysine in peptide linkage to α-aminoadipic-δ-semialdehyde. Proc Natl Acad Sci 61: 708

Rosenbloom J, Cywinski A (1976) Biosynthesis and secretion of tropoelastin by chick aorta cells. Biochem Biophys Res Commun 69: 613

Ross R (1971) The smooth muscle cell. II Growth of smooth muscle in culture and formation of elastic fibers. J Cell Biol 50: 172–186

Ross R, Bornstein P (1969) The elastic fiber. I The separation and partial characterization of its macromolecular components. J Cell Biol 40: 366–381

Rucker RB, Murray J, Lefevre M, Lee J (1977) Putative forms of soluble elastin and their relationship to the synthesis of fibrous elastin. Biochem Biophys Res Commun 75: 358

Rucker RB, Tom K, Tanaka M, Haniu M, Yasunobu KT (1975) Chick tropoelastin isolation and partial chemical characterization. Biochem Biophys Res Commun 66: 287

Ryhanen L, Graves PN, Bressan GM, Prockop DJ (1978) Synthesis of an elastin component of molecular weight about 70,000 by polysomes from chick embryo aortas. Arch Biochem Biophys 185: 344

Saboria JL, Segura M, Flores M, Garcia R, Palmer E (1979) Differential expression of gizzard actin genes during chick embryogenesis. J Biol Chem 254: 1119

Sandberg LB, Weissman N, Gray WR (1971) Structural features of tropoelastin related to the sites of crosslinks in aortic elastin. Biochemistry 10: 52

Sandberg LB, Weissman N, Smith DW (1969) The purification and partial characterization of a soluble elastin-like protein from copper-deficient porcine aorta. Biochemistry 8: 2940

Serafini-Fracassini A, Field JM, Armitt C (1975) Characterization of the microfibrillar component of bovine ligamentum nuchae. Biochem Biophys Res Commun 65: 1146-1152

Shibahara S, Davidson J, Smith K, Boyd C, Tolstoshev P, Crystal R (1980) Modulation of elastin mRNA levels in developing sheep lung and nuchal ligament. Fed Proc 36: 989

Siegel RC, Pinnell SR, Martin GR (1970) Crosslinking of collagen and elastin. Properties of lysyl oxidase. Biochemistry 9: 4486.

Sykes BC, Partridge SM (1974) Salt-soluble elastin from lathyritic chicks. Biochem J 141: 567

Tanzer ML, Housley T, Berube L, Fairweather R, Franzblau C, Gallop PM (1973) Structure of two histidine-containing crosslinks from collagen. J Biol Chem 248: 393

Thomas J, Elsden DF, Partridge SM (1963) Degradation products from elastin. Nature 200: 651-652

Uitto J, Hoffmann H, Prockop DJ (1976) Synthesis of elastin and procollagen by cells from embryonic aorta. Arch Biochem Biophys 173: 187

Urry DW (1974) Arterial mesenchyma and arteriosclerosis interaction of elastin. Adv Exp Med Biol 43: 211

Discussion

Rosenquist. In the morning sessions we were clearly told that glycosaminoglycans and collagen in different areas of the body and of different types have functions other than those classically given for them, for example, strength in the case of collagen. I heard recently some information about a sudden increase in elastic connective tissue in kidneys that are being rejected immunologically (transplanted kidney). This doesn't seem to have anything to do with what we know about the function of elastin. Could you comment on whether or not you feel that elastin in different areas or of different kinds has different functions from what we are usually given to believe is its only function, that is, stretching?

Foster. I think the function of elastic fibers is universal, that is, elasticity. However, elastic fibers may interact with different components of the extracellular matrix and may be orientated differently, depending on how that elasticity functions in a particular tissue. If we are dealing with aortic tissue, the radial tension is going to be distributed in such a way that the arrangement of elastin in lamellae is the best structure to resist or to confine that tension. If we look in a ligament, the direction of tension is a linear parallel arrangement, and I think the elastin structure reflects that. It is morphological orientation rather than the property of elasticity that changes with elastic fibers. I am not familiar with any report concerning elastic fibers in kidney tissue.

Bustos. The increase in ratio that you showed in the cell-free system and the organ culture could be due to an increase in the numerator or a decrease in the denominator. Did you determine this individually and then determine the ratio or was your system giving you the ratio itself?

Foster. The total amount of tropoelastin (a + b) does not change dramatically during chick aortic development (11 - 18 day embryos). This would suggest that the amount of functional mRNA coding for tropoelastin b increases, wherase the mRNA for tropoelastin a decreases.

Yu. Dr. Foster clearly demonstrated the difference between the elastin synthesis in the lung and the aorta. I don't know

much about the anatomy of the lung of the chicken, but I understand that it differs in elastic recoil from blood vessels. Your
difference might be due to the developmental stage you are looking at.

Foster. I am not an expert at avian respiratory physiology.
However, I do know that the breathing mechanism of the chicken
is very different. We have done a complete study in various
anatomic subdivisions of the pig lung, and the ratio is like that
of the chick. It seems to be a characteristic of pulmonary tissues -- a to b is 1 to 1, and we have looked at both fetal and
adult pigs.

Glagov. Can I raise another hypothesis that you may have
already tested, about why there's a spurt in the aorta at day 12
or 13 and yet, even on day 18, there is not a spurt in the
lungs? Can it be that by day 12 or 13 there are signals coming
to the aorta, because of the maturation of the circulatory system, that aren't coming to the lungs? If you look at the lungs
after birth, you may get the same kind of spurt once the lungs
start to breathe and this stimulus activates the altered ratio;
whatever the significance of that altered ratio happens to be.

Foster. We are exploring that possibility using glucocortico-
steroids, specifically dexamethasone, which (Rosenbloom J,
Cywinski A [1976] Biosynthesis and secretion of tropoelastin by
chick aorta cells. Biochem Biophys Res Commun 69: 613-620)
causes a precocious maturation of aortic elastin; they did not
look at the lung.

Proteolytic Mechanisms
and Pulmonary Emphysema

GERARD M. TURINO, STEPHEN KELLER, TUKARAM V. DARNULE,
MOHAMED M. OSMAN, and INES MANDL

Pulmonary emphysema causes between 40,000 and 45,000 deaths per year in the United States. However, most people with this chronic illness, whose natural history extends over many years, are physically disabled by severe breathlessness for much of their late adult life. It is estimated that in the United States, several million people are disabled from some form of airway obstructive disease - including pulmonary emphysema (Task Force Report 1980).

While emphysema has been recognized from the time of Laennec (1826), little was known of its etiology until the last 10 - 15 years. It was known that emphysema was a destructive change in the parenchyma of the lung, resulting in loss of alveolar spaces and occasionally formation of large coalescent air-containing cysts or bullae, and that obstruction to airflow in the lung was the predominant physiologic abnormality (Rohrer 1915). However, no physiologic or biochemical concepts of the time served to explain the origin of this anatomic derangement and destruction. Attempts to induce such alveolar destruction by experimental models of airway obstruction were unsuccessful (Boren 1965; Eiseman et al. 1959; Haidak et al. 1950), and clinical medicine provided numerous examples of long-standing airway obstruction that did not result in generalized alveolar destruction, i.e., allergic asthma and cystic fibrosis of the pancreas.

This was the state of understanding of pulmonary emphysema in 1961, when the World Health Organization convened a committee of medical scientists, mainly from England and the United States, to formulate definitions of various forms of lung disease (WHO Techn. Report 1961). This committee defined pulmonary emphysema as a disease that resulted in distension and destruction of alveolar-containing portions of the lung. Recognition of the disease is therefore based upon anatomic criteria rather than physiologic or clinical evidence, and this form of lung disease is set quite apart from chronic bronchitis, which was defined by the presence of cough and sputum, and from asthma, which was defined by episodic bronchial obstruction, usually associated with allergy.

To continue the chronology, the stage was set for current investigations into the etiologic mechanisms of pulmonary emphysema by a series of observations in different laboratories, both in the United States and abroad.

It was recognized in the early 1960s that proteolytic enzymes, which could be directed against certain structural components of the lung parenchyma, could be a useful tool in defining the role of structural elements, such as cartilage or elastin or collagen, in pulmonary mechanics (Turino et al. 1961, 1964, 1968). Papain was originally used for this purpose, since its effects could be directed against bronchial cartilage, and subsequently pancreatic elastase and clostridial collagenases, as well as testicular hyaluronidase, were also used.

Concomitant with these applications of proteolytic enzymes in pulmonary physiology, it was demonstrated that intratracheal instillation of crude papain resulted in alveolar wall destruction (Gross 1964). The morphologic appearance of the lungs after such treatment (Fig. 1) resembled the pulmonary emphysema seen in humans. The significance of these findings was heightened by the observation that family members with a deficiency of serum alpha$_1$-antitrypsin, a serum inhibitor of proteolytic en-

Proteolytic Mechanisms and Emphysema 249

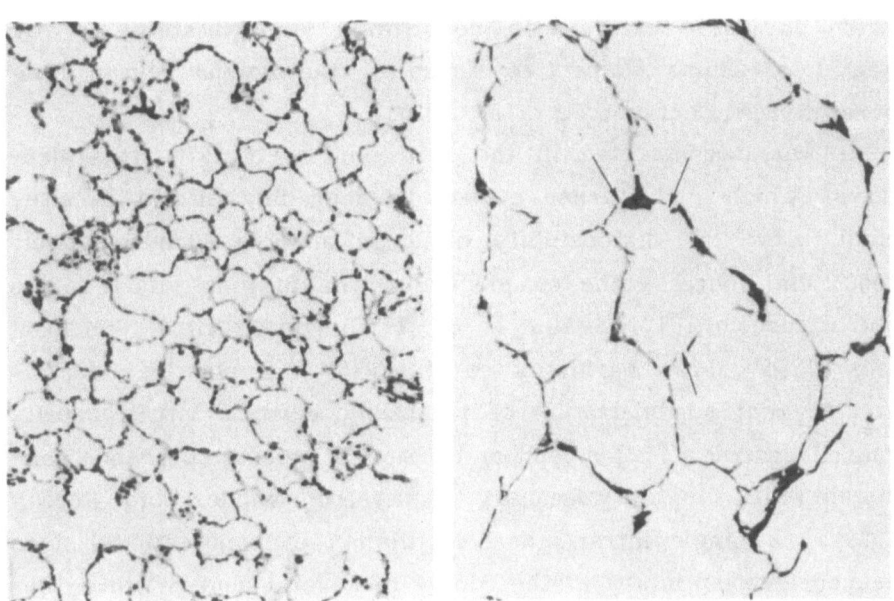

FIG. 1. Light microscopy of pulmonary emphysema in a dog lung
three weeks after repeated doses of intratracheal papain (on the
right). Note the rupture of alveolar septae (arrows) and the
larger size of air spaces. On the left is a normal lung shown at
the same magnification (from Osman et al. 1980). X 165

zymes, had a high incidence of pulmonary emphysema (Laurell
and Eriksson 1963). These observations, coupled with the realization that more had to be learned of the cellular and tissue
structure-function relationships in the lung, set the stage for
current directions of research on pulmonary elastin and etiologic
mechanisms of pulmonary emphysema.

Pulmonary Elastin

Estimates of elastin content of human lung have varied widely
(1.3% - 47% of dry lung weight) as a result in part of the different methods of analysis, variable methods of sampling of lung,
and different ages of subjects (Lowry et al. 1941; Pierce and
Hocott 1960; Wright et al. 1960; Fitzpatrick et al. 1962; Scarselli

and Repetto 1959; John and Thomas 1972). More recent estimates indicate that elastin constitutes approximately 30% by
weight of crude connective tissue of the normal human lung
parenchyma (Chrzanowski et al. 1980).

It was demonstrated in the 1960s and early 1970s that elastases, which had marked effects in degrading elastin in situ,
could alter the distensibility of large airways (Turino et al.
1968) and increase the compliance of the lung in vivo (Turino
and Lourenco 1972; Snider et al. 1977) and in vitro (Johanson
and Pierce 1972; Karlinsky et al. 1976). It also was demonstrated that administration of pancreatic elastase intratracheally
caused destruction of alveoli and a morphological appearance consistent with human pulmonary emphysema (Snider and Korthy
1978). A single intratracheal instillation of pancreatic elastase
caused alveolar injury in the course of several hours, which then
progressed for several months without administration of additional
proteolytic enzyme (Kaplan et al. 1973; Snider and Sherter 1977).
The basis of this progression of injury, however, remains unknown.

Such studies focused attention on elastin in lung parenchyma
as the critical component in preserving alveolar structure. Alteration of collagen in large airways (Turino 1968) or in whole
lungs in vitro (Johanson and Pierce 1972; Karlinsky et al. 1976)
by administration of clostridial collagenase did not produce emphysema anatomically or an increase in lung compliance. Additional evidence for the primary role of elastin destruction in the
development of emphysema came from the observation of Blackwood et al. (1973) that the ability of various proteolytic enzymes
to induce pulmonary emphysema experimentally in animals was
correlated positively with elastolytic activity of the enzyme.

Following the demonstration of marked effects of pancreatic
elastase on lung distensibility, it became of interest to quantitate
corresponding changes in lung elastin content in experimental
emphysema. Thus, in pulmonary emphysema, induced in hamsters by intratracheal administration of elastase (Kuhn et al.

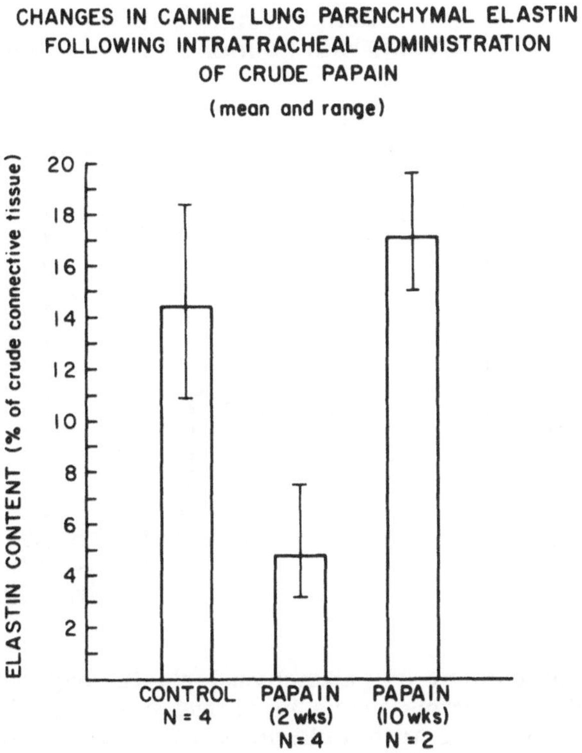

CHANGES IN CANINE LUNG PARENCHYMAL ELASTIN
FOLLOWING INTRATRACHEAL ADMINISTRATION
OF CRUDE PAPAIN

(mean and range)

FIG. 2. Mean lung parenchymal elastin levels (height of the bar) expressed as percent crude connective tissue occurring in dogs after development of diffuse pulmonary emphysema induced by administration of intratracheal papain. Three months after instillation of papain showing the levels returned to normal (from Osman et al. 1980).

1976), and in rats by i.v. administration of elastase (Mandl et al. 1977), lung parenchymal elastin was abnormally low. Similarly, in dogs, in which emphysema had been induced by intratracheal administration of papain, lung elastin was low (Osman et al. 1980). In both hamsters and dogs, after the development of emphysema and reduced levels of lung elastin, there was resynthesis of elastin so that parenchymal lung elastin content was returned to normal within 2 - 3 months after administration, despite the presence of emphysema microscopically (Fig. 2). Also, elastin continued to appear damaged and disorganized.

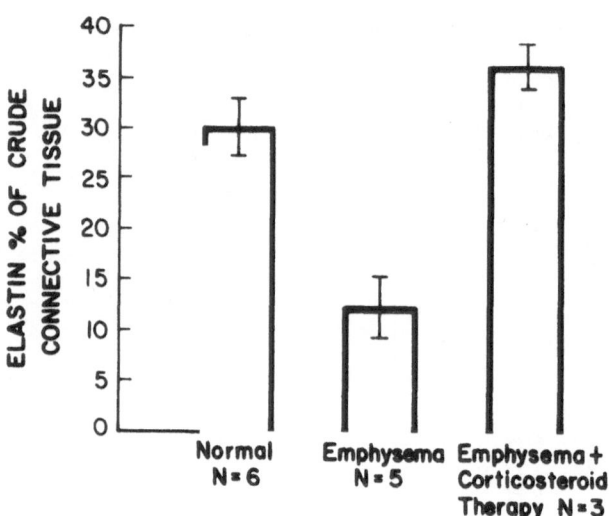

FIG. 3. The content of parenchymal elastin expressed as percent of crude connective tissue in normal human subjects as compared with 5 patients with pulmonary emphysema and 3 patients with pulmonary emphysema who had received corticosteroid therapy for many months prior to death (from Chrzanowski et al. 1980).

Human lungs having the morphologic changes of emphysema also showed elastin damage microscopically (Wright 1961). However, chemical determinations showed no significant differences between lung elastin in normal lungs and that obtained at post-mortem from patients with emphysema (Pierce et al. 1961; Fitzpatrick 1967; Pecora et al. 1967). More recently, a new method of quantifying elastin in lung parenchyma has been developed (Keller et al. 1980) that depends upon measurement of desmosine and isodesmosine as specific amino acid markers for elastin. By this method, 30% of the total connective tissue of normal human adult lung parenchyma (large bronchi, blood vessels and pleura removed) is elastin. Patients with pulmonary emphysema, not on corticosteroid therapy, had elastin proportions ranging between 9% and 20% of total connective tissue (Fig. 3). However, normal values of lung elastin have been found in patients who received oral corticosteroids for several months prior to death. The latter observation in such patients receiving corticosteroids is consistent with the recently demonstrated evidence of stimulation of elastin synthesis in chick aortas by corticosteroids and the depression of collagen synthesis in the same laboratory model (Eichner and Rosenbloom 1979). Further studies should be done using animals to evaluate the effects of corticosteroid administration on the development and progression of elastase-induced emphysema, as well as on lung distensibility and airway function.

Reductions in lung elastin content in human emphysema were demonstrated in patients with the abnormal alpha$_1$-antitrypsin phenotype ZZ as well as the normal MM. Also, the amino acid composition of elastin isolated from lungs of patients with emphysema was the same as that of elastin in normal lungs (Chrzanowski et al. 1980). The demonstration of low lung elastin in human emphysema is consistent with the hypothesis that lung elastin is the vulnerable connective tissue component in this disease and that in the process of development of emphysema, the anatomic continuity of elastin is disrupted, resulting in the destruction of alveoli. The low levels of lung parenchymal elastin in advanced disease suggest that either the mechanisms for resynthesis by the cells capable of resynthesizing elastin or the conditions for its synthesis are inadequate to restore lung elastin to normal values, as was observed in emphysema experimentally induced by intratracheal elastase or papain.

Proteolytic Damage in vivo: Neutrophil Elastase

As early as 1968, Janoff and Scherer demonstrated the presence of elastase activity in human neutrophils. Also, neutrophils from the blood of dogs and humans, which had been concentrated, homogenized, and nebulized into the lungs of dogs, have produced pulmonary emphysema similar to that induced by papain (Marco et al. 1971). Similar, but less severe, changes were ob-

served when homogenized suspensions of macrophages were nebulized into lungs. Subsequently, it was demonstrated that elastase, isolated and purified from both dog and human neutrophils,
also produced emphysema when instilled into the airways (Weinbaum et al. 1978).

In vitro, elastases have more general proteolytic actions. It
has been shown that neutrophil elastase is capable of degrading
arterial wall elastin (Janoff and Scherer 1968), lung elastin
(Janoff et al. 1972), cartilage matrix (Janoff 1970), and basement membrane (Bray and LeRoy 1976). Ohlsson and Ohlsson
(1974) have isolated elastase from human neutrophils and demonstrated that proteoglycans and fibrinogen can be degraded by
these enzymes. More recently, McDonald et al. (1979) have
demonstrated that pancreatic elastases can degrade fibronectin.
Fibronectin, a component of basement membranes of the lung,
may be vulnerable to the action of neutrophil elastases, and
could, therefore, provide a mechanism by which elastase de-
grades alveolar basement membrane.

It is noteworthy that the elastolytic activity of lysosomal
homogenates of neutrophils from patients with clinically diagnosed
chronic obstructive lung disease is significantly higher than that
of neutrophils from normal subjects (Fig. 4) (Rodriguez et al.
1979; Galdston et al. 1977). The latter observation may be the
result of chronic pulmonary infection in such patients rather
than a primary abnormality, but may well be a pathogenetic factor in established chronic obstructive lung disease contributing
to damage of alveoli.

Proteolytic Damage in vivo: Alveolar Macrophase Elastase

Elastase activity has been demonstrated in both peritoneal
macrophages (Werb and Gordon 1975) and alveolar macrophages
(Rodriguez et al. 1977; Green et al. 1979). There is also evidence that human alveolar macrophages possess receptors for
human neutrophil elastase (Campbell et al. 1979). Receptor

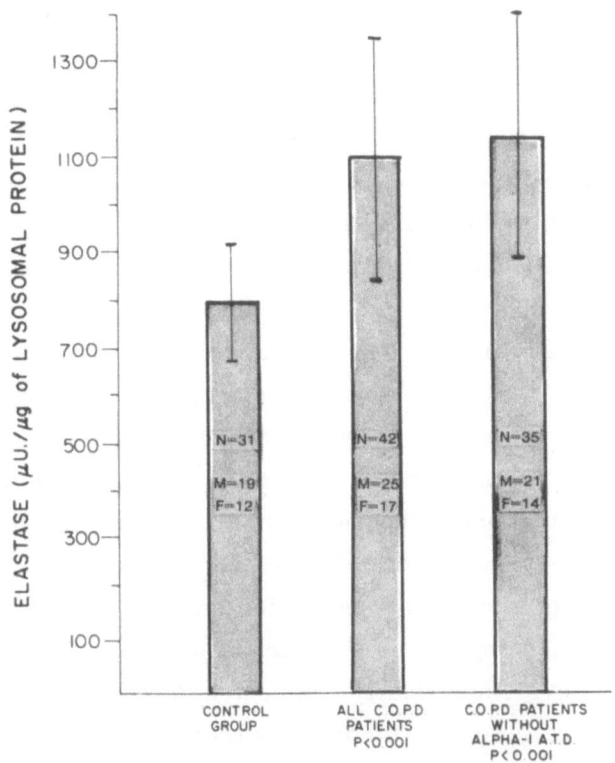

FIG. 4.   Levels of neutrophil elastase activity in normal subjects
(left bar), in patients with chronic obstructive lung disease and
MM phenotype (right bar) and patients including those with
alpha$_1$-antitrypsin phenotypes other than M (middle bar).   The
height of the bar is the mean value for lysosome elastase activity.   The brackets are standard deviation.   The mean level of
elastase activity of patients is statistically significantly higher
than in the normal subjects (from Rodriguiez et al. 1979).

binding, and the subsequent internalization of neutrophil elas-

tase, is not dependent on the presence of alpha$_2$-macroglobulin.

Thus, demonstration of elastase activity in alveolar macrophages

lavaged from human and animal lungs in early studies may have

been due to the presence of phagocytized neutrophil elastase in

these preparations.   Nonetheless, there is evidence that a mono-

cyte cell line (a human histiocytic cell, U 937) is capable of syn-

thesizing elastase that is not of neutrophil origin (Senior et al.

1980). Also, secretion of elastase-like enzymes has been demonstrated in monocytes from human peripheral blood exposed to
immune complexes (Ragsdale and Arned 1979). Lavie, Zucker-
Franklin, and Franklin (1980) have demonstrated elastase-type
proteases on the surface of human blood monocytes. These elastase-like enzymes bear some characteristics of neutrophil elastase, but whether they are synthesized de novo in the macrophage or derived from phagocytized neutrophil elastases is unknown.

The precise amounts of elastase activity that exist in the non-
stimulated and stimulated alveolar macrophages in smokers and
nonsmokers as well as in patients with chronic obstructive lung
disease require further study. Gadek et al. (1978) have demonstrated that neutrophils and macrophages interact so that macrophages secrete a chemotactic factor for neutrophils upon exposure to cigarette smoke that could increase the numbers of elas-
tase-secreting neutrophils in alveolar tissue.

Thus far, evidence clearly implicates neutrophil elastases as
having access to lung and having a well demonstrated capacity to
degrade lung elastin and to produce experimental emphysema.
The evidence for the presence of significant levels of elastase
activity in human alveolar macrophages is less consistent (Hinman
et al. 1980) but over all it is likely that alveolar macrophages
possess elastase activity, although the precise amount is uncertain.

Serum Anti-Protease Activity and Cigarette Smoke

While it has been recognized that smokers develop pulmonary
emphysema at a vastly greater frequency than the general population, until recently there were few insights into how cigarette
smoke could affect elastin synthesis and destruction in the lung.
Two lines of evidence have evolved that indicate that exposure
to tobacco smoke may have its effect through a direct suppression of the inhibitory function of alpha$_1$-antiprotease in the lung.

Carp and Janoff (1978) have demonstrated that exposure of human serum to the water soluble components of tobacco smoke results in a significant reduction in inhibitory capacity against pancreatic elastase. The reduction in inhibitory capacity is reversible by exposure of serum to anti-oxidants such as thymol and hydroquinone. These observations suggest that oxidation may alter the inhibitory action of $alpha_1$-antiprotease, and such oxidations occur on the methionine residues of the $alpha_1$-antiprotease inhibitor.

The second line of evidence is a demonstration of reduced elastase inhibitory capacity of alveolar fluid lavaged from the lungs of rats exposed to tobacco smoke (Janoff et al. 1979) and from the lungs of smokers as compared with nonsmokers (Gadek et al. 1979). This effect of tobacco smoke on alveolar $alpha_1$-antiprotease in such patients is coupled with an increase of the numbers of neutrophils and macrophages that exist in the lung in smokers and that can elaborate elastases. There is also evidence that the elastase secretion per unit cell is increased in neutrophils in chronic obstructive lung disease (Rodriguez et al. 1979) and that in smokers the alveolar macrophages may be activated to secrete increased amounts of elastase as compared with alveolar macrophages from nonsmokers (Rodriguez et al. 1977; Eliraz et al. 1977).

Immunogenicity of Human Lung Elastin in Emphysema

Some recent studies have evolved from the realization that alveolar elastin is a predominant target tissue in the development of pulmonary emphysema. Since breakdown of lung elastin by elastases in situ should lead to elastin fiber degradation products in the circulating blood, attempts are being made to detect such peptides in the blood of animals with experimental emphysema induced by elastases and in human beings with emphysema. Assays for elastin degradation products have been developed along three lines:

RIA for Elastin Peptides

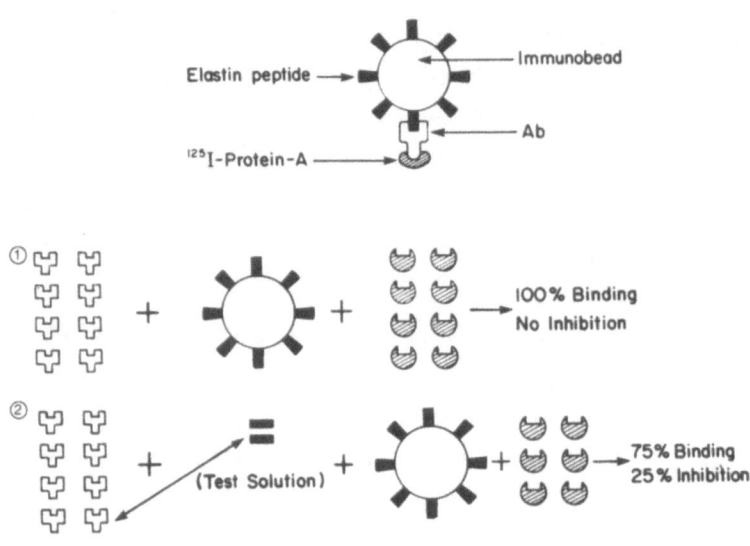

FIG. 5. Schematic representation of indirect radioimmunoassay technique used to measure elastin peptides in serum. The unknown levels of antigenic elastin peptides compete for antibody with elastin peptides bound to immunobeads. Soluble antibody-antigen complexes are removed by centrifugation, leaving insoluble antibody-antigen complexes bound to immunobeads to combine with ^{125}I-labelled Staphylococcus A protein. In the presence of serum containing elastin peptides fewer antibodies are present in the insoluble complex and the difference in ^{125}I label binding to these complexes indicates the amount of antigenic peptides in the serum.

1) The development of antibodies to human lung elastin peptides that have been isolated after treatment of human lung elastin with pancreatic elastase (Darnule et al. 1977). Antibody production from such preparations has been found to be of high titer in guinea pigs (Darnule et al. 1980a). The most antigenic of the peptides are those of the lower molecular weight fractions in the range of 14,000 daltons which contain desmosine and isodesmosine (Darnule et al. 1980b). The radioimmunoassay depends upon the measurement of radioactive-iodine-labeled staphylococcus protein A bound to standardized elastin peptides on

immuno-beads which compete with elastin peptides in unknown serum for analysis (Fig. 5),

2) Development of antibodies in rabbits to the amino acid desmosine, which is specific for elastin. The radioimmunoassay utilizes radioactively labeled desmosine as the antigen to detect desmosine in blood or urine (Harel and Janoff 1980; King et al. 1980),

3) Development of antibodies to insoluble lung elastin and lung elastin peptides. The assay was carried out by the use of hemagglutination for detection of the presence of elastin fragments in body fluids such as fluid from lavage or serum (Kucich et al. 1980).

Thus far in preliminary data, significantly higher concentrations of desmosine have been demonstrated in the urine of smokers and in patients with chronic obstructive lung disease as compared with nonsmokers and normal lungs (Harel and Janoff 1980). Also, higher concentrations of elastin peptides have been detected in blood serum of rats for up to 96 hours after production of experimental emphysema by intratracheal instillation of pancreatic elastase (Darnule et al. 1980c).

Some obvious concerns in these studies are 1) the specificity of circulating elastin peptides as a reflection of elastin degradation from lung as opposed to other sites of elastin degradation such as aorta and other large arteries, 2) fluctuations of elastin peptides in serum or urine brought on by smoking alone as compared with the presence of anatomic emphysema, and 3) possible decreases in elastin peptides entering the circulation in the later stages of emphysema when more marked alveolar destruction and reduced synthesis and degradation of elastin result in a smaller substrate pool of elastin in the lung. The use of radioimmunoassays to detect elastin peptides in serum or desmosine in urine will require much more information on the individual, day-to-day fluctuations in the values measured in order to properly evaluate the significance of differences in elastin peptides in the circulating blood or desmosine in urine between individuals. Also,

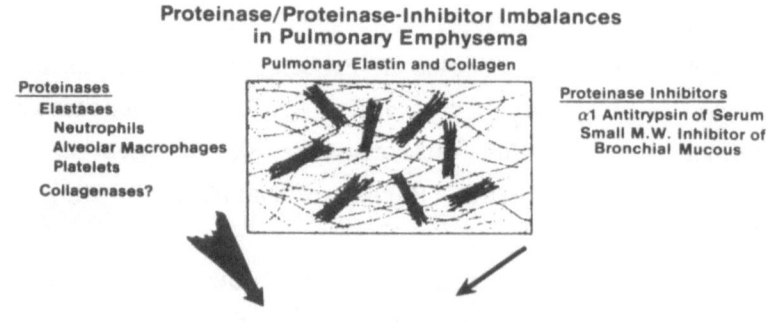

FIG. 6. Schematic representation of protease-antiprotease balance in the lung which can determine lung parenchymal destruction in pulmonary emphysema.

newer methods of enzyme-linked immunoassays (ELISA) may offer advantages over the use of radio-labeled antigens. In any event, such techniques for determining elastin degradation in vivo could greatly assist clinical investigators in detecting the development of pulmonary emphysema early in the disease and in developing methods of prevention of lung parenchymal damage.

Pathophysiologic Pathways to Pulmonary Emphysema

Alveolar destruction in human lungs that results in the clinical and anatomic manifestations of pulmonary emphysema thus evolves as a consequence of imbalances between the concentration of elastases, such as those derived from neutrophils, macrophages, and platelets, and the inhibition of these elastases by inhibitors in serum, such as alpha$_1$-antiprotease and alpha$_2$-macroglobulin (Fig. 6). While bronchial secretions in humans do contain a small molecular weight inhibitor, this inhibitor is located largely in bronchial mucous and may not play a role in the protection of alveoli against elastase injury.

In the case of emphysema associated with alpha$_1$-antiprotease deficiency of the ZZ phenotype, the imbalance would occur because of deficiency in production and/or reduced secretion of alpha$_1$-antiprotease from the liver of such patients. But these genetic deficiencies that lead to critically low concentrations of alpha$_1$-antiprotease inhibitor in blood occur in only a small proportion of patients with emphysema. The larger proportion of patients are normal individuals with MM alpha$_1$-antiprotease phenotype who are smokers. On clinical grounds, smoking becomes a critical factor in defining the mechanism of this imbalance. In this regard, exposure to cigarette smoke and a decrease in the function of alpha$_1$-antiprotease inhibitor in the lung, and most critically in the alveolar lining, becomes the predominant factor. This effect of tobacco smoke in such patients, coupled with increases in the number of neutrophils and macrophages that exist in the lung, tips the balance of proteolytic enzyme activity in favor of destruction of lung elastin.

Such a concept at least provides a working hypothesis upon which to extend investigations into the etiology of emphysema and to devise modes of prevention and therapy. That is, it may be possible to counteract the effects of cigarette smoke, or alternatively to provide inhibitor substances for those who are deficient, by devising exogenous sources or by stimulation of synthesis of natural inhibitor by the liver. These are avenues for future investigation.

Acknowledgment

The work was supported in part by grants from the National Institutes of Health, HS15832, from the Health Research Council of the State of New York and from the Helen R. Gordon Fund of the Columbia University College of Physicians and Surgeons.

REFERENCES

Blackwood EC, Hosannah Y, Perman E, Keller S, Mandl I (1973) Experimental emphysema in rats. Elastolytic titer of inducing enzyme as determinant of response. Proc Soc Exp Biol Med 144: 450

Boren HG (1965) Experimental emphysema. Basis, review and critique. Amer Rev Resp Dis 92: 1

Bray BA, LeRoy EC (1976) Human alveolar basement membrane. Chemical and immunological comparisons with glomerular basement membrane and trophoblast basement membrane. Microvasc Res 12: 77-89

Campbell EJ, White RR, Senior RM, Rodriguez RJ, Kuhn C (1979) Receptor mediated binding and internalization of leucocyte elastase by alveolar macrophages in vitro. J Clin Invest 64: 824

Carp H, Janoff A (1978) Possible mechanisms of emphysema in smokers. In vitro suppression of serum elastase inhibitory capacity by fresh cigarette smoke and its prevention by antioxidants. Amer Rev Resp Dis 118: 617

Chrzanowski PJ, Keller S, Cerreta JM, Mandl I, Turino GM (1980) Elastin content in normal and emphysematous lung. Am J Med (in press)

Darnule TV, Likhite V, Turino GM, Mandl I (1977) Immune response to peptides produced by enzymatic digestion of microfibrils and elastin of human lung parenchyma. Conn Tissue Res 5: 67-73

Darnule TV, Likhite V, Darnule AT, Turino GM, Mandl I (1980a) Enhancement of humoral immune response against human lung elastin peptides. Experientia (in press)

Darnule TV, Darnule AT, Likhite V, Turino GM, Mandl I (1980b) Antigenic determinants in human lung elastin peptides. Conn Tiss Res 7: 269

Darnule TV, Osman M, Darnule AT, Mandl I, Turino GM (1980c) Immunological detection of lung elastin peptides in the serum of rats with elastase induced emphysema. Amer Rev Resp Dis 121 (part 2): 331

Eichner R, Rosenbloom J (1979) Collagen and elastin synthesis in developing chick aorta. Arch Biochem Biophys 198: 414–423

Eiseman B, Petty T, Silen W (1959) Experimental emphysema. Amer Rev Resp Dis 80 (Suppl, July): 147

Eliraz A, Kimbel P, Weinbaum G (1977) Canine alveolar macrophage and neutrophil exposure to cigarette: regulation of elastase secretion. Chest 72: 259

Fitzpatrick M (1967) Studies of human pulmonary connective tissue. Chemical changes in structural proteins with emphysema. Amer Rev Resp Dis 96: 254–265

Fitzpatrick M, Hospelhorn VD (1962) Studies on human pulmonary connective tissue. 1. Amino acid composition of elastin isolated by alkaline digestion. J Lab Clin Med 60: 799

Gadek JE, Fells GA, Crystal RG (1979) Cigarette smoking induces functional antiprotease deficiency in the lower respiratory tract of humans. Science 206: 1315

Gadek J, Humminghake G, Zimmerman R, Crystal R (1978) Mechanisms controlling release of neutrophil chemotactic factor by alveolar macrophages. Amer Rev Resp Dis 117: 65

Galdston M, Melnick EL, Goldring RM, Levytska V, Curasi CA, Davis AL (1977) Interactions of neutrophil elastase, serum trypsin inhibitory activity and smoking history as risk factors for chronic obstructive pulmonary disease in patients with MM, MZ and ZZ phenotypes for $alpha_1$-antitrypsin. Amer Rev Resp Dis 116: 837

Green MR, Lin JS, Berman LB, Osman MM, Cerreta JM, Mandl I, Turino GM (1979) Elastolytic activity of alveolar macrophages in normal dogs and human subjects. J Lab Clin Med 94: 549

Gross P, Babyak MA, Tolker E, Kaschak, M (1964) Enzymatically produced pulmonary emphysema. A preliminary report. J Occup Med 6: 481

Haidak EL, Gregory JJ, Beautyman W (1950) Artificial tumors in dog bronchus and their implications in production of experimental emphysema. Proc Soc Exp Biol Med 105: 66

Harel S, Janoff A (1980) Radioimmunoassay for desmosine: potential clinical test for elastin degradation in emphysema. Amer Rev Resp Dis 121 (part 2): 349

Hinman LM, Stevens CA, Matthay RA, Gee JBL (1980) Elastase and lysozyme activities in human alveolar macrophages. Am Rev Resp Dis 121: 263

Janoff A (1970) Mediators of tissue damage in the leukocyte lysosomes. X. Further studies on human granulocyte elastase. Lab Invest 22: 228

Janoff A, Carp H, Lee DK (1979) Cigarette smoke inhalation decreases alpha$_1$-antitrypsin activity in rat lung. Science 206: 1313

Janoff A, Sandhaus RA, Hospelhorn VD, Rosenberg R (1972) Digestion of lung proteins by human leucocyte granules in vitro. Proc Soc Exp Biol Med 140: 516

Janoff A, Scherer J (1968) Mediators of inflammation in leukocyte lysosomes. IX Elastinolytic activity in granules of human polymorphonuclear leukocytes. J Exp Med 128: 1137

Johanson WG Jr, Pierce AK (1972) Effects of elastase, collagenase and papain on structure and function of rat lungs in vitro. J Clin Invest 51: 288-293

Kaplan PD, Kuhn C, Pierce JA (1973) The induction of emphysema with elastase. 1. The evolution of the lesion and the influence of serum. J Lab Clin Med 82: 349

Karlinsky JB, Snider GL, Franzblau C, Stone PJ, Hoppin FG (1976) In vitro effects of elastase and collagenase of mechanical properties of hamster lungs. Amer Rev Resp Dis 113: 769

Keller S, Mandl I, Turino GM (1980) Determination of the relative amounts of elastin in lung tissues. (submitted for publication)

King GS, Mohan VS, Starcher BC (1980) Radioimmunoassay for desmosine. Conn Tiss Res 7: 263

Kucich U, Christner P, Rosenbloom J, Weinbaum G (1980) An analysis of the organ and species immunospecificity of elastin. Conn Tiss Res (in press)

Kuhn C, Yo S-Y, Chraplyvy M, Linder HE, Senior RM (1976) The induction of emphysema with elastase. II. Changes in connective tissue. Lab Invest 34: 372-380

Laennec RTH (1826) Traite de L'Auscultation Mediate, 2 ed, JJ Chaude, Paris

Laurell CB, Eriksson S (1963) The electrophoretic $alpha_1$-globulin pattern of serum in $alpha_1$-antitrypsin deficiency. Scand J Clin Lab Invest 15: 132

Lavie G, Zucker-Franklin D, Franklin E (1980) Elastase-type proteases on the surface of human blood monocytes: possible role in amyloid formation. J Immunol 125: 175

Lowry OH, Gilligan DR, Katersky EM (1941) The determination of collagen and elastin in tissues with results obtained in various normal tissues from different species. J Biol Chem 139: 795

Mandl I, Darnule TV, Fierer JA, Keller S, Turino GM (1977) Elastin degradation in human and experimental emphysema. In: Sandberg LB, Gray WR, Franzblau C (eds) Elastin and elastic tissue. Plenum Press, New York

Marco V, Mass B, Meranze DR, Weinbaum G, Kimbel P (1971) Induction of experimental emphysema in dogs using leukocyte homogenates. Amer Rev Resp Dis 104: 595

McDonald JA, Baum BJ, Rosenberg DM, Kelman JA, Brin SC, Crystal RG (1979) Destruction of a major extracellular adhesive glycoprotein (fibronectin) of human fibroblasts by neutral proteases from polymorphonuclear leucocyte granules. Lab Invest 40: 350

Ohlsson U, Ohlsson I (1974) The neutral proteases of human granulocyte elastases. Eur J Biochem 42: 519

Osman M, Leuenberger P, Cerreta J, Keller S, Mandl I, Turino GM (1980) Pulmonary elastin content in dogs with papain induced emphysema. Proc Soc Exp Biol Med (in press)

Pecora LJ, Manne WR, Baum GL, Feldman DP, Recavarren J (1967) Biochemical study of ground substances in normal and emphysematous lungs. Amer Rev Resp Dis 95: 623–630

Pierce JA, Hocott JB (1960) Studies on the collagen and elastin content of human lungs. J Clin Invest 39: 8

Pierce JA, Hocott JB, Ebert RV (1961) The collagen and elastin content of lung in emphysema. Ann Int Med 55: 210–221

Ragsdale CG, Arend WP (1979) Neutral protease secretion by human monocytes – effect of surface bound immune complexes. J Exp Med 149: 954

Rodriguez JR, Seals JE, Radin A, Lin JS, Mandl I, Turino GM (1979) Neutrophil lysosomal elastase activity in normal subjects and in patients with chronic obstructive pulmonary disease. Amer Rev Resp Dis 119: 409

Rodriguez RJ, White RR, Senior RM, Levine EA (1977) Elastase release from human alveolar macrophages: comparison between smokers and nonsmokers. Science 198: 313–314

Rohrer F (1915) Der Strömungswiderstand in den menschlichen Atemwegen und der Einfluss der unregelmässigen Verzweigung des Bronchial-systems auf den Atmungsverlauf in verschiedenen Lungenbezirken. Pflueger Arch ges Physiol 162: 225–299

Scarselli V, Repetto M (1959) The elastin content of lung in relation to age. Ital J Biochem 8: 169

Senior RM, Ladis JA, Campbell EJ, Koren HS (1980) Elastase activity associated with a human macrophage-like cell line. Clin Res 28: 531A

Snider GL, Korthy AL (1978) Internal surface area and number of respiratory air spaces in elastase induced emphysema in hamsters. Amer Rev Resp Dis 117: 685

Snider GL, Sherter CB (1977) A one year study of the evolution of elastase induced emphysema in hamsters. J Appl Physiol Respir Environ Exercise Physiol 43: 721

Snider GL, Sherter CB, Koo KW, Karlinsky JB, Hayes JA, Franzblau C (1977) Respiratory mechanics in hamsters following treatment with endotracheal elastase or collagenase. J Appl Physiol 42: 206

Task Force Report: Epidemiology of Respiratory Diseases (July 1979) Dept. of Health and Human Services, Publication NIH Publication #81-2019 - October 1980

Turino GM, Goldring RM, Katz LA (1961) The effect of experimental bronchomalacia on pulmonary mechanics. J Clin Invest 40: 1086

Turino GM, Lourenco RV (1972) The connective tissue basis of pulmonary mechanics. In: Mitman C (ed) Pulmonary emphysema and proteolysis. Academic Press, New York, p. 59

Turino GM, Lourenco RV, McCracken GH (1964) The role of connective tissue in pulmonary mechanics. J Clin Invest 43: 1297

Turino GM, Lourenco RV, McCracken GH (1968) Role of connective tissue in large pulmonary airways. J Appl Physiol 25: 645

Weinbaum G, Sloan B, Meranze DR, Kimbel P (1978) A model of experimental emphysema using a completely homologous system. Amer Rev Resp Dis 117: 411

Werb Z, Gordon S (1975) Elastase secretion by stimulated macrophages. J Exp Med 142: 361

WHO Techn Rep Ser (1961) No. 213, 15 Report of an expert committee on chronic cor pulmonale

Wright GW, Kleinerman J, Zorn EM (1960) The elastin and collagen content of normal and emphysematous human lungs (abstract). Am Rev Respir Dis 81: 938

Wright RR (1961) Elastic tissue of normal and emphysematous lungs. A tridimensional histologic study. Am J Path 39: 355-368

Discussion

Rhodes. I would like to make a comment, rather than ask a question, and suggest that possibly the destruction of the normal alveolar morphology, in addition to reflecting the loss of elastin, would also indicate a loss of basement membrane collagen. Kang and his colleagues (Mainardi CL, Dixit SN, Kang AH [1980] Degradation of Type IV [basement membrane] collagen by a proteinase isolated from human polymorphonuclear leukocyte granules. J Biol Chem 255: 5435-5441) have recently shown that elastase is very active in degrading Type IV collagen.

Turino. In our laboratory, Dr. Bonnie A. Bray has demonstrated fibronectin in human lung alveolar parenchyma in the basement membrane (Bray BA [1978] Presence of fibronectin in basement membrane and acid structural glycoproteins from human placenta and lung. Ann NY Acad Sci 312: 142-150; Bray BA [1979] Cold insoluble globulin [fibronectin] in connective tissues of adult human lung and in trophoblast basement membrane. J Clin Invest 62: 745-752), perhaps in association with collagen. It has also been demonstrated by work from Crystal's laboratory that fibronectin is particularly susceptible to elastase degradation (McDonald JA, Baum BJ, Rosenberg DM, Delman JA, Brin SC, Crystal RG [1979] Destruction of a major extracellular adhesive glycoprotein [fibronectin] by neutral proteases from polymorphonuclear leucocyte granules. Lab Invest 40: 350). It may be that one mechanism by which elastase breaks down basement membrane is through degrading fibronectin. Also Bray (Bray BA, LeRoy EC [1976] Human alveolar basement membrane. Chemical and immunological comparisons with glomerular basement membrane and trophoblast basement membrane. Microvas Res 12: 77-89) showed that the basement membrane, in vitro, is susceptible to elastase even though its major action is degradation of elastin.

Histochemical Investigations of Elastin, Collastin, and Other Collagens

HOLDE PUCHTLER, FAYE SWEAT WALDROP,
and SUSAN N. MELOAN

Conventional staining technics for connective tissues, e.g., elastica stains, Van Gieson's picro-fuchsin, and trichrome methods, were introduced between 1880 and 1910, but their chemical mechanism and significance remained obscure. Interpretations of staining patterns were based on tradition rather than chemical data. Histochemical studies during the 1960s demonstrated that elastica stains, e.g., resorcin-fuchsin, were not specific (Puchtler et al. 1961) and that there were striking differences between collagens (Puchtler and Sweat 1963, 1964a; Joiner et al. 1965; Smith et al. 1966); at that time all human collagen was still supposed to have the formula $(\alpha1)_2\alpha2$. In addition, perusal of nineteenth century literature indicated that much early knowledge of connective tissue and arteriosclerosis has been forgotten. Many of these data have been rediscovered during the past twenty years.

Current concepts of connective tissue and arteriosclerosis research have been comprehensively discussed by other contributors to this volume. This chapter is a review of various aspects of the histochemistry of elastin and collagen and their occurrence in arteriosclerosis. The historical context of various concepts are also considered. Emphasis is placed on the work of scientists who blazed the trails or dared to critically analyze fashionable hypotheses, rather than on current literature which is widely known and readily available.

Definitions

Elastica stain(s). This term denotes the conventional stains resorcin-fuchsin, orcein, aldehyde-fuchsin, and Verhoeff's iron hematein. It is purely descriptive and has no chemical connotations.

Elastic tissue, fibers, or membranes. Any tissue component colored by the above stains. These terms do not convey any information concerning the chemical composition of such material.

History and Histochemistry of Elastica Stains

Resorcin-fuchsin

History. Resorcin-fuchsin was introduced by Weigert in 1898. He gave detailed instructions for preparation of the dye, but limited his description of results to a one sentence statement that elastic fibers appear dark blue, almost black, on a light background. Weigert, who contributed so much to histologic technic, did not publish any further work or comment on this method. According to von Czyhlarz (1897), Weigert gave a sample of resorcin-fuchsin to Professor Rieder for testing. Rieder passed the dye on to Jores, whose interpretations of the resorcin-fuchsin stain went to press before Weigert's paper appeared in print (Jores, 1898). Because resorcin-fuchsin colored many fibers which did not react with other elastica stains, including orcein, Jores (1898) declared resorcin-fuchsin far superior to other reactions for elastin. He had to concede that there were significant morphologic and histochemical differences between elastin membranes and supposedly elastic lamellae and fibers, but insisted these obvious discrepancies were unimportant; any structure which bound resorcin-fuchsin was, by definition, elastic tissue. In contrast to Weigert, Jores was not an expert on dye chemistry and microscopic technics; yet, current concepts of the selectivity and significance of elastica stains are based on Jores' (1898) opinions.

The specificity of resorcin-fuchsin for elastin was questioned repeatedly (Thomé 1901; Lehrell 1903; Oppenheim 1918; Wolff 1928; Tunbridge et al. 1952; Gillman et al. 1955; Partridge 1958), but these critical studies were largely ignored. Wolff (1928) suggested the term pseudo-elastica for collagenous fibers which bind resorcin-fuchsin. This term was chosen also by Gillman et al. (1957) and Gillman (1959), who described numerous differences between elastin membranes and pseudo-elastica. Yet, Jores' (1898) hypothesis concerning the reliability of this stain for identification of elastin is still widely accepted.

Binding of Resorcin-fuchsin by Collagens. Fullmer and Lillie (1957) observed binding of resorcin-fuchsin and other elastica stains by acetylated collagen. Acetylation or formation of other esters in tissue sections produced also strong coloration of basement membranes and glycogen (Puchtler et al. 1961; Puchtler and Sweat 1964a). Further studies indicated similarities in reactivity of resorcin-fuchsin and disperse dyes for cellulose acetate and suggested formation of hydrogen bonds between phenolic hydroxyl groups of the dye and suitable binding sites in tissues (Puchtler et al. 1961). Deamination with Van Slyke's reagent induced moderate dye binding by basement membranes; collagen and reticulum fibers did not react (Puchtler et al. 1961; Puchtler and Sweat 1963). After pretreatment of sections with periodic acid and $NaHSO_3$, resorcin-fuchsin stained basement membranes and ring fibers intensely and selectively (Puchtler and Sweat 1964a,b; King et al. 1968). This reaction is the method of choice for demonstration of basement membrane cristae (Harper et al. 1970). The lack of selectivity of resorcin-fuchsin for elastin is indicated also by its affinity for certain mucins, agar, and gelatin (Puchtler et al. 1961).

Binding of resorcin-fuchsin and other elastica stains by collagen samples pretreated with buffers, acids, alkali, or enzymes received much attention during the 1950s (Tunbridge et al. 1952; Burton et al. 1955; Keech et al. 1956; Tunbridge 1956; Partridge 1958; Hall 1959, 1961). When such treatments were applied to tissue sections, collagen and reticulum fibers stained strongly with resorcin-fuchsin, but basement membranes did not react (Kuhns et al. 1961; Puchtler and Sweat 1963, 1964a). The solvent in the phenylhydrazine procedure for blocking of carbonyl groups also induced uptake of the elastica stain by collagen and reticulum fibers (Sweat and Puchtler 1964). Such pretreated collagen not only acquired affinity for elastica stains, but also lost its periodicity and became associated with amorphous material, i.e., pretreated collagen was indistinguishable from elastin by electron microscopy (Burton et al. 1955; Keech et al. 1956; Tunbridge 1956; Hall 1959). Similar abnormal fibrils and amorphous masses with affinity for elastica stains were found in pathologically altered collagen (Tunbridge et al. 1952; Burton et al. 1955; Tunbridge 1957; Hall 1959; Sirsat and Khanolkar 1962). Yet, in various electron microscopic studies, e.g., of skin, lung, and arteries, structures consisting of aperiodic fibrils or filaments associated with amorphous matrix are usually classified as elastin, especially when they react with elastica stains. The outstanding work done in Great Britain during the 1950s has been largely ignored.

Parenthetically, during purification of elastin, samples are often treated with resorcin-fuchsin or other elastica stains to ascertain the complete removal of collagen. However, under these conditions, remaining collagen and reticulum fibers bind elastica stains as avidly as elastin. Hence the amino acid composition of "elastin" regarded as pure on the basis of elastica stains can vary widely from sample to sample; the presence of collagen would explain also varying amounts of hydroxyproline.

Binding of resorcin-fuchsin by collagen of premature infants (Joiner et al. 1968), collagenous fibers in the elastica interna (Rodgers et al. 1967b), in arteriosclerosis (Jackson et al. 1968),

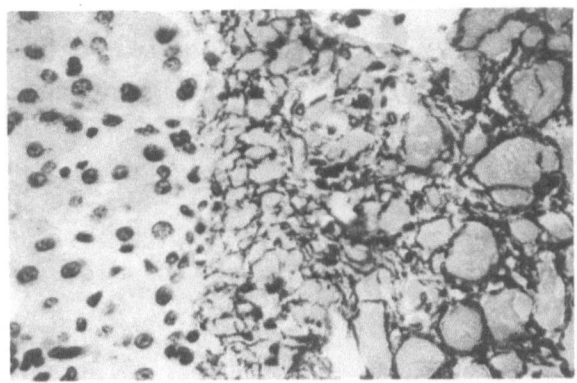

FIG. 1. Liver, stained with orcein-methylene blue. Fine connective tissue fibers between collagen bundles are strongly colored; reticulum fibers between hepatocytes (at left) do not react. Human autopsy material, methacarn fixation. X 400

and in lung (Younker et al. 1980) will be discussed in context with other elastica stains (see below).

Orcein

The history and supposed selectivity of the orcein stain have already been reported (Puchtler and Meloan 1979) and will therefore be reviewed only briefly. Orcein is one of the oldest textile dyes and was widely used in ancient Egypt (Caley 1927). It was introduced into histology in 1878 as a stain for cytoplasm and neurocytes (Gierke 1884). Unna (1890, 1891) recommended Tänzer's acid orcein solution as a stain for elastic tissue, but three years later Unna (1894a) retracted all claims concerning the selectivity of acid orcein for elastin because it colored also certain collagen fibers. He suggested the term collastin for collagen fibers with staining properties of elastin. According to Unna (1894a), procedures for elastin will also visualize collastin; further studies are required to distinguish between these tissue components. Furthermore, acid orcein was known to color also mast cells (Unna 1894b) and mucus (Zimmermann 1898). Orcein in absolute ethanol was recommended as a selective stain for col-

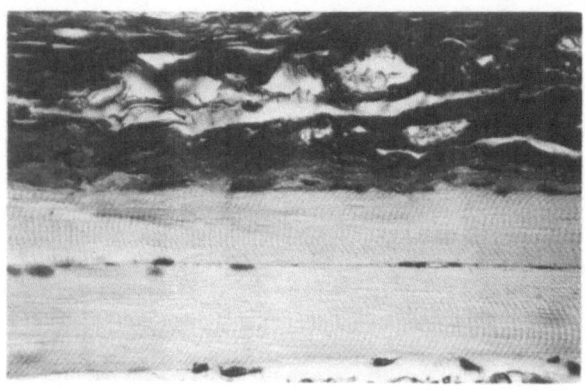

FIG. 2. Muscle, Duchenne-type muscular dystrophy, stained as Fig. 1. Collagen adjoining muscle fibers is strongly colored by the elastica stain. Cross-striation of muscle fibers is barely recognizable. Human autopsy material, methacarn fixation. X 400

lagen (Unna 1894b; Dmitrijeff 1897). Neutral solutions of orcein were also widely employed for staining of collagen (Hoyer 1900; Lehrell 1903). Yet, though Unna (1894a, b) and others proved that orcein is definitely not specific for elastin, many current textbooks still list orcein as a stain for demonstration of elastin.

Differences in intensity of staining by different dye batches are usually due to variations in composition. Chemical studies demonstrated up to 13 fractions in commercial orcein (Engle and Dempsey 1954; Friedberg and Goldstein 1969), including anionic, cationic and non-ionic compounds (Pearse 1968).

Investigations in this laboratory demonstrated binding of orcein by fine fibers between and around coarse collagen bundles (Fig. 1), certain collagen fibers in arterial lesions and in tissues from premature infants, and collagen from patients with various diseases, e.g., Duchenne-type generalized muscular dystrophy (Fig. 2) and eclampsia (Puchtler and Meloan 1979). Binding of orcein by experimentally altered collagen is similar to that of resorcin-fuchsin (Hall 1959, 1961). Upon autoclaving, glutaraldehyde-fixed tendon also showed affinity for orcein and other elastica stains (Grant 1965). The similar staining properties of orcein and resorcin-fuchsin are probably due to their meta-dioxy-benzene components. Apparently, both dyes can form hydrogen bonds with suitable binding sites of collagen, as suggested by Partridge (1958).

Comparative studies of sections stained with orcein and resor-cin-fuchsin indicated that Wolff's (1928) pseudo-elastica is identi-cal with Unna's (1894a) collastin (Puchtler and Meloan 1979). A review of the literature showed that the term pseudo-elastica is employed in context with resorcin-fuchsin, whereas the designa-tion collastin is associated with the orcein stain. Since the term collastin is much more informative and was coined decades before the name pseudo-elastica was introduced, the term collastin will be used to denote collagenous structures which bind the elastica stains resorcin-fuchsin, orcein, aldehyde-fuchsin, and Verhoeff's iron hematein.

Aldehyde-fuchsin

In 1950 Gomori introduced aldehyde-fuchsin as a stain for elastic tissue, beta cells of pancreas, certain basophils in pitui-tary, and some kinds of mucus. As previously reported (Pucht-ler et al. 1979), Gomori (1953, personal communication) observed these staining properties of aldehyde-fuchsin incidentally during investigations of the Feulgen reaction and did not regard alde-hyde-fuchsin as a specific reagent for elastin. Though this stain has been studied extensively, its composition, mechanism and histochemical significance are still obscure. A discussion of the voluminous literature is beyond the scope of this review. Bangle (1954) suggested that aldehyde-fuchsin is a Schiff base formed by reaction of acetaldehyde with basic fuchsin. This hypothesis has been widely accepted, but infrared spectroscopic studies did not confirm a Schiff base structure (Buehner et al. 1979). Considerations of the relations between dye structure, color, and reactivity also did not favor a Schiff base or azometh-ine structure. Chemical studies demonstrated that the dye solu-tion contained up to 11 compounds (von Denffer and Heidbrink

1974) and considerable alterations of aldehyde-fuchsin solutions occurred during aging (Ortman et al. 1966) that seemed to parallel changes in staining properties.

Aldehyde-fuchsin is not a new dye as widely assumed, but was prepared by Lauth in 1861 (Schiff 1865) and is thus one of the earliest synthetic dyes. It was known as "Aldehydblau" (Schiff 1866) and could easily be converted to Aldehyde Green, the first synthetic green dye (Gattermann and Wichmann 1889). Both dyes were known to histologists (Magnus 1910). The composition of Aldehyde Blue was studied by Schiff (1866), who did not find any azomethine or Schiff base structures. Correlation of Schiff's (1866) findings with modern chemical data suggests that a variety of compounds are formed under the conditions of aldehyde-fuchsin preparation (Puchtler et al. 1979).

Aldehyde-fuchsin colors elastin and collastin in the same shade, i.e., it is definitely not specific for elastin, but its reaction mechanisms are not yet understood. In certain respects the staining properties of aldehyde-fuchsin differ significantly from those of resorcin-fuchsin (Puchtler et al. 1979). Histochemical studies are complicated by the fact that aldehyde-fuchsin is not a chemical entity, but a mixture of poorly known compounds.

Verhoeff's Iron Hematein

Verhoeff (1908) introduced an iron hematein formula containing Lugol's solution for demonstration of elastic tissue; sections were differentiated until desired staining patterns were obtained. As stated by Verhoeff (1908): "If the differentiation has been carried too far, the sections may be restained..." In other words, there is no chemical or histochemical end-point; staining patterns can be adjusted arbitrarily to support preconceived notions as to which structures should be classified as elastin. Verhoeff (1908) did not attempt to prove the selectivity of his stain for elastic tissue, but recommended it also for staining of mordanted myelin sheaths, i.e., structures considered devoid of elastin. Although no chemical or histochemical evidence that

Verhoeff's (1908) iron hematein is specific for elastin has ever been presented, it is widely used for this purpose in this country. However, Verhoeff's elastica stain has not been accepted in continental Europe, e.g., it is not listed in the Enzyklopädie der mikroskopischen Technik (1910) nor in the classical works by Langeron (1921), Romeis (1948), or Roulet (1948).

Parenthetically, the widely used term iron hematoxylin is incorrect. The pale yellow hematoxylin does not noticeably contribute to the staining patterns; only hematein can form strongly colored chelates with metals.

Chemical and Histochemical Investigations. Extensive studies by Arshid et al. (1954 a,b) demonstrated that iron hematein is not a basic dye, as sometimes suggested by microscopists, but contains cationic, anionic, and non-ionic olated chelates. Binding of these complexes occurs by hydrogen bond formation via phenolic hydroxyl groups of the dye and by van der Waals forces; Coulomb forces contribute to the uptake of ionic chelates.

In histochemical investigations of Verhoeff's (1908) elastica stain, staining and differentiation times were strictly standardized to eliminate individual variations (Puchtler and Waldrop 1979). Without differentiation, Verhoeff's iron hematein stained almost all tissue structures. After differentiation, nuclei, elastin, collastin, and myelin sheaths remained intensely colored. Omission of Lugol's solution from the dye bath greatly enhanced the selectivity; in differentiated sections, elastin, myelin sheaths, and nuclei were strongly stained, but collastin was decolorized. Similar reaction patterns were obtained when HCl was added to Verhoeff's (1908) dyebath. Verhoeff's (1908) formula differs from other iron hematein stains in its high hematein content. This high dye concentration proved to be critical for staining of elastin and myelin sheaths.

During the last decade, Verhoeff's (1908) elastica stain was recommended for electron microscopic identification of elastin (Brissie et al. 1975; Hance and Crystal 1975; Cotta-Pereira et

al. 1977; Sage and Gray 1977). The selectivity of this stain
seems to be tacitly taken for granted, though the intense coloration of nuclei by Verhoeff's (1908) elastica stain should cast
doubt on its alleged specificity. Apparently, Brissie et al.
(1974) first recommended Verhoeff's (1908) stain for ultrastructural studies of elastin. However, perusal of their technical
data showed that these authors employed a variation which differed significantly from Verhoeff's formula. When applied to
paraffin sections, this variant stained all tissue structures more
intensely and was more resistant to differentiation than Verhoeff's original stain. Clearly, the modified technic used in electron microscopy is as unspecific as Verhoeff's (1908) classical
stain (Puchtler and Waldrop 1979). Comparison of published
electron micrographs of elastic fibers, e.g., in skin, and of experimentally altered collagen shows striking similarities of these
structures. For example, supposedly elastic fibers with lucent
holes and/or frayed periphery resemble the "moth-eaten" collagen
fibers obtained by Keech et al. (1956). Furthermore, the
amount and location of supposedly elastic fibers are very different from those of histochemically demonstrable elastin (see below). Apparently, binding of iron hematein under the conditions
of electron microscopic technics does not convey any information
concerning the chemical composition of stained material. Electron
microscopic studies of myelin sheaths stained with Verhoeff's
(1908) elastica stain seem to be lacking.

Clearly, Verhoeff's (1908) elastica stain is definitely not specific for elastin. However, at the current state of the art, it is
the method of choice for demonstration of myelin sheaths in un-
mordanted formalin-fixed central nervous tissues. Differentiation
can be eliminated by counterstaining with picro-Sirius Red F3BA
(Sweat et al. 1964a). In contrast to other stains for myelin
sheaths, which require 24 hours to several weeks, the Verhoeff
elastica stain - picro-Sirius Red F3BA procedure can be performed in 30 minutes. It was therefore suggested to reclassify

Verhoeff's (1908) elastica stain as a method for myelin sheaths (Puchtler and Waldrop 1979).

Fluorescence Microscopic Distinction Between Elastin and Collastin

Since conventional staining technics are definitely not specific for elastin, it was considered desirable to develop new technics for distinction between elastin and collastin. Connective tissue fibers exhibiting strong autofluorescence are usually regarded as elastic tissue (Kretschmann 1963). However, many collagen fibers in tissues of premature infants and in various lesions are as strongly fluorescent as elastin (Puchtler et al. 1966, 1973a; Joiner et al. 1968; Jackson et al. 1968). Hence, in order to demonstrate elastin selectively, the autofluorescence of collagens must be quenched.

Binding of heteropolyacids by collagen was clarified by Kühn et al. (1958) and Kühn (1960), who demonstrated the importance of guanidyl groups. Since collagen and elastin differ greatly in the number and spacing of arginine side-chains, it was deemed feasible to develop a fluorescence microscopic technic for distinction between elastin and collagen based on differences in amino acid composition of these proteins (Puchtler et al. 1966, 1973a). Phosphomolybdic acid (PMA) was considered preferable to phosphotungstic acid (PTA), because PMA bound to tissues can be reduced to molybdenum blue (Puchtler and Isler 1958; Puchtler and Sweat 1963); this facilitates correlation of light and fluorescence microscopic observations. Collagen fibers are colored deep blue; elastin remains unstained (Puchtler et al. 1966; Jackson et al. 1968).

PMA and PTA both quench the autofluorescence of collagens, but have little or no effect on the primary fluorescence of elastin; the fluorescent elastin core of elastic fibers and membranes stands out clearly against the dark background (Puchtler et al. 1966). The elastica interna of medium-sized arteries showed mosaic-like fluorescence patterns and a gradual decrease of fluo-

rescent material; small arteries were nonfluorescent (Rodgers et
al. 1967a). In arteriosclerotic lesions only elastin membranes
remained fluorescent; fibers supposedly formed by splitting or
duplication of such membranes were nonfluorescent (Puchtler et
al. 1966, 1973a; Jackson et al. 1968).

These fluorescence microscopic observations are in agreement
with chemical and physical data. In studies of aorta and pulmonary arteries, Farrar et al. (1965) observed discrepancies
between histologic and chemical data; the elastica stain suggested
much more elastin than could be found by chemical analysis.
Lansing (1952) found no significant change in elastin content of
aorta between 20 and 100 years. According to physical investigations by Moret (1964), changes in the elasticity of arteries
during aging and in arteriosclerosis are caused by an increase of
collagen in the vessel wall; elastin is not involved.

Fluorescence microscopic studies of sections of skin and lung
treated with PMA demonstrated much less elastin than suggested
by elastica stains. Electron microscopic studies without elastica
stains demonstrated few elastin fibers in skin (Gross and Schmitt
1948; Tunbridge et al. 1952); most of the material colored by
elastica stains proved to be abnormal collagen (Tunbridge 1956,
1957). These observations are supported by findings that elastogenesis in skin is completed soon after birth (Stadler and Orfanos 1978). Fluorescence microscopic observations on lung are
in agreement with data by Farrar et al. (1965) and McLaughlin
(1966) that lung contains considerably fewer elastic fibers than
indicated by elastica stains.

Elastin Cores and Schwalbe's Sheaths

Early Elastica Stains
Jores (1898) recommended resorcin-fuchsin mainly because
this dye colored much more connective tissue fibers than other
stains for elastin. This emphasis on quantity rather than specificity raised the question as to what was stained by earlier meth-

ods for elastin, especially whether or not these technics were selective for structures visualized by the PMA fluorescence microscopic technic for elastin.

Staining methods listed by Gierke (1884) and in the Enzyklopädie der mikroskopischen Technik (1910) were tested. Sections were treated with these technics, current elastica stains, histochemical reactions, and PMA for fluorescence microscopy of elastin. Comparison of reaction patterns indicated that the early elastin stains colored elastin cores of elastic membranes and fibers as described by Mall (1896) and others, but showed little or no affinity for collastin and other tissue structures (Meloan and Puchtler 1979). Evidently, reactions for elastin used during the second half of the nineteenth century were much more selective than currently popular elastica stains, e.g., Verhoeff's iron hematein. However, these technics and contemporary histochemical concepts of elastin were discarded when resorcin-fuchsin and other elastica stains were introduced around the turn of the century.

Several findings by nineteenth century scientists have now been confirmed by investigations with electron microscopy, e.g., the presence of a rather amorphous elastin core and microfibrillar layer of elastic fibers and membranes, but the earlier chemical and histochemical studies have not been mentioned. It appears therefore timely to review major findings.

Chemical Concepts of Elastic Tissue from 1852 to 1950

In 1852 Zollikofer complained that elastic tissue was rarely mentioned by chemists, although it was considered important by anatomists and physiologists. According to Zollikofer, elastic fibers were characterized by their high degree of elasticity (hence the name), their yellow color, and their brittleness. Thus, the name originally referred to a mechanical property, not a specific chemical composition. In chemical studies, Zollikofer (1852) was surprised by the absence of glycine from elastic tissue of ligamentum nuchae, since the close relationship of elastin and collagen was the subject of much discussion. Throughout the nineteenth and early twentieth centuries chemical knowledge of elastin remained limited. Collagen, elastin, gelatin, keratin, and mucin were classified as gelatinoids (Witthaus 1887). Von Richter (1899) regarded elastin as a disintegrated albumin molecule and grouped it with gelatin and keratin. These concepts of contemporary elastin chemistry should be remembered in evaluations of the specificity of orcein (Unna 1891) and resorcin-fuchsin (Jores 1898) stains.

The first amino acid analysis of elastin was published by Abderhalden and Schittenhelm (1904). Their data were only slowly accepted because they showed significant differences between the amino acid composition of elastin and collagen (Wells 1933). In 1928 Richter-Anschütz still described elastin as a gelatin-producing substance. There was little progress in the following decades. According to Kendrew (1954), many chemical and physical studies of elastin were vitiated by contamination with collagen. Modern elastin chemistry began in the early 1950s, largely through the work of Partridge and co-workers (Partridge 1962).

Schwalbe's Sheaths or Membranes of Schwalbe

Morphologic differences between periphery and core of elastic fibers had been observed since the 1830s (Schwalbe 1876). In sections treated with silver impregnation technics, von Recklinghausen (1862) described in elastic fibers black rods that were surrounded by a thin membrane. In 1870, von Ebner reported structural and microchemical differences between the center and the periphery of elastic fibers (Schwalbe 1876). On the basis of his chemical and histochemical studies Schwalbe (1876) concluded that material hitherto regarded as pure elastin consisted of at least two chemically distinct components, namely a longitudinally striated sheath and an almost homogeneous elastin core. In recognition of Schwalbe's contribution to the histochemistry of elastic tissue, the sheaths were termed Schwalbe's sheaths (Young 1892) or membranes of Schwalbe (Mall 1896). Only the core was regarded as elastin (Toldt 1884); Schwalbe's sheaths were considered analogous to, though not chemically identical with, sheaths of other tissue structures, e.g., sarcolemma of muscle.

In his extensive studies of elastic tissue, Mall (1896) confirmed that "there is no longer any doubt that the elastic fibers are composed of two substances -- the interior which stains intensely with magenta, and the membrane which does not." Furthermore, the membranes of Schwalbe appeared to be heterogeneous; "...membranes are often found which seem to be composed of delicate fibrils, and which suggest that at least two substances are present in them" (Mall 1896). Elastic membranes of aorta and large arteries showed analogous structures. As described by Mall (1896), "the Henle's fenestrated membrane is therefore composed of three layers -- an upper and a lower transparent membrane in which there are no openings, ... and a middle layer which stains with magenta, and is identical with the interior of elastic fibers." Thus, there are no passageways between the media and intima; the supposed pores rather resemble sealed windows with panes on the inside and outside of the wall. Considering the status of contemporary elastin chemistry, these achievements of early histochemists and morphologists are truly remarkable.

The concept of an elastin core enclosed by a chemically different fibrillar layer was widely accepted (von Zwingmann 1891) and taught in contemporary textbooks (Toldt 1884; Böhm and von Davidoff 1904; von Ebner 1902). The chemical nature of Schwalbe's sheaths could not be determined with certainty. For some time Mall regarded this material related to reticulum fibers, but later withdrew this concept (Young 1892). However, when elastin cores were digested, the empty membranes of Schwalbe and adjoining connective tissue fibers often seemed to be continuous (Mall 1896). Similar pictures can be obtained with histochemical technics which leave elastin unstained, e.g., with resorcin-fuchsin and other elastica stains in absolute ethanol-HCl

(Puchtler et al. 1976) or solvent dyeing technics (Younker et al. 1978; Waldrop et al. 1980).

Lansing et al. (1952) quoted Mall's (1896) work and confirmed the differential staining of the periphery and interior of elastic fibers; furthermore, these authors observed a complex fibrillar organization of elastic fibers treated with elastase. During the 1960s electron microscopists gradually rediscovered Schwalbe's (1876) sheath, i.e., a layer of longitudinally aligned fibrils enclosing a core of rather amorphous elastin (More et al. 1962; Greenlee et al. 1966; Ross and Bornstein 1969). The amino acid composition of the microfibrillar component differs from that of the central amorphous elastin (Gallop et al. 1972). These findings confirm earlier observations by Schwalbe (1876), Mall (1896), and others. But in contrast to nineteenth century authors, who accorded the fibrillar layer the status of an entity unrelated to elastin, electron microscopists apparently tend to regard the fibrillar layer as an integral part of elastic fibers and membranes, i.e., bundles of microfibrils without amorphous elastin are usually classified as elastic tissue or precursors of elastic fibers and membranes.

Current elastica stains color not only the elastin core and Schwalbe's sheath, but also a variety of other tissue components. In order to evaluate hypotheses based on these technics, e.g., resorcin-fuchsin and Verhoeff's iron-hematein, it was essential to determine which structures, besides elastin, bind elastica stains.

Binding of Elastica Stains by Collagen

Transition of the Elastica Interna

It is widely assumed that internal elastic membranes of all arteries contain elastin. However, differences in structure and composition between internal elastic membranes of small and sizable arteries have been described by early histologists (Koelliker 1854; Toldt 1884). For example, trichrome stains color the elastica interna of sizable arteries, e.g., renal interlobar arteries, bright red, while the elastica interna of small arteries is colored blue and is thus indistinguishable from collagen (Oppenheim 1918; Wolff 1928). An analogous color change from blue to red is seen with Mallory's PTAH stain (Rodgers et al. 1967a). Histochemical studies demonstrated gradual replacement of the elastin core by material with the reactivity of collagen. The occurrence of this transition varied from organ to organ; e.g., in kidney it commenced in arteries 400 μm in diameter, in spleen it became noticeable in arteries 750 μm in diameter. Arteries less than 100 μm in diameter lacked elastin. The elastica interna of renal arterioles and small arteries exhibited basement membrane-like properties; this material was continuous with glomerular basement membranes (Rodgers et al. 1967a). In spleen the basement membrane-like material extended upward into arteries 30 - 40 μm in diameter (Rodgers et al. 1968). Clearly, coloration of the elastica interna by elastica stains does not convey any information concerning its composition.

These findings have been confirmed by fluorescence microscopy (Puchtler et al. 1973a). Current studies with solvent dyeing technics indicate that part of the material which gradually replaces elastin is histochemically similar to Schwalbe's sheaths, i.e., it may contain microfibrils (see below). These observations are in agreement with electron microscopic data that microfibrils often become embedded in amorphous material. The lack of elastin in the elastica interna of small arteries has been noted in electron microscopic studies (Fawcett 1959; Hogan and Feeney 1963). The transition from elastic to muscular arteries is well established. The histochemical studies by Rodgers et al. (1967a) indicate a further decrease and finally loss of elastin. However, changes in composition with decreasing size of the artery are not limited to connective tissue; studies by Laszt (1972) indicate changes in enzyme content and contractility of vascular muscle towards the periphery.

Relations between size of arteries and types of arteriosclerotic lesions have been noted (Zacharjewskaja 1930; Ophüls 1933).

Friedenwald (1933) described hyalin in retinal vessels without elastin. Hogan and Feeney (1963) suggested that the absence of elastin may be responsible for the negligible atherosclerosis in such vessels. In histochemical studies of the renal arterial system, atherosclerosis was seen only in vessels with an elastica interna containing a prominent elastin core (Rodgers et al. 1967a). Current studies indicate similar relations in coronary arteries.

Original Definition of the Internal Elastic Membrane. The absence of elastin from the internal elastic membrane of large segments of the arterial system raised the question of how this structure acquired its misleading name. Apparently, the term was coined by Koelliker (1854), who wrote: "The tunica intima consists of only two laminae, an epithelium and a peculiar, glistening, less transparent membrane, which I shall term the elastic internal tunic." This internal elastic membrane became recognizable in arteries more than 62 µm in diameter, but was very delicate and did not attain its full development in arteries less than 130 - 180 µm in diameter; it could not be determined whether or not the elastica interna was continuous with capillary basement membranes (Koelliker 1854). Clearly, Koelliker (1854) did not consider the collastin and basement membrane-like material in small arteries as an elastica interna; the full development in arteries 130 - 180 µm in diameter coincides with the appearance of elastin.

Koelliker's (1854) statement "we find in the new-born child not a single true elastic fiber" may seem peculiar because elastica stains color numerous structures, even in tissues of premature infants weighing 400 - 500 g. However, current studies show that elastic fibers and membranes of premature infants consist of conspicuous Schwalbe's sheaths surrounding traces of elastin; the elastin cores become more prominent with maturation. Correlation of Koelliker's (1854) writings with current histochemical and electron microscopic data suggests that Koelliker did not regard Schwalbe's sheaths as true elastic fibers.

Identification of elastin in tissues of children is further complicated by the fact that other fibers also bind elastica stains.

Collastin in Tissues of Infants

In 1964 Joiner observed binding of resorcin-fuchsin by collagen fibers in tissues of premature infants (Joiner et al. 1965). Such fibers, e.g., in the adventitia of arteries, showed the staining, polarization, and fluorescence microscopic properties of collagen, but also bound elastica stains, i.e., they exhibited the characteristics of collastin. Uptake of resorcin-fuchsin tended to decrease with increasing weight and age of infants (Joiner et al. 1968). Chemical data indicated progressive cross-linking of collagen during maturation (Grassmann 1960; Hormann 1962). Since experimental splitting of interchain bonds of collagen induces binding of elastica stains (Partridge 1958; Puchtler and Sweat 1963, 1964a), it seemed permissible to assume that binding of resorcin-fuchsin by collagen of infants occured at free bonding sites of incompletely cross-linked collagen; hence the term immature collagen was suggested (Joiner et al. 1968).

TABLE 1. Binding of Resorcin-Fuchsin by Collagen of Infants

Weight of infants	Age of infants	Staining of collagen
390 – 1650 g	2 days – 1 week	+ + + + +
1740 – 3000 g	9 days – 5 months	+ + + +
3050 – 4000 g	3 days – 5 months	+ + +
4510 – 6785 g	1 month – 5 months	+ +
8500 – 10000 g	10 months – 1 year	+

Below one year of age, binding of resorcin-fuchsin decreased with increasing weight rather than chronological age (Table 1). For example, collagen from a three-month-old infant weighing 1960 g stained as intensely as collagen from a one–day–old child weighing 2000 g. Apparently, maturation of collagen progressed similarly under intra- and extrauterine conditions (Joiner et al. 1968). Binding of resorcin-fuchsin by collagen ceased at approximately two years of age. These studies were terminated before type III collagen was discovered. Correlation of histochemical observations and chemical data on the distribution of collagen types suggests that the decrease in resorcin-fuchsin binding by collagen of infants parallels changes in the ratio of type III:type I collagen.

Collagen from children with malformations of the heart bound more resorcin-fuchsin than collagen from children of comparable weight and age who died from acute diseases. There seemed to be relations between severity of cardiac lesions and intensity of coloration of collagen. This supposition is supported by observations that collagen from children who underwent cardiac surgery a year or more before death showed only slightly increased binding of the elastica stain (Joiner et al. 1968). Chemical data concerning type III collagen in patients with severe congenital malformation of the heart could not be found in the literature available for this study. Collagen from children with certain chronic diseases, e.g., Marfan's syndrome, retained its affinity for resorcin-fuchsin (Joiner et al. 1968). Chemical studies by Krieg and Müller (1977) showed much more type III collagen in adventitia of patients with Marfan's syndrome than in controls. Data by Prockop et al. (1979) indicate a collagen with few cross-links.

In adults, collagen fibers with affinity for elastica stains were found at sites of collagen formation, e.g., in hepatic cirrhosis (Sesta et al. 1965) and in arteriosclerosis (Jackson et al. 1968). Chemical studies demonstrated type III collagen in these lesions (Gay et al. 1975a; Remberger et al. 1975; McCullagh et al. 1980). However, although staining patterns and data on the distribution of type III collagen show considerable correspondence, they are not identical. A major exception is reticulum fibers, which bind antibodies to type III collagen, but do not react with elastica stains, even in premature infants weighing less than 500 g. These discrepancies raise questions concerning the definition and identification of reticulum fibers.

Silver Impregnation Methods for Reticulum Fibers. In immunofluorescence studies of type III collagen, reticulum fibers are usually identified by silver impregnation technics; the specificity of these stains is apparently taken for granted. Silver nitrate solutions have long been used for staining of a variety of tissues (Gierke 1884); the early literature on silver impregnation technics has been reviewed by Puchtler and Meloan (1978). Bielschowsky's silver impregnation technic for neurofibrils proved suitable also for fine connective tissue fibers (Maresch 1905). Maresch (1905) emphasized that this stain was not specific for reticulum fibers, but colored also other structures. Since then, a wide variety of silver impregnation methods have been introduced, but their chemical mechanism remained obscure.

Foot (1927) defined reticulum fibers as fine connective tissue fibers that become impregnated with silver. Reticulin is often used as a synonym for reticulum fibers, though, by definition, reticulin denotes the residue after extraction of collagen from such fibers (Siegfried 1892; Young 1892). The confusion was compounded when basement membranes were also classified as reticulin (Windrum et al. 1955; Robb-Smith 1952), i.e., the reticulin of histologists included type III and type IV collagens and associated compounds. Histochemical studies demonstrated that silver impregnation methods for reticulum fibers are definitely not specific for a certain connective tissue fiber, but color also basement membranes, I bands of striated muscle, various structures in central nervous tissue, and cell borders of epithelium (Puchtler and Waldrop 1978). Furthermore, these silver compounds did not react with the collagen of reticulum fibers, but with associated material. In short, silver impregnation technics have no chemical or histochemical significance, but color a medley of tissue structures.

Moreover, these unspecific silver impregnation technics obliterate the ring fibers of spleen, which are still missing from current textbooks. Ring fibers were well known during the second half of the nineteenth century; the early literature was reviewed by King et al. (1968). Sokoloff (1888) and Kultschitzky (1895) distinguished sharply between reticulum and ring fibers and regarded the latter as the equivalent of basement membranes in other blood vessels. On the basis of silver impregnation stains, Foot (1927) declared ring fibers a part of the reticulum. This misconception was widely accepted and ring fibers vanished from the literature until they were described again by Lillie (1951). King et al. (1968) investigated ring fibers in normal and pathologically altered spleens and confirmed that they are indeed modified basement membranes adapted to the special function of venous sinuses. Thus splenic "reticulin" contains type III and type IV collagens.

Dye Binding by Reticulum Fibers. Difficulties in staining of reticulum and other fine connective tissue fibers are due to shortcomings of histologic technics. The mechanisms of dye binding by collagen have been elucidated by leather chemists (Otto 1962). We have applied these chemical principles to the staining of human collagen. Comparative studies of various dyes under the conditions of Van Gieson's technic demonstrated relations between dye configuration and substantivity for fine connective tissue fibers (Puchtler and Sweat 1964a). Owing to its propeller-like structure, Acid Fuchsin in Van Gieson's picrofuchsin is unsuitable for staining of loosely arranged fibers associated with an interfibrillar matrix. Dyes with elongated molecules, which can align themselves parallel to filaments, impart strong coloration to delicate connective tissue fibers. Picro-Sirius Red F3BA was found optimal for light and polarization microscopic studies of collagen and reticulum fibers (Sweat et al. 1964a; Puchtler and Sweat 1964a). When fibers and elongated dye molecules are aligned parallel, their birefringence is additive; thus, picro-Sirius Red F3BA greatly enhances the birefringence of reticulum fibers (Puchtler and Sweat 1964a; Puchtler et al. 1966, 1973b). Substitution of blue dyes with elongated molecules in Lillie's allochrome procedure greatly improved the light fastness of stained connective tissue fibers (Sweat et al. 1964b).

Older trichrome technics, e.g., Mallory's procedure and Heidenhain's azan, require differentiation with its inherent variations and are therefore unreliable. Gomori's one-step trichrome technic also is unsatisfactory for fine connective tissue fibers; an analysis of this procedure showed that its pH is considerably above the values recommended for dyeing of collagen. However, adjustment of the pH of the trichrome solution to the optimum for dye uptake by collagen greatly enhances coloration of reticulum and other fine connective tissue fibers (Sweat et al. 1968).

Collastin in Arterial Lesions

History. Early observations and conflicting theories concerning the connective tissue of arteries were reviewed by Schultz (1849). Koelliker (1854) discussed the great proneness of the intima to become thickened and described layers which consisted of sometimes homogeneous, sometimes striated or fibrillar material with the characteristics of connective tissue. These layers were designated as striped lamellae. That the term connective tissue denoted collagen is indicated by Koelliker's (1854) reference to Eulenberg (1836), who obtained gelatin from the intima. These layers became the subject of numerous investigations. Langhans (1866) and Talma (1879) described striped lamellae in arteries of infants. In his extensive investigations of fiber formation in the intima with age and in arteriosclerosis, Thoma (1883, 1891) regarded these layers as collagenous material. Böhm and von Davidoff (1904) suggested the term inner fibrous layer for intimal connective tissue adjoining the elastica interna.

Dmitrijeff (1897) deplored that all authors discussed formation of collagen in the intima, but did not mention elastic fibers. He ascribed this omission to shortcomings of staining methods. Although Unna (1894a) had retracted all claims concerning the

selectivity of orcein for elastic tissue, Dmitrijeff (1897) declared
it to be specific and described elastic fibers in intimas treated
with this stain. He suggested formation of elastic fibers by
fibroblasts and by modified endothelial cells, but did not postu-
late splitting or duplication of the elastica interna. Dmitrijeff's
(1897) theory of elastin formation by intimal cells is still widely
accepted.

The hypothesis of splitting or duplication of elastic membranes
was advocated by Jores (1898), who postulated splitting of the
internal elastic membrane into several lamellae and formation of
elastic fibers independent of the elastica interna. He had to
admit striking morphologic and histochemical differences between
the elastica interna and the lamellae and fibers supposedly derived from it, but declared these discrepancies unimportant.
Thus, the hypothesis of splitting or duplication of the internal
elastic membrane and formation of elastic fibers in the intima was
based solely on the assumption that the elastica stains orcein and
resorcin-fuchsin are specific for elastin. The concept of splitting or fraying was extended to elastic membranes of large arteries, e.g., aorta. Jores' (1898) hypothesis still survives in current literature.

Splitting or duplication of the internal elastic membrane in
arteries of children was described by Hallenberger (1906), Argaud (1908), Bindi (1908), and many later authors. Schmiedl
(1907) and Levene (1956) observed splitting of the elastica interna in newborn infants. However, such splitting could be
found only in arteries treated with elastica stains. In duplicate
sections treated with trichrome methods only the internal elastic
membrane of sizable arteries was colored red; the lamellae and
fibers supposedly derived from it were stained blue like collagen
(Oppenheim 1918; Wolff 1928). Wolff (1928) stressed the histochemical differences between these structures and deplored that
the concept of splitting of elastic membranes was tacitly taken
for granted. As discussed above, Wolff (1928) suggested the
term pseudo-elastica for collagenous material which bound elastica

stains.   Extensive studies by Gillman (1959) also indicated processes other than splitting of elastic membranes and confirmed
the appearance of pseudo-elastica.

Histochemical Studies.   Investigations by Joiner et al. (1966)
showed that supposedly elastic lamellae and fibers in arterial
intima of children were histochemically similar to, if not identical
with, collagen in tissues of premature infants.   During the first
year such collagen fibers appeared between the internal elastic
membrane and the endothelium and gradually formed a continuous
layer, the inner fibrous layer of Böhm and von Davidoff (1904).
There is also a thin stratum of collagen between the elastica interna and the media.   Because of their affinity for elastica
stains, these birefringent collagen fibers have sometimes been
regarded as part of the elastica interna, and it was suggested
that elastic membranes consist of a central isotropic band framed
on each side by a birefringent layer (Kretschmann 1963).   However, in polarization microscopic studies of arteries stained with
picro-Sirius Red F3BA, the birefringent bands could be identified as collagen (Joiner et al. 1966).   These observations confirm
findings by Velican (1962), who reported disappearance of birefringent material in the intima of infants after incubation with
collagenase.

    Further development of the inner fibrous layer was variable
(Joiner et al. 1967).   In general, between 1 and 16 years of age
the single collagenous band increased in thickness.   However,
two or more layers were found in segments of some arteries of
most infants more than a few months old.   The collastin in these
multiple layers imitated splitting or duplication of the internal
elastic membrane.   Besides collastin, such thickened intimas contained also collagen fibers without affinity for elastica stains.
These differences in reactivity seemed to indicate maturation of
collagen (Jackson et al. 1968), but may denote different types of
collagen.   Perhaps the process is analogous to alterations in the
ratio of type I:type III collagen observed in skin and other tissue of infants.   Multiple layers of collastin and other collagens

were infrequent below 16 years of age, but were seen in an 18-month-old infant. Such lesions were indistinguishable from hyperplastic arteriosclerosis of adults.

Arterial Lesions in Adults. In some adults the inner fibrous layer remained a single narrow band until middle age. Collastin found in thickened intimas and in arteriosclerotic lesions was histochemically indistinguishable from fibers found in adventitia of premature infants and in arterial intima of children (Jackson et al. 1968). These observations of immature, i.e., embryonic-type, collagen were intriguing because Risse (1853) described as the first alteration in the intima the formation of connective tissue which closely resembled embryonic collagen. But during the 1960s our histochemical observations of an embryonic-type collagen in arterial intima of adults were ruled unacceptable by arbiters of arteriosclerosis research. However, our findings acquired new meanings when type III collagen -- which was first discovered in infants (Miller et al. 1971) -- was identified in arteries (Chung and Miller 1974; Chung et al. 1974; Miller and Matukas 1974). Immunofluorescence studies demonstrated type III collagen in the subendothelial layer (Gay et al. 1975b, 1976) and in the intimal fibro-muscular layer (McCullagh et al. 1980).

Besides collastin, histochemical studies indicated at least two other collagens in arterial intima: firstly, fibers resembling collagen of adults, e.g., in adventitia (Jackson et al. 1968), and secondly, a peculiar collagenous material around myointimal cells. This layer exhibited a strong PAS reaction, but differed from renal glomerular basement membranes in its birefringence and affinity for certain dyes; this material was gradually replaced by adult-type collagen fibers (Waldrop et al. 1971). Chung et al. (1976) isolated from intima a protein which exhibited several features commonly regarded characteristic for basement membranes and suggested that it may be derived from endothelial basement membranes. Perhaps this collagen contributes to the unusual microscopic properties of the pericellular layer.

Comparative studies of arteries of children and adults indicated a gradual development of collagenous and cellular layers; there was no clear demarcation of physiologic and pathologic thickening of the intima. These histochemical observations suggest that the process of collagen synthesis, which leads to formation of the presumably normal inner fibrous layer, continues in many children and adults and results in the deposition of two or more layers. Perhaps collagen formation in the intima is temporarily arrested in some individuals and activated again later in life. Thus, collagen formation in hyperplastic arteriosclerosis may be an accentuation of a physiologic process (Puchtler et al. 1966).

Throughout these studies, elastin was observed only in elastic membranes of aorta and other elastic arteries and in the elastica interna and externa of sizable arteries. No elastin could be found in thickened intimas (Joiner et al. 1966, 1967; Puchtler et al. 1966, 1973a, 1976; Jackson et al. 1968). The identification of chemically distinct collagens in intima and media (Chung et al. 1976) and the absence of elastin from the intima called attention to theories of the origin of myointimal cells and formation of the musculo-elastic layer.

Supposedly Physiologic Intima Cushions. Alterations in arteries of children have often been interpreted as physiologic intima cushions. Histochemical studies showed wide variations in number, size, and distribution of intimal cushions or plaques; there were no correlations between age of patients and number or severity of these alterations. Intimal cushions never occurred adjacent to normal media, but seemed to form gradually over areas of medial damage (Rodgers et al. 1967b). It seems therefore unlikely that such intimal cushions are physiologic. In "blind" studies intimal cushions in arteries of children were indistinguishable from arteriosclerotic lesions in adults (Clark et al. 1973a,b). Comparison of these histochemical observations with data on intimal alterations by Remak (1850) and later authors indicates that these lesions are not physiologic, but represent early stages of preclinical arteriosclerosis. When medial lesions are small, there is sometimes scar formation that may mimic regression of intimal cushions.

Myoendothelial Cells and Musculo-elastic Layer

According to Wissler (1968), Altschul (1950) and later authors called attention to smooth muscle cells in thickened intima. The discovery of the musculo-elastic layer has been ascribed to Dock in 1946 (Blumenthal and Alex 1967). In fairness to Dock it should be emphasized that he did not claim to have discovered these structures. On the contrary, Dock (1946) quoted Benninghoff's (1930) comprehensive review, i.e., Dock was evidently familiar with the extensive early literature. Reports on arteriosclerosis research during the last decades rarely quote work published between the 1840s and the 1930s. Thus a century of research on myointimal cells and the musculo-elastic layer has been almost lost from memory. It appears therefore fitting to review achievements of early scientists in context with more recent data.

Myoendothelial Cells. In 1847 Koelliker noted the similarity of intimal epithelial cells and smooth muscle and regarded this epithelium as contractile (Koelliker 1854), but revised his concepts when vascular epithelial cells were classified as endothelium in 1865. Parenthetically, in the 1840s Koelliker discovered also myoepithelial cells in skin; thus, the notion of a myoepithelium lining the arterial lumen may not have seemed extraordinary. Von Ebner (1902) mentioned the demonstration of contraction of endothelial cells by Stricker and Gobulew "thirty years earlier," i.e., around 1870. However, these observations received little attention until electron microscopic studies of endothelium showed numerous well organized filaments indicative of contractile functions (Hibbs et al. 1958; Fawcett 1959; Hama 1960). Histochemical investigations demonstrated myofibrils in endothelial cells at various sites (Puchtler et al. 1969). The presence of myosin in these cells was proved in immunofluorescence studies (Becker and Nachman 1973). Recent histochemical studies have suggested that myofibrils of medial muscle and myoendothelial cells are not identical, but differ in their reactivity under various experimental and pathologic conditions. The existence of several chemically distinct myosins has been established (Pollard and Weihing 1974; Painter et al. 1975). However, detailed chemical data on myosins in medial muscle and myoendothelial cells could not be found in the literature available to us.

Myointimal Cells. Remak (1850) described longitudinally arranged smooth muscle cells in the intima. These myointimal cells were found in infants, especially at sites of bifurcation or branching of arteries, seemed to become more numerous with age, and were prominent in arteriosclerotic lesions; deposition of lipids commenced in these cells (Trompetter 1876; Westphalen 1886; Bregmann 1890; Fuchs 1902). Langhans (1866) found cell divisions and young cells mainly near the surface of the intima, but regarded the subendothelial cells as fibroblasts rather than myoblasts. This hypothesis coexisted with the concept of myointimal cells until electron microscopists demonstrated smooth muscle cells in thickened intima and arteriosclerosis (Haust et al. 1960; Reale and Ruska 1965).

Origin of Myointimal Cells: a) Migration theory: Migration of smooth muscle cells from the media into the intima was mentioned by Bonnet (1896) and supported by Merkel (1903) and Benda (1921), but its origin could not yet be traced. Von Winiwarter (1879) suggested the opposite, namely migration of intimal cells into the media, but only at sites with a defective elastica interna. Incidentally, prior to the introduction of the elastica stains in the 1890s, cells were not supposed to penetrate intact elastic membranes in either direction because the apparent openings in fenestrated membranes were covered by Schwalbe's sheaths. However, the migration hypothesis seems to have become so dominant in recent arteriosclerosis research that other findings are rarely mentioned.

b) Transformation theory: Henle (1843) suggested transformation of endothelial into subendothelial cells; this theory was
widely supported (Virchow 1856; Trompetter 1876; Friedländer
1876; Talma 1879; von Winiwarter 1879; Mehnert 1888). Proliferation of endothelial cells was observed also in repair processes,
e.g., after ligation (Riedel 1876; Auerbach 1877; Zahn 1884),
puncture or incision of arteries (Pfitzer 1879; Crawford 1956),
and necrosis of the media (Waterman 1908). Migration of medial
muscle cells into the intima was regarded improbable because
these cells showed no tendency to move into defects of the media;
scars formed after incision of arteries contained only connective
tissue. In systematic studies of vascular transplants, Borst and
Enderlen (1909) found proliferation of endothelial cells and their
transformation into intimal smooth muscle cells; participation of
the media in the formation of myointimal cells could be ruled out.

These findings are supported by recent observations. Haust
et al. (1960) considered derivation of myointimal cells from endothelium.   McCullagh and Ehrhart (1974) found heavy incorporation of ^{3}H-proline in endothelium lining thickened intima and suggested that endothelial cells may be active in plaque growth.
The dissimilarity in enzyme equipment of medial muscle and myointimal cells (Borgers et al. 1972) and the detection of distinct
collagen chains (Chung et al. 1976) also supports the transformation rather than the migration theory. In experimental studies
by Spaet et al. (1980), medial muscle cells never crossed the
internal elastic membrane.

In histochemical studies, myoendothelial cells in normal arteries were separated from the media by a continuous elastica interna and inner fibrous layer. In areas of slight alterations of
the media, the adjoining inner fibrous layer became thickened.
Gradually, two or more layers of myoendothelial cells separated
by collagen fibers were formed; in some arteries such transitions
were seen proximal and distal to intimal plaques (Puchtler et al.
1969). In early stages of plaque formation the elastica interna
remained intact. With increasing severity of lesions, the elastica

interna became fragmented and segments disappeared; in such areas the border of media and intima was no longer clearly identifiable (Puchtler et al. 1976).

Musculo-elastic Layer. Pfitzer (1879) and Zahn (1884) observed homogeneous material and collagenous fibers between layers of intimal cells. According to Thoma (1883, 1891), during childhood the layer of cells and connective tissue spreads gradually from large to medium-sized arteries. Myointimal cells were found also between supposedly elastic fibers, hence the name musculo-elastic layer (Westphalen 1886; Mehnert 1888; Grünstein 1895; Gilbert 1903). When the musculo-elastic layer is confined to small areas, it is usually referred to as an intimal cushion (see above). Such formations have been regarded as a reaction to hemodynamic and other stresses (Waterman 1908). The early literature on the musculo-elastic layer was reviewed by Jores (1903, 1924). However, as already mentioned, a wide variety of special stains and histochemical and fluorescence microscopic technics did not reveal any elastin in thickened intimas or arteriosclerotic lesions, though the adjoining elastica interna of large and sizable arteries exhibited the characteristics of elastin (Puchtler et al. 1966, 1973a, 1976; Jackson et al. 1968). Clearly, myointimal cells of the musculo-elastic layer are associated with collastin, not elastin.

New Reactions for Elastin, Schwalbe's Sheaths, and Collagens

Current elastica stains are not only inadequate for critical studies of elastin, but are actually very misleading. Earlier elastica stains used during the second half of the nineteenth century, e.g., the magenta method for elastin cores (Mall 1896), are somewhat capricious and have very low light fastness, i.e., they fade within a few weeks or months. Numerous variations of existing methods were tested in this laboratory, but none permitted sharp distinction between elastin and collastin. In previous studies, data from textile and leather dyeing were invaluable for the development of new technics, e.g., for myosins (Puchtler et al. 1969, 1974), polarization microscopy of stained collagens (Puchtler and Sweat 1964a; Puchtler et al. 1973b), and infrared fluorescence microscopy of stained sections (Meloan and Puchtler 1974; Paschal et al. 1978). It seemed therefore promising to test the usefulness of concepts of textile dyeing for selective demonstration of elastin and associated structures. Dyeing from organic solvents appeared well suited for the conditions of microscopic histochemistry. These procedures will be referred to as solvent dyeing.

Dye Binding from Organic Solvents

Textile Dyeing. Textile chemists found organic solvents superior to water in some areas of dye application (Waller and Lewis 1957; Milićević 1970; Love 1978). However, the effects of various solvents on dye binding are not yet fully understood. The chemistry and properties of alcohols are reviewed by Monick (1968). There is very little difference in the hydrogen bonding of methanol, ethanol, n-propanol and n-butanol; hence, effects of these solvents must be due to other factors (Crowley et al. 1966). Dye binding in organic solvents by polyamide fibers decreases with increasing length of the carbon chain of alcohols, but dye binding by polyester and polyacrylic fibers increases (Jörg 1972). According to Sumner (1964) effects of hydrophilic organic solvents are due to their interaction with dye molecules. Solvation of ionic dyes in higher alcohols is insufficient for most technical purposes, but these solvents prove very suitable for neutral premetallized and other non-ionic dyes (Harris and Guion 1972; Riedel 1975).

Effects of Solvents on Elastica Stains. Resorcin-fuchsin, orcein, and aldehyde-fuchsin solutions contain 70% - 95% ethanol. When methanol is substituted for ethanol, resorcin-fuchsin colors also nuclei (Meloan and Puchtler 1975). Elastica stains in absolute ethanol do not react with elastin cores of elastic fibers and membranes, but Schwalbe's sheaths and certain connective tissue

fibers are nicely colored; elastin can be counterstained in contrasting colors (Puchtler et al. 1976). Fibers supposedly derived from elastin membranes and numerous fibers formed in
hepatic cirrhosis continue to bind resorcin-fuchsin (Waldrop et
al. 1977). In tissues of premature infants, collagen fibers bind
elastica stains, e.g., in skin and adventitia of arteries (Puchtler
et al. 1976).

However, resorcin-fuchsin and other elastica stains in absolute ethanol are undesirable for identification of Schwalbe's
sheaths and collastin because many light and electron microscopists still consider Verhoeff's iron hematein and other traditional
technics as specific for elastin. It was therefore deemed desirable to employ dyes which either have no firm association with
components of connective tissue or have not previously been applied to human tissues.

Solvent Dyeing with Sulfonated Dyes. In pilot studies a variety of wool and cotton dyes were applied to human tissues from
various alcohols (Younker et al. 1978). Staining patterns were a
function of the solvent and the dye configuration. For example,
solutions of various dyes in dissolved methanol stained elastic
membranes and fibers selectively (Fig. 3); when applied in ethanol, the same dyes left elastin unstained but reacted nicely with
Schwalbe's sheaths and/or certain connective tissue fibers (Fig.
4). With few exceptions, elastin did not bind dyes in ethanol or
higher alcohols. Effects of higher alcohols on dye uptake by
collagens varied from dye to dye. Comparative studies indicated
coloration of different collagen fibers when the same dye, e.g.,
Fast Wool Cyanone G, was applied from ethanol, propanol, buta-
nol, and benzyl alcohol. In experiments to date, staining properties of elastin apparently resembled those of polyamide fibers
which lack polar side-chains. Coloration of collagen by high
molecular milling dyes tended to increase rather than decrease
with increasing carbon chain length of the alcohol.

Under the conditions of solvent dyeing, dye configuration is a
critical factor. Even closely related dyes, e.g., Bordeaux Red

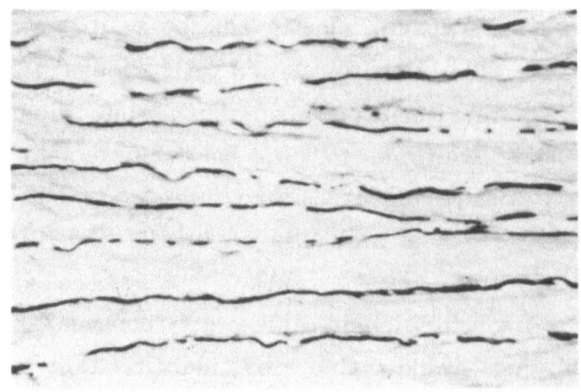

FIG. 3. Aorta, stained with Fast Wool Cyanone G in methanol. Elastin membranes are stained selectively. Some elastin membranes, e.g., above center, show fragmentation and loss of segments. Human autopsy material, methacarn fixation. X 400

and Ponceau 6R, which differ only in the position of one sulfonic acid group, produced different staining patterns when applied under identical conditions (Younker et al. 1978). The importance of nonpolar forces for dye binding has long been stressed by chemists (Derbyshire and Peters 1955; Zollinger 1965). These forces, rather than ionic bonds, determine dye uptake from the solvents tested. Sulfonated dyes with identical configuration showed a decrease in substantivity with increasing number of sulfonic acid groups (Younker et al. 1978). Such inverse relations between affinity and number of ionic groups are well known in textile and leather dyeing (Vickerstaff 1954; Otto 1962).

Premetallized 2:1 (Dye:Metal) Dyes Without Ionizing Groups. The reactivity of premetallized dyes of the Isolan series varied widely from dye to dye. Isolan Blue RLS proved valuable for demonstration of Schwalbe's sheaths and for combination stains (Waldrop et al. 1979). Isolan Black GL colored Schwalbe's sheaths intensely, but stained also numerous connective tissue fibers. When dissolved in ethanol or higher alcohols, neither dye reacted with elastin.

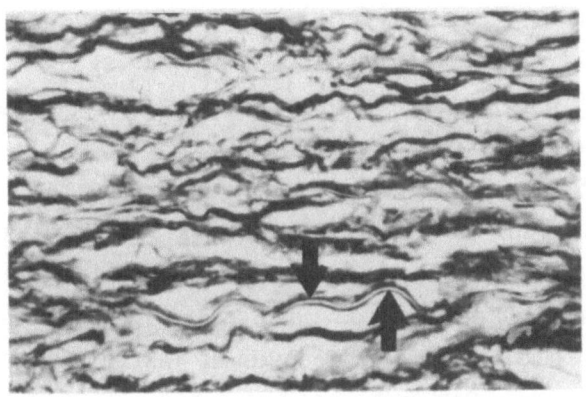

FIG. 4. Aorta, stained with Isolan Blue RLS in ethanol. Schwalbe's sheaths (arrows) and material between elastic membranes are colored. The elastin core framed by Schwalbe's sheath remains unstained. Human autopsy material, methacarn fixation. X 630

Since these dyes lack ionizing groups, they cannot form salt-type linkages; thus, dye binding must be due to other factors. Hydrogen bonds and nonpolar forces proved to be essential for binding of 2:1 metal complex dyes (McGregor 1961). Substantivity of such dyes is a function of their configuration. The role of van der Waals forces in textile dyeing is well established (Derbyshire and Peters 1955; Zollinger 1965). Marshall and Horobin (1973) demonstrated similar mechanisms in the binding of metal complex dyes by mammalian tissues. Further studies are required to clarify the interactions of various 2:1 metal complex dyes with elastin and other tissue structures under the conditions of solvent dyeing.

Combination Stains. To facilitate studies of elastin, Schwalbe's sheaths and associated structures in various lesions, it was desirable to visualize these tissue components in the same section. The selectivity of reactions for elastin was ascertained by fluorescence microscopy (Puchtler et al. 1973a); Schwalbe's sheaths were identified by morphologic criteria. Judicious matching of dye pairs which color elastin and Schwalbe's sheath, respectively, from the same solvent permitted simultaneous demonstration of these structures in contrasting colors. These one-step reactions do not require differentiation and are therefore histochemically significant. If desired, collagen can be pretreated with picro-Sirius Red F3BA (Sweat et al. 1964a) to show collagen, elastin, Schwalbe's sheaths, and associated structures side by side.

Parenthetically, many dyes used in this investigation are textile dyes. Comparative studies of some textile and biologic dyes carrying the same Colour Index designations showed considerable discrepancies. As demonstrated by Rosenthal et al. (1965), some batches of biologic dyes contain impurities not present in the corresponding textile brand. In this study, several biologic dyes with the Colour Index number of Fast Wool Cyanone G or Levanol Fast Cyanine 5RN contained compounds which stained structures other than elastin when the dyes were dissolved in methanol, i.e., dye brands from different suppliers are not readily interchangeable.

Applications of Solvent Dyeing

Skin. Elastin fibers occurred in the middle and deep layers of the dermis. These fibers consisted of an elastin core and a conspicuous Schwalbe's sheath. Elastin fibers were only rarely seen in the stratum papillare. There were far fewer elastin fibers than suggested by elastica stains (Waldrop et al. 1980). These observations confirm fluorescence microscopic findings (Puchtler et al. 1973a) and are in agreement with electron microscopic data (Gross and Schmitt 1948; Hannay 1951; Tunbridge et al. 1952). As already mentioned, elastogenesis in skin is completed soon after birth (Stadler and Orfanos 1978). Solvent dyeing technics confirmed earlier findings that the supposed increase of elastic tissue with age and in various lesions is an increase in collastin, i.e., altered collagen (Tunbridge 1956, 1957). The material studied to date did not show an increase in elastin.

Solvent dyeing technics indicated fibers with the characteristics of Schwalbe's sheaths, but without an elastin core. Since these fibers bind elastica stains, they are usually classified as elastic tissue. They differ from collastin in their low affinity for certain collagen stains.

Arteries. Elastin membranes framed by distinct Schwalbe's sheaths were found in the media of elastic arteries and in the elastica interna and externa of sizable arteries. In medium-sized arteries elastin was gradually replaced as described by Rodgers et al. (1967a). Besides collagen, material with the reactivity of Schwalbe's sheath appeared in the elastin core; this material probably corresponds to microfibrils within amorphous elastin described by electron microscopists. The elastica interna of small arteries was composed of Schwalbe's sheath and collagenous material; elastin could not be found.

There was no increase in elastin with age or in arteriosclerotic lesions. On the contrary, as shown in Fig. 3, elastin membranes became fragmented and segments disappeared. Defects were bridged by remnants of Schwalbe's sheath and/or collastin. Since these structures bind elastica stains, such lesions are usually interpreted as an increase, rather than a decrease, in elastin (Fig. 5). Loss of elastin from elastic membranes adjoining the aortic intima commenced during childhood, and the border between media and intima became blurred. Fragmentation of elastin membranes and lacunae filled with fibrous material, presumably collagen, have been observed also at the ultrastructural level (Karrer and Cox 1961). These morphologic observations are in agreement with chemical data which showed a decrease in elastin and an increase in collagen (Brown et al. 1974; Johnson et al. 1980).

No splitting, fraying, or duplication of elastin membranes could be found in sections treated with solvent dyeing technics. The fibers and lamellae formed along elastin membranes consisted of collastin and material with the reactivity of Schwalbe's sheath. However, the role of Schwalbe's sheath in these processes is not

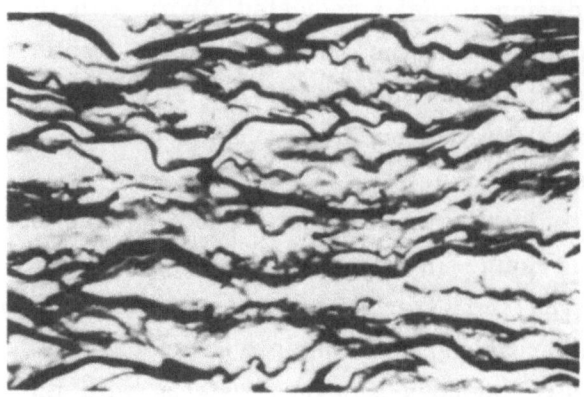

FIG. 5. Aorta, stained with resorcin-fuchsin. Elastin, Schwalbe's sheaths, and material between elastic membranes are equally intensely colored; elastin and collastin are indistinguishable. Human autopsy material, methacarn fixation. X 630

yet clear. As multiple layers were formed, the elastin core of the original elastic membrane disappeared, i.e., there was a decrease rather than an increase in elastin. Thus, solvent dyeing technics confirm that the supposed splitting or duplication of elastin membranes is a staining artefact, as demonstrated by Wolff (1928) and other authors during the past 50 years.

Lung. Concepts concerning the distribution and function of elastic tissue in lung are based largely on elastica stains. In electron microscopic studies, supposedly elastic tissue stained with Verhoeff's (1908) method and lead showed at least three different structural forms (Yu and Still 1977). Since Verhoeff's elastica stain is definitely not specific, it appears probable that at least part of the stainable material did not contain elastin. This assumption is supported by chemical studies which showed considerably less elastin than indicated by elastica stains (Farrar et al. 1965; McLaughlin 1966). Similar discrepancies were found in fluorescence microscopic studies (Puchtler et al. 1973a); many elastic fibers are apparently collastin (Puchtler et al. 1976).

To obtain further information concerning the nature of these fibers, various solvent dyeing technics were applied to sections

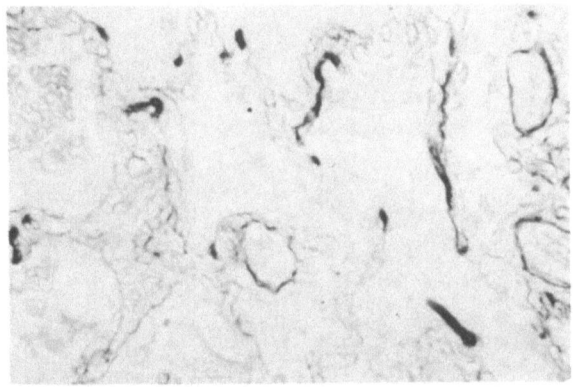

FIG. 6. Lung, stained with resorcin-fuchsin. Fibers in alveolar walls and around blood vessels and bronchi are strongly stained and are therefore regarded as elastic tissue. Human autopsy material, methacarn fixation. X 400

of human lungs (Younker et al. 1980). These reactions visualized elastin in elastic membranes of pulmonary arteries and elastic fibers in pleura. However, supposedly elastic fibers around bronchi (Karrer 1958) and in alveolar walls, which stained nicely with resorcin-fuchsin (Fig. 6) or other elastica stains, exhibited the reactions of collastin or of Schwalbe's sheaths. For example, Isolan Blue RLS in ethanol or amyl alcohol did not react with elastin, e.g., in elastic membranes of pulmonary arteries (Fig. 7), but fibers in alveolar walls (Fig. 8) and around bronchi were strongly colored. Similar patterns were obtained with a variety of chemically different dyes (Younker et al. 1980). Comparison of elastin membranes and elastic fibers in the same section ruled out differences in staining due to variation in processing. Thus, the observed differences in reactivity are histochemically significant. Apparently, lung contains much less elastin than suggested by elastica stains.

Other Connective Tissue Components. As discussed above, Schwalbe's sheath apparently corresponds to the layer of microfibrils around the elastin core. Filaments resembling those associated with elastin fibers were found also at various other sites,

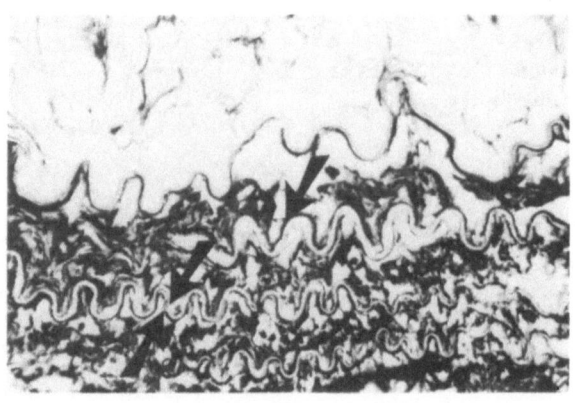

FIG. 7. Lung branch of pulmonary artery, stained with Isolan
Blue RLS in amyl alcohol. Numerous connective tissue fibers react readily with the dye, but elastin membranes remain unstained
(arrows). Human autopsy material, methacarn fixation.   X 400

e.g., in lung (Karrer 1962; Low 1962; Haust 1965). Correlation
of electron microscopic data with patterns of solvent dyeing
raised the question whether or not material with the reactivity of
Schwalbe's sheath, e.g., between collagen fibers and along and
between elastin membranes, may represent bundles of microfibrils. Since such fibers bind elastica stains, as does Schwalbe's
sheath, histologists have probably regarded these structures as
elastic fibers or as collastin.

Various types of collagen cannot yet be visualized selectively
by light microscopy, e.g., B chains in lung (Haralsen et al.
1980) and C and D chains of basement membranes (Kefalides
1980). Wolff et al. (1971) demonstrated in connective tissue a
group of acidic structural proteins which differ from collagen
and elastin. Histochemical studies seem to be lacking. Further
investigations are needed to determine whether or not such proteins may be visualized by certain solvent dyeing technics.

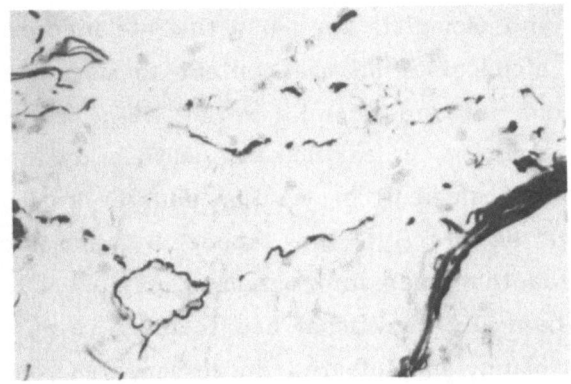

FIG. 8. Lung, same section as Fig. 7. In contrast to elastin membranes in the pulmonary artery (Fig. 7), supposedly elastic fibers in alveolar walls and around blood vessels and bronchi are distinctly colored. Human autopsy material, methacarn fixation. X 400

The Future of Dyes in Microscopy

During the last decades, application of the chemistry of dyeing to histochemistry has often been regarded as vastly inferior to electron microscopy and immunofluorescence. However, electron microscopists embraced Verhoeff's (1908) elastica stain and enlarged its nonspecific staining patterns. Yet, increasing the magnification from x 500 to x 50,000 cannot be expected to impart chemical significance to an unspecific stain. The use of Verhoeff's (1908) iron hematein in combination with immunofluorescence technics for various types of collagen also does not bestow any chemical specificity upon this procedure. The scientific value of such applications of dyes has been summarized by Baker (1960): "Dabbling with dyes by persons ignorant of the chemistry of what they are doing has no counterpart in the rest of science and indeed cannot be regarded as a scientific activity."

The great pioneers of histology and histochemistry during the second half of the nineteenth century were well versed in con-

temporary chemistry of dyes and dyeing. The ways of professional dyers and biologists parted in the late nineteenth century,
when many histologists became content to use available procedures they did not understand (Gierke 1884; Baker 1960). The
tremendous progress in textile and leather dyeing during the
past 50 years received little attention and the wealth of physico-
chemical data has rarely been tapped by microscopists. Our
studies proved that such information is invaluable for the development of chemically significant new technics, e.g., for amyloid,
collagens, myosins, and infrared fluorescence microscopy.

The potential usefulness of various new dye classes has not
yet been explored. Pilot studies indicated the value of premetallized dyes without ionizing groups and of reactive (covalent bond
forming) dyes for selective demonstration of certain tissue structures, e.g., myosins, glia fibers, and keratin formation. Light-
fast fluorescent brighteners are ideal for fluorescence microscopy,
e.g., of amyloid. Considering the relations between dye configuration and substantivity for certain tissue components, it seems
safe to assume that studies of additional milling and direct dyes
with different structures will result in new reactions for identification of various connective tissue components and their alterations in arterial and other lesions.

Acknowledgments

This investigation was supported in part by Biomedical Research Support Grant # 5 S07 RR05365-19. The material covered
in this review includes much work and new ideas contributed by
former coworkers. We thank Drs. Y. Akamatsu, R. H. Badarud-
din, R. Bates, J. H. Brown, M. G. Carter, A. D. Clark, J. T.
Harper, J. G. Jackson, D. W. Joiner, J. T. King, J. G. Kuhns,
L. D. Paschal, J. C. Rodgers, S. I. Rosenthal, J. J. Sesta,
H. G. Skelton, E. J. Smith, P. Woo, and T. D. Younker for
their collaboration and many interesting discussions and Mr. H.
M. Conner for his assistance in obtaining specimens. We also
wish to thank Dr. R. N. Rao, Director of Anatomical Pathology,

Medical College of Georgia, for free access to the extensive tissue collection of his division, and Dr. T. D. Younker for his translation of Schultze's (1849) Latin work.

We are deeply indebted to Dr. A. B. Chandler, Chairman, Department of Pathology, Medical College of Georgia, for ideal working conditions and for the academic freedom to investigate various problems and to publish freely even when experimental data do not support current dogmas. It is a rare and invaluable privilege to work under a chairman who provides a haven for the great traditions of medical science. We also wish to thank Dr. A. B. Chandler, the Dean's Research Committee, Medical College of Georgia, and the Medical Research Foundation of Georgia for their generous financial support.

The senior author wishes to express her gratitude to Dr. H. B. O'Rear, Vice Chancellor for Health Affairs, University System of Georgia, and formerly President, Medical College of Georgia, and Dr. L. D. Stoddard for accepting a deaf scientist in 1959, and to enable her to continue a career in research. Special thanks are due to Dr. W. H. Moretz, President, Dr. Lois T. Ellison, Provost, and Dr. F. Goodale, Dean, School of Medicine, Medical College of Georgia, for their support and for their stand on behalf of handicapped students. The Medical College of Georgia is unique in its willingness to provide opportunities for the handicapped. Many thanks are due to Dr. J. R. Teabeaut, II, for finding a niche for a deaf teacher in his educational program.

Last, but not least, we thank Dr. T. H. Schiebler, Managing Editor, and the Editorial Board of <u>Histochemistry</u> for their willingness to provide a forum for discussion of new or contradictory data. At a time when dogmas are protected by anonymous reviewers, the great traditions of free scientific debate maintained in <u>Histochemistry</u> are invaluable for progress in the fields discussed in this report.

REFERENCES

Abderhalden E, Schittenhelm A (1904) Die Abbauprodukte des Elastins. Hoppe Seylers Z Physiol Chem 41: 293-298

Altschul R (1950) Selected studies on arteriosclerosis. Thomas, Springfield

Argaud R (1908) Recherches sur l'histotopographie des éléments contractiles et conjonctifs des parois artérielles chez les mollusques et les vertébrés. J Anat Physiol 44: 328-414

Arshid FM, Desai JN, Duff DJ, Jain SK, Macneal IR (1954a) A study of certain natural dyes. I. J Soc Dyers Colour 70: 392-401

Arshid FM, Connelly RF, Desai JN, Fulton RG, Giles CH, Kefalas JC (1954b) A study of certain natural dyes. II. J Soc Dyers Colour 70: 402-412

Auerbach B (1877) Ueber die Obliteration der Arterien nach Ligatur. Inaug Diss, Bonn

Baker JR (1960) Principles of biological microtechnique. Methuen, London

Bangle R (1954) Gomori's paraldehyde-fuchsin stain. I. J Histochem Cytochem 2: 291-299

Becker CG, Nachman RL (1973) Contractile proteins in endothelial cells, platelets smooth muscle. Am J Pathol 71: 1-22

Benda C (1921) Die Gefässe. In: Aschoff L (ed) Pathologische Anatomie, 5th edn, Vol 2. Fischer, Jena

Benninghoff A (1930) Blutgefässe und Herz. In: von Möllendorff, W (ed) Handbuch der mikroskopischen Anatomie des Menschen, Vol 6, Part 1. Springer, Berlin, pp 1-232

Bindi F (1908) Sul compartemento del tessuto elastico nelle arterie in rapporto a varie età della vita. Morgagni (Milano) 1: 197-213

Blumenthal HT, Alex M (1967) Arteriosclerosis of the coronary circulation. In: Blumenthal HT (ed) Cowdry's arteriosclerosis: a survey of the problem. Thomas, Springfield

Böhm AA, von Davidoff M (1904) A textbook of histology including microscopic technic, 2nd edn. Saunders, Philadelphia

Bonnet (1896) Ueber den Bau der Arterienwand. Dtsch Med Wochenschr 22: 2-3

Borgers M, Schaper J, Schaper W (1972) Ultrastructural cytochemistry of coronary smooth muscle. In: Betz E (ed) Vascular smooth muscle. Springer, New York, pp 116-118

Borst, Enderlen (1909) Über Transplantation von Gefässen und ganzen Organen. Dtsch Z Chir 99: 54-163

Bregmann E (1890) Ein Beitrag zur Kenntnis der Angiosclerose. Inaug Diss, Dorpat

Brissie RM, Spicer SS, Hall BJ, Thompson NT (1974) Ultrastructural staining of thin sections with iron hematoxylin. J Histochem Cytochem 22: 895-907

Brissie RM, Spicer SS, Thompson NT (1975) The variable fine structure of elastin visualized with Verhoeff's iron hematoxylin. Anat Rec 181: 83-94

Brown RG, Walker RE, Aeschbacher HU, Boer AH, Smith MC (1974) Age related changes in the composition of the aorta of the groundhog, Marmota Monax. Growth 38: 295-300

Buehner TS, Nettleton GS, Longley JB (1979) Staining properties of aldehyde fuchsin analogs. J Histochem Cytochem 27: 782-787

Burton D, Hall DA, Keech MK, Reed R, Saxl H, Tunbridge RE, Wood MJ (1955) Apparent transformation of collagen fibrils into 'elastin'. Nature 176: 966-969

Caley ER (1927) The Stockholm Papyrus. J Chem Ed 4: 979-1002

Chung E, Miller EJ (1974) Collagen polymorphism: characterization of molecules with the chain composition $[\alpha 1(III)]_3$ in human tissue. Science 183: 1200-1201

Chung E, Keele EM, Miller EJ (1974) Isolation and characterization of the cyanogen bromide peptides from the $\alpha 1(III)$ chain of human collagen. Biochem 13: 3459-3464

Chung E, Rhodes K, Miller EJ (1976) Isolation of three collagenous components of probable basement membrane origin from several tissues. Biochem Biophys Res Commun 71: 1167-1174

Clark AD, Puchtler H, Waldrop FS (1973a) Intimal hyperplasia in the renal arterial system of children and adolescents. J SC Med Assoc 69: 24

Clark AD, Puchtler H, Waldrop FS (1973b) Investigation of "intimal cushions" in the renal arterial system of children and young adults. Bull Ga Acad Sci 31: 93

Cotta-Pereira G, Rodrigo FG, David-Ferreira JF (1977) The elastic system fibers. In: Sandberg LB, Gray WR, Franzblau C (eds) Elastin and elastic tissue. Plenum Press, New York - London, pp 19-30

Crawford T (1956) The healing of puncture wounds in arteries. J Pathol Bacteriol 72: 547-552

Crowley JD, Teague GS, Lowe JW (1966) A three-dimensional approach to solubility. J Paint Technol 38: 269-280

Derbyshire AN, Peters RH (1955) An explanation of dyeing mechanisms in terms of nonpolar bonding. J Soc Dyers Colour 71: 530-536

Dmitrijeff A (1897) Die Veranderung des elastischen Gewebes der Arterienwande bei Arteriosklerose. Beitr Pathol Anat Allg Pathol 22: 207-247

Dock W (1946) The predilection of atherosclerosis for the coronary arteries. J Am Med Assoc 131: 875-878

Ehrlich R, Krause R, Mosse M, Rosin H, Weigert K (eds) (1910) Enzyklopädie der mikroskopischen Technik. Urban & Schwarzenberg, Berlin

Engle RL, Dempsey EW (1954) The separation of orcein into four fractions by chromatography and the staining qualities of each fraction. J Histochem Cytochem 2: 9-20

Eulenberg A (1836) De Tela Elastica. Formis Neitackianis, Berolini

Farrar JF, Blomfield J, Reye RDK (1965) The structure and composition of the maturing pulmonary circulation. J Pathol Bacteriol 90: 83-96

Fawcett DW (1959) The fine structure of capillaries, arterioles and small arteries. In: Reynolds SRM, Zweifach BW (eds) The microcirculation. The University of Illinois Press, Urbana, pp 1-27

Foot NC (1927) On the endothelium of the venous sinuses of the human spleen. Anat Rec 36: 91-102

Friedberg SH, Goldstein DJ (1969) Thermodynamics of orcein staining of elastic fibers. Histochem J 1: 361-376

Friedenwald JS (1933) Retinal arteriosclerosis. In: Cowdry EV (ed) Arteriosclerosis. MacMillan, New York, pp 363-395

Friedländer C (1876) Ueber Arteriitis obliterans. Centralbl Med Wiss 1876: 65-70

Fuchs RF (1902) Zur Physiologie und Wachstumsmechanik des Blutgefäss-Systems. Fischer, Jena

Fullmer HM, Lillie RD (1957) The staining of collagen with elastic tissue stains. J Histochem Cytochem 5: 11-14

Gallop PM, Blumenfeld OO, Seifter S (1972) Structure and metabolism of connective tissue proteins. Ann Rev Biochem 41: 617-672

Gattermann L, Wichmann G (1889) Ueber Aldehydblau. Ber Dtsch Chem Ges 22: 227-236

Gay S, Fietzek PP, Remberger K, Eder M, Kühn K (1975a) Liver cirrhosis: immunofluorescence and biochemical studies demonstrate two types of collagen. Klin Wochenschr 53: 205-208

Gay S, Balleisen L, Remberger K, Fietzek PP, Adelmann BC, Kühn K (1975b) Immunohistochemical evidence for the presence of collagen type III in human arterial walls, arterial thrombi, and in leucocytes incubated with collagen in vitro. Klin Wochenschr 53: 899-902

Gay S, Walter P, Kühn K (1976) Characterization and distribution of collagen types in arterial heterografts originating from the calf carotis. Klin Wochenschr 54: 889-894

Gierke H (1884) Färberei zu mikroskopischen Zwecken. Z wiss Mikrosk 1: 497–557

Gilbert W (1903) Untersuchungen über den Bau der Intima der Aorta unter normalen und pathologischen Verhältnissen. Georgi, Bonn

Gillman T (1959) Reduplication, remodeling, regeneration, repair and degeneration of arterial elastic membranes. Arch Pathol 67: 624–642

Gillman T, Penn J, Bronks D, Roux M (1955) Abnormal elastic fibers. Arch Pathol 59: 733–749

Gillman T, Hathorn M, Penn J (1957) Micro-anatomy and reactions to injury of vascular elastic membranes and associated polysaccharides. In: Tunbridge RE, Keech M, Delafresnaye JF, Wood GC (eds) Connective tissue. Thomas, Springfield

Gomori G (1950) Aldehyde-fuchsin: a new stain for elastic tissue. Am J Clin Pathol 20: 665–666

Grant RA (1965) Preparation of elastin-like material from collagen by crosslinking followed by heat treatment. Biochem J 97: 5c–7c

Grassmann W (1960) Kollagen und Bindegewebe. Sven Kem Tidskr 72: 275–302

Greenlee TK, Ross R, Hartman JC (1966) The fine structure of elastic fibers. J Cell Biol 30: 59–71

Gross J, Schmitt FO (1948) The structure of human skin collagen as studied with the electron microscope. J Exp Med 88: 555–567

Grünstein N (1895) Histologische Untersuchungen über den Bau der menschlichen Aorta in verschiedenen Altersstufen. Bach, Bonn

Hall DA (1959) The fibrous components of connective tissue with special reference to the elastic fiber. Int Rev Cytol 8: 211–251

Hall DA (1961) The chemistry of connective tissue. Thomas, Springfield

Hallenberger O (1906) Über die Sklerose der Arteria radialis. Arch Klin Med 87: 62-86

Hama K (1960) The fine structure of some blood vessels of the earthworm Eisenia foetida. J Biophys Biochem Cytol 7: 717-724

Hance AJ, Crystal RG (1975) The connective tissue of lung. Am Rev Resp Dis 112: 657-711

Hannay FW (1951) Some clinical and histopathological notes on pseudoxanthoma elasticum. Br J Dermatol 63: 92-99

Haralson MA, Mitchell WM, Rhodes RK, Gay S, Kresina TF, Miller EJ (1980) Synthesis of B chain collagen by Chinese hamster lung cells. Fed Proc 39: 1789

Harper JT, Puchtler H, Meloan SN, Terry MS (1970) Histochemical study of basement membrane cristae in human kidneys. Lab Invest 22: 500

Harris FO, Guion TH (1972) New approach to solvent dyeing with nonionic dyes. Text Res J 42: 626-627

Haust MD (1965) Fine fibrils of extracellular space (microfibrils). Am J Pathol 47: 1113-1137

Haust MD, More RH, Movat HZ (1960) The role of smooth muscle cells in the fibrogenesis of arteriosclerosis. Am J Pathol 37: 377-389

Henle J (1843) Traité d'anatomie generale ou histoire des tissue et de la composition chimique du corps humain. Bailliere, Paris

Hibbs RG, Burch GE, Phillips JH (1958) The fine structure of the small blood vessels of normal human dermis and subcutis. Am Heart J 56: 662-670

Hogan MJ, Feeney L (1963) The ultrastructure of the retinal vessels. II. The small vessels. J Ultrastruct Res 9: 29-46

Hörmann H (1962) Zur Frage der Quervernetzung von Kollagen. Leder 13: 79-86

Hoyer H (1900) Zur Histologie der capillaren Venen in der Milz. Anat Anz 17: 490-497

Jackson JG, Puchtler H, Sweat F (1968) Investigation of staining, polarization and fluorescence microscopic properties of pseudo-elastic fibers in the renal arterial system. J R Microsc Soc 88: 473-485

Joiner DW, Puchtler H, Sweat F (1965) Investigation of the cross-linking of collagen in infants. Lab Invest 14: 577

Joiner DW, Puchtler H, Gropp S (1966) Investigation of a collagen-like fibrous layer between the internal elastic membrane and intima in arteries of infants and its possible relation to hyperplastic arteriosclerosis. Lab Invest 15: 1141

Joiner DW, Puchtler H, Gropp S (1967) Lesions resembling hyperplastic arteriosclerosis in infants: staining, polarization and fluorescence microscopic studies. Lab Invest 16: 651

Joiner DW, Puchtler H, Sweat F (1968) Staining of immature collagen by resorcin-fuchsin in infant kidneys. J R Microsc Soc 88: 461-471

Johnson WTM, Himelstein AL, Farmer DB, Horwitz O (1980) Chemical changes on aging in aortic and venus intima in relationship to atherosclerosis. Fed Proc 39: 428

Jores L (1898) Ueber die Neubildung elastischer Fasern in der Intima bei Endarteriitis. Beitr Path Anat Allg Pathol 24: 458-474

Jores L (1903) Wesen und Entwicklung der Arteriosklerose auf Grund anatomischer und experimenteller Untersuchungen. Bergmann, Wiesbaden

Jores L (1924) Arterien. In: Henke F, Lubarsch O (eds) Handbuch der speziellen pathologischen Anatomie und Histologie. Springer, Berlin, pp 608-786

Jorg F (1972) Vergleichende messtechnische und mikroskopische Studien uber das farberische Verhalten von Polyamid- und Polyester-Fasern aus organischen Losungsmitteln. Melliand Textilber 53: 1041-1048

Karrer HE (1958) The fine structure of connective tissue in the tunica propria of bronchioles. J Ultrastruct Res 2: 96-121

Karrer HE, Cox J (1961) An electron microscopic study of the aorta in young and in aging mice. J Ultrastruct Res 5: 1-27

Keech MK, Reed R, Wood MJ (1956) Further observations on the transformation of collagen fibrils into "elastin": an electron microscope study. J Pathol Bacteriol 71: 477-493

Kefalides F (1980) The "C" and "D" chains of basement membrane collagen arise from the same precursor type IV chain. Fed Proc 39: 1791

Kendrew JC (1954) Elastin. In: Neurath H, Bailey K (eds) The proteins, Vol II, Pt B. Academic Press, New York, pp 946-949

King JT, Puchtler H, Sweat F (1968) Investigation of ring fibers in human spleens. Arch Pathol 85: 237-245

Koelliker A (1854) Manual of human microscopical anatomy. Lippincott, Grambo & Co, Philadelphia

Kretschmann HJ (1963) Fluoreszenz-polarisationsmikroskopische Analyse der Ultrastruktur von Elastiklamellen und Elastikfasern. Z Zellforsch 60: 7-68

Krieg T, Muller PK (1977) The Marfan's syndrome. Exp Cell Biol 45: 207-221

Kühn K (1960) Über den Ursprung des Querstreifungsmusters bei Kollagen. Leder 11: 110-117

Kühn K, Grassmann W, Hofmann U (1958) Die elektronenmikroskopische "Anfärbung" des Kollagens und die Ausbildung einer hochunterteilten Querstreifung. Z Naturforsch 13b: 154-160

Kuhns JG, Puchtler H, Sweat F (1961) Conversion of collagen and reticulum fibers into "elastic fibers". J La State Med Soc 115: 443

Kultschitzky N (1895) Zur Frage über den Bau der Milz. Arch Mikrosk Anat Entwicklungsgesch 46: 673-695

Langeron M (1921) Précis de Microscopie, 3rd edn. Masson et Cie, Paris

Langhans T (1866) Beiträge zur normalen und pathologischen Anatomie der Arterien. Virchows Arch 36: 187-226

Lansing AG (1952) The role of elastic tissue in the formation of the arteriosclerotic lesion. Ann Intern Med 36: 39–49

Lansing AI, Rosenthal TB, Alex M, Dempsey EW (1952) The structure and chemical characterization of elastic fibers as revealed by elastase and by electron microscopy. Anat Rec 114: 555–575

Laszt L (1972) Regulation der Gefässmuskelkontraktion durch zwei in der Gefässwand vorkommende vasoaktive Stoffe. In: Betz E (ed) Vascular smooth muscle. Springer, Berlin, pp 47–48

Lehrell F (1903) Histochemische Untersuchungen uber das bindegewebige Gerüst der Milz der Wirbeltiere. Int Monatsschr Anat Physiol 20: 171–206

Levene CI (1956) The early lesions of atheroma in the coronary arteries. J Pathol Bacteriol 72: 79–82

Lillie RD (1951) The allochrome procedure. Am J Clin Pathol 21: 484–487

Love RB (1978) The use of nonaqueous solvents in dyeing. Pt 1. J Soc Dyers Colour 94: 440–447

Low FN (1962) Microfibrils: fine filamentous components of the tissue space. Anat Rec 142: 131–137

Magnus (1910) Aldehydgrün. In: Ehrlich R, Krause R, Mosse M, Rosin H, Weigert K (eds) Enzyklopädie der mikroskopischen Technik. Urban & Schwarzenberg, Berlin, p 14

Mall FP (1896) Reticulated tissue, and its relation to the connective tissue fibrils. Johns Hopkins Hospital Rep 1: 171–208

Maresch R (1905) Ueber Gitterfasern der Leber und die Verwendbarkeit der methode Bielschowskys zur Darstellung feinster Bindegewebsfibrillen. Centralbl Allg Pathol Anat 16: 641–649

Marshall PN, Horobin RW (1973) The mechanism of action of "mordant" dyes – a study using preformed metal complexes. Histochemie 35: 361–371

McCullagh KG, Ehrhart LA (1974) Increased arterial collagen synthesis in experimental canine atherosclerosis. Atherosclerosis 19: 13–28

McCullagh KG, Duance VC, Bishop KA (1980) The distribution of collagen I, III, and V AB in normal and atherosclerotic human aorta. J Pathol 130: 45-55

McGregor R (1961) Developments in dyeing theory. Rev Text Prog 13: 322-331

McLaughlin RT (1966) Collagen and elastin assay on various mammalian and human lungs. Am Rev Resp Dis 94: 632-634

Mehnert E (1888) Ueber die topographische Verbreitung der Angiosclerose nebst Beiträgen zur Kenntnis des normalen Baues der Aeste des Aortenbogens und einiger Venenstämme. Inaug Diss, Dorpat

Meloan SN, Puchtler H (1974) Observations on infrared fluorescence of stained sections. J SC Med Assoc 70: 81

Meloan SN, Puchtler H (1975) A methanol resorcin-fuchsin stain for elastic tissues and nuclei. Stain Technol 50: 367-370

Meloan SN, Puchtler H (1979) A re-investigation of early elastica stains. Anat Rec 193: 170-171

Merkel H (1903) Die Beteiligung der Gefässwand an der Organisation des Thrombus, mit bes. Berücksichtigung des Endothels. Junge, Erlangen

Milićević B (1970) Solvent dyeing: theory and practice. Text Chem Color 2: 87-98

Miller EJ, Matukas VJ (1974) Biosynthesis of collagen: the biochemists view. Fed Proc 33: 1197-1204

Miller EJ, Epstein EH, Piez KA (1971) Identification of three genetically distinct collagens by cyanogen bromide cleavage of insoluble human skin and cartilage collagen. Biochem Biophys Res Commun 42: 1024-1029

Monick JA (1968) Alcohols: the chemistry, properties and manufacture. Reinhold, New York

More RH, Balis J, Bencosme SA, Haust MD (1962) Electron microscope study of the elastic tissue in human aortas. Fed Proc 21: 121

Moret PR (1964) Modifications de l'élasticité artérielle avec l'âge. Cardiol Suppl 15: 40-75

Ophuls W (1933) The pathogenesis of arteriosclerosis. In: Cowdry EV (ed) Arteriosclerosis. MacMillan, New York, pp 249-270

Oppenheim F (1918) Uber den histologischen Bau der Arterien in der wachsenden und alternden Niere. Frankf Z Pathol 21: 57-84

Ortman R, Forbes WF, Balasubramanian A (1966) Concerning the staining properties of aldehyde basic fuchsin. J Histochem Cytochem 14: 104-111

Otto G (1962) Das Farben des Leders. Roether, Darmstadt

Painter RG, Sheetz M, Singer SJ (1975) Detection and ultrastructural localization of human smooth muscle myosin-like molecules in human nonmuscle cells by specific antibodies. Proc Natl Acad Sci USA 72: 1359-1363

Partridge SM (1958) Elastin-like structures from collagen. In: Stainsby C (ed) Recent advances in gelatin and glue research. Pergamon, New York, pp 255-256

Partridge SM (1962) Elastin. Adv Protein Chem 17: 227-302

Paschal LD, Puchtler H, Meloan SN (1978) Demonstration of lesions of striated muscle by infrared fluorescence microscopy. Lab Invest 38: 359

Pearse AGE (1968) Histochemistry, theoretical and applied, 3rd edn, Vol 1. Brown, Boston

Pfitzer R (1879) Ueber den Vernarbungsvorgang an durch Schnitt verletzten Blutgefassen. Virchows Arch 77: 397-420

Pollard TD, Weihing RR (1974) Actin and myosin and cell movement. CRC Crit Rev Biochem 2: 1-65

Prockop DJ, Kivirikko KI, Tuderman L, Guzman NA (1979) The biosynthesis of collagen and its disorders. N Engl J Med 301: 13-23, 77-85

Puchtler H, Isler H (1958) The effect of phosphomolybdic acid on the stainability of connective tissue by various dyes. J Histochem Cytochem 6: 265-270

Puchtler H, Meloan SN (1978) Demonstration of phosphates in calcium deposits. Histochemistry 56: 177-185

Puchtler H, Meloan SN (1979) Orcein, collastin and pseudo-elastica. Histochemistry 64: 119-130

Puchtler H, Sweat F (1963) Influence of various pretreatments on the staining properties of connective tissue fibers. Ann d'Histochim 8: suppl 189-198

Puchtler H, Sweat F (1964a) Histochemical specificity of staining methods for connective tissue fibers. Histochemie 4: 24-34

Puchtler H, Sweat F (1964b) A selective stain for renal basement membranes. Stain Technol 39: 163-166

Puchtler H, Waldrop FS (1978) Silver impregnation methods for reticulum fibers and reticulin. Histochemistry 57: 177-187

Puchtler H, Waldrop FS (1979) On the mechanism of Verhoeff's elastica stain. Histochemistry 62: 233-247

Puchtler H, Sweat F, Bates R, Brown JH (1961) On the mechanism of resorcin-fuchsin staining. J Histochem Cytochem 9: 553-559

Puchtler H, Sweat F, Jackson JG, Joiner DW (1966) Collagen-like staining, polarization and fluorescence microscopic properties of "elastic fibers" in hyperplastic arteriosclerosis. In: Comte P (ed) Biochemistry and physiology of connective tissue. Société Ormeco et l'Imprimerie du Sud-Est, Lyon, pp 691-700

Puchtler H, Sweat F, Terry MS, Conner HM (1969) Investigation of staining, polarization and fluorescence microscopic properties of myoendothelial cells. J Microsc 89: 95-104

Puchtler H, Waldrop FS, Valentine LS (1973a) Fluorescence microscopic distinction between elastin and collagen. Histochemie 35: 17-30

Puchtler H, Waldrop FS, Valentine LS (1973b) Polarization microscopic studies of connective tissue stained with picro-Sirius Red F3BA. Beitr Pathol 150: 174-187

Puchtler H, Waldrop FS, Carter MG, Valentine LS (1974) Investigation of staining, polarization and fluorescence microscopic properties of myoepithelial cells. Histochemistry 40: 281-289

Puchtler H, Meloan SN, Pollard GR (1976) Light microscopic distinction between elastin, pseudo-elastica (type III collagen?) and interstitial collagen. Histochemistry 49: 1–14

Puchtler H, Meloan SN, Waldrop FS (1979) Aldehyde-fuchsin: historical and chemical considerations. Histochemistry 60: 113–123

Reale E, Ruska H (1965) Die Feinstruktur der Gefässwände. Angiologia 2: 314–366

Remak R (1850) Histologische Bemerkungen über die Blutgefässwände. Müllers Arch Anat Physiol Wiss Med 1850: 79–101

Remberger K, Gay S, Fietzek PP (1975) Immunhistochemische Untersuchungen zur Kollagencharakterisierung in Lebercirrhosen. Virchows Arch 367: 231–240

Richter-Anschütz (1928) Chemie der Kohlenstoffverbindungen oder organische Chemie, 12th edn, Vol 1. Akademische Verlagsgesellschaft, Leipzig

Riedel B (1876) Die Entwicklung der Narbe im Blutgefässe nach der Unterbindung. Dtsch Z Chir 6: 462–473

Riedel G (1975) Loslichkeit von Farbstoffen in organischen Lösungsmitteln. Defazet Dtsch Farben Z 29: 435–436

Risse A (1853) Observationes quaedam de arteriarum statu normali atque pathologico. Dalkowski, Regiomonti

Robb-Smith AHT (1952) The nature of reticulin. In: Ragan C (ed) Connective tissues, transaction of the third conference. Macy, New York, pp 92–116

Rodgers JC, Puchtler H, Gropp S (1967a) Transition from elastin to collagen in internal elastic membranes. Arch Pathol 83: 557–566

Rodgers JC, Puchtler H, Gropp S (1967b) Staining, polarization and fluorescence microscopic studies of medial sclerosis in the renal arterial system. Lab Invest 16: 651

Rodgers JC, Puchtler H, Gropp S (1968) Histochemical, polarization and fluorescence microscopic studies of hyaline arteriolosclerosis in spleens. Lab Invest 18: 332–333

Romeis B (1948) Mikroskopische Technik, 15th edn. Leibniz, Munich

Rosenthal SI, Puchtler H, Sweat F (1965) Paper chromatography of dyes: method to investigate vagaries of staining. Arch Pathol 80: 190-196

Ross R, Bornstein P (1969) The elastic fiber. Part I. J Cell Biol 40: 366-381

Roulet F (1948) Methoden der pathologischen Histologie. Springer, Vienna

Sage EH, Gray WR (1977) Evolution of elastin structure. In: Sandberg LB, Gray WR, Franzblau C (eds) Elastin and elastic tissue. Plenum, New York, pp 291-309

Schiff H (1865) Note sur l'action des aldéhydes sur la rosaniline. Compt R Acad Sci 61: 45-75

Schiff H (1866) Eine neue Reihe organischer Diamine. Justus Liebigs Ann Chem 140: 92-137

Schmiedl H (1907) Die histologischen Veränderungen der Arteria mesenterica superior in den verschiedenen Lebensaltern. Z Heilk 28: 165-193

Schultze MJS (1849) De Arteriarum Notione, Structura, Constitutione Chemica et Vita. Kunike, Gryphiae

Schwalbe G (1876) Beiträge zur Kenntnis des elastischen Gewebes. Z Anat Entwicklungsgesch 2: 236-273

Sesta JJ, Puchtler H, Gropp S (1965) Comparison of the staining properties of collagen fibers in hepatic cirrhosis and young physiological collagen. Lab Invest 14: 577

Siegfried M (1892) Über die chemischen Eigenschaften des reticulierten Gewebes. Brockhaus, Leipzig

Sirsat SM, Khanolkar VR (1962) Structural alterations of collagen in diseased states. In: Ramanathan N (ed) Collagen. Interscience, New York, pp 327-349

Smith EJ, Puchtler H, Sweat F (1966) Investigation of the chemical mechanism of trichrome stains. Lab Invest 15: 1141-1142

Sokoloff N (1888) Über die venöse Hyperämie der Milz. Virchows Arch 112: 209-236

Spaet TH, Tiell ML, Cintron JR, Won J (1980) Can selective arterial medial injury produce intimal hyperplasia? Fed Proc 39: 1071

Stadler R, Orfanos CL (1978) Reifung und Alterung der elastischen Fasern. Arch Dermatol Res 262: 97-111

Sumner HH (1964) Dyeing theory. Rev Text Prog 16: 255-270

Sweat F, Puchtler H (1964) On a side effect of the acetic acid solvent in the phenylhydrazine procedure for the blocking of carbonyl groups. J Histochem Cytochem 12: 392

Sweat F, Puchtler H, Rosenthal SI (1964a) Sirius Red F3BA as a stain for connective tissue. Arch Pathol 78: 69-72

Sweat F, Puchtler H, Woo P (1964b) A light-fast modification of Lillie's allochrome stain. Arch Pathol 78: 73-75

Sweat F, Meloan SN, Puchtler H (1968) A modified one-step trichrome stain for demonstration of fine connective tissue fibers. Stain Technol 43: 227-231

Talma S (1879) Ueber Endarteriitis chronica. Virchows Arch 77: 242-268

Thoma R (1883) Ueber die Abhängigkeit der Bindegewebsneubildung in der Arterienintima von den mechanischen Bedingungen des Blutumlaufs. Virchows Arch 93: 443-505

Thoma R (1891) Ueber Gefäss- und Bindegewebsneubildung in der Arterienwand. Beitr pathol Anat Allg Pathol 10: 433-448

Thomé R (1901) Die Kreisfasern der capillaren Venen in der Milz. Anat Anz 19: 271-280

Toldt C (1884) Lehrbuch der Gewebelehre, 2nd edn. Enke, Stuttgart

Trompetter J (1876) Ueber Endarteriitis. Georgi, Bonn

Tunbridge RE (1956) The relationship of elastin and collagen (morphological studies). Experientia Suppl 4: 15-18

Tunbridge RE (1957) The Heberden oration. Lancet 272: 29

Tunbridge RE, Tattersall RN, Hall DA, Astbury WT, Reed R (1952) The fibrous structure of normal and abnormal human skin. Clin Sci 11: 315-323

Unna PG (1890) Uber die Taenzersche Orceinfarbung des elastischen Gewebes. Monatsh Prakt Dermat 12: 366-367

Unna PG (1891) Notiz betreffend die Tanzersche Orceinfarbung des elastischen Gewebes. Monatsh Prakt Dermat 12: 394-396

Unna PG (1894a) Basophiles Kollagen, Kollastin und Kollacin. Monatsh Prakt Dermat 19: 465-475

Unna PG (1894b) Die spezifische Farbung des Kollagens. Monatsh Prakt Dermat 18: 509-520

Velican C (1962) Biology of the sclerotic process. Part VIII. Morfol Norm Patol (Bucharest) 7: 373-378

Verhoeff FH (1908) Some new staining methods of wide applicability; including a rapid differential stain for elastic tissue. J Am Med Assoc 50: 876-877

Vickerstaff T (1954) Dye structure and affinity. In: The physical chemistry of dyeing. Oliver and Boyd, London, pp 412-415

Virchow R (1856) Gesammelte Abhandlungen zur wissenschaftlichen Medizin. Meidinger, Frankfurt, pp 492-507

von Czyhlarz ER (1897) Ueber ein Pulsionsdivertikel der Trachea. Centralbl Allg Pathol Anat 8: 721-728

von Denffer H, Heidbrink V (1974) Dunnschichtchromatographische Untersuchungen verschiedener Aldehydefuchsine. Acta Histochem (Jena) 48: 62-68

von Ebner V (1902) A. Koelliker's Handbuch der Gewebelehre, Vol 3, 6th edn. Engelmann, Leipzig

von Recklinghausen F (1862) Die Lymphgefasse und ihre Beziehungen zum Bindegewebe. Hirschwald, Berlin

von Richter V (1899) Organic chemistry, 3rd American from 8th German edn. Blakiston, Philadelphia

von Winiwarter F (1879) Ueber eine eigentumliche Form von Endarteriitis und Endophlebitis mit Gangran des Fusses. Langenbecks Arch Chir 23: 202-226

von Zwingmann A (1891) Das elastische Gewebe der Aortenwand und seine Veranderungen bei Sklerose und Aneurysma. Schnakenburg, Dorpat

Waldrop FS, Puchtler H, Valentine LS (1971) Histochemical studies of myoendothelial cells and their role in collagen formation in early arteriosclerosis. J Reticuloendothel Soc 9: 632-633

Waldrop FS, Meloan SN, Puchtler H, Pollard GR (1977) Histochemical demonstration of different collagens in arteriosclerosis and other sites of collagen formation. Lab Invest 36: 351-352

Waldrop FS, Younker TD, Puchtler H (1979) Effects of dye structure and solvents on the binding of premetallized dyes. Ga J Sci 37: 107

Waldrop FS, Younker TD, Puchtler H (1980) New methods for distinction between elastin and collastin. Anat Rec 196: 251

Waller J, Lewis GW (1957) Dyeing. Rev Text Prog 9: 328-357

Waterman N (1908) Einige Bermerkungen zur Frage: Arteriosklerose nach Adrenalin-Injektion. Virchows Arch 191: 202-208

Weigert C (1898) Ueber eine Methode zur Färbung elastischer Fasern. Centralbl Allg Pathol Pathol Anat 9: 289-292

Wells HG (1933) The chemistry of arteriosclerosis. In: Cowdry EV (ed) Arteriosclerosis. MacMillan, New York, pp 323-353

Westphalen H (1886) Histologische Untersuchungen über den Bau einiger Arterien. Mattiesen, Dorpat

Windrum GM, Kent PW, Eastoe JE (1955) The constitution of human renal reticulin. Br J Exp Pathol 36: 49-59

Wissler RW (1968) The arterial medial cell, smooth muscle or multifunctional mesenchyme. J Atheroscler Res 8: 201-213

Witthaus RA (1887) The medical student's manual of chemistry, 2nd edn. Wood, New York

Wolff CK (1928) Elastica und Pseudoelastica der grossen Arterien. Virchows Arch 270: 37-50

Wolff I, Fuchswans W, Weiser M, Furthmayr H, Timpl R (1971) Acidic structural proteins of connective tissue: characterization of their heterogeneous nature. Eur J Biochem 20: 426-431

Young LA (1892) The fibres of retiform tissue. J Physiol 13: 332-334

Younker TD, Waldrop FS, Puchtler H (1978) Dye binding by collagens and elastin: effects of dye configurations and solvents. J SC Med Assoc 74: 59

Younker TD, Waldrop FS, Puchtler H (1980) Investigation of elastin and collastin in human lungs. Anat Rec 196: 253

Yu SY, Still MF (1977) Ultrastructural changes of elastic tissue in hamster lung during elastase-emphysema. In: Sandberg LB, Gray WR, Franzblau C (eds) Elastin and elastic tissue. Plenum, New York-London, pp 39-56

Zacharjewskaja MA (1930) Klinische und histologische Untersuchungen über die Arteriosklerose der Nieren. Virchows Arch 276: 380-446

Zahn FW (1884) Untersuchung über die Vernarbung von Querrissen der Arterienintima und Media nach vorheriger Umschnürung. Virchows Arch 96: 1-15

Zimmermann KW (1898) Beiträge zur Kenntnis einiger Drüsen und Epithelien. Arch Mikrosk Anat Entwicklungsgesch 52: 552-706

Zollinger H (1965) The dye and the substrate: the role of hydrophobic bonding in dyeing processes. J Soc Dyers Colour 81: 345-350

Zollikofer H (1852) Beiträge zur Kenntnis des elastischen Gewebes. Justus Liebigs Ann Chem 82: 162-180

Discussion

Oegema. Would you tell us what your favorite stain is now for elastin?

Puchtler. Well, we don't really have a favorite stain; we have only been working on solvent dyes for a few years. As I have shown, Unna (Unna PG [1891] Notiz betreffend die Tänzersche Orceinfärbung des elastischen Gewebes. Monatsh Prakt Dermat 12: 394-396) recommended orcein and retracted it three years later (Unna PG [1894a] Basophiles Kollagen, Kollastin und Kollacin. Monatsh Prakt Dermat 19: 465-475), but everybody ignored his retraction, and it is still listed as an elastin stain.

Banga (Banga I [1953] Thermal contraction of collagen and its
dissolution with elastase.   Nature 172: 1099) retracted earlier
claims for the specificity of elastase because it digests denatured
collagen 10 times faster than elastin.   This retraction also has
been widely ignored. We don't want to add to this list and,
therefore, we are very careful about publishing. Usually, Mrs.
Waldrop, Mrs. Meloan and I repeat staining methods again and
again, making new solutions, using different tissues. We let it
sit for a few months, and then repeat it until we are sure that
it will work in the hands of other people.

We are still working on solvent dyeing. For example, Niagara
Blue – Fast Wool Red gives a very deep red elastin. It tends to
stain nuclei sometimes, depending on the dye batch. The blue
dye is not selective for Schwalbe's sheath, but will stain a lot of
collagen.   Isolan Blue RLS, which cannot form ionic bonds, is a
2:1 metal complex dye, that is, two dye molecules form a chelate
with ionic groups in tissues, only binding via van der Waals and
London dispersion forces.   It is very selective for Schwalbe's
sheath, that is the microfibrillar layer. We get similar staining
in some other areas and are currently trying to figure out what
is the microfibrillar material that electron microscopists have seen
in various organs, but which so far has been ignored or could
not be shown by light microscopists.

Cowden.   Do you have any particular recommendations for
fluorescent stains for elastin or collagen that are selective for
either class?

Puchtler.   We cannot yet recommend a fluorescent dye for
collagen.   For elastin, the phosphomolybdic acid method seems to
be the most reliable. We reported the method to the International Congress of Leather Chemists Societies in Lyon in 1965 to
get their critical comments, and it was well received; everybody
was really delighted how simple it was. We published the method
in 1973 in Histochemie, now Histochemistry (Puchtler H, Waldrop
FS, Valentine LS [1973] Fluorescence microscopic distinction between elastin and collagen.   Histochemie 35: 17-30).   One only

needs to treat the section with phosphomolybdic acid, then dehydrate, mount in a nonfluorescent mountant and put under ultraviolet-blue light. Ultraviolet-blue is usually preferable to ultraviolet alone, because blue light near 400 nanometers is also absorbed and adds to the intensity of fluorescence. We have been trying to get something similar for collagen, but haven't found anything yet; the problem is fading of fluorescence. The elastin also shows some fading when it is exposed too long to ultraviolet-blue light.

Part III
Holde Puchtler: An Appreciation

The Symposium on Connective Tissues honoring Dr. Puchtler was concluded with a banquet attended by her pupils, friends, and colleagues. During this occasion, her contributions to medical science and to the Department of Pathology and to the Medical College of Georgia were recognized.

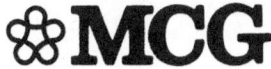 **MCG**

PROCLAMATION

Whereas HOLDE PUTCHLER, M.D., HAS GIVEN 21 years of dedicated and faithful service to the Medical College of Georgia; and

Whereas Dr. Putchler has during those years made significant professional contributions to the world's knowledge of histochemistry; and

Whereas Dr. Putchler has been a most excellent teacher to future generations of physicians and researchers and;

Whereas Dr. Putchler has been an inspiration to all of us through her ability and courage.

Now therefore be it resolved that the Medical College of Georgia go on record as expressing its sincere appreciation to Dr. Putchler for all of her capable, conscientious service and dedication to health care. We look forward to many more years of contributions from this outstanding scientist and teacher.

SIGNED THIS DAY *Sept. 30, 1980*

BY _____
PRESIDENT WILLIAM H. MORETZ, M.D.

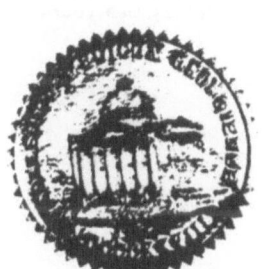

GREETINGS:

DR. HOLDE PUCHTLER

Historians look at past events and the great men and women of the era.
They try to decide - did the times make the person, or did the person
make the times?

It is an interesting debate. However, it is my belief that there is something special within certain people which will cause them to succeed in
whatever venture they choose. Further, this kind of person, more often
than not, will have positive effects on mankind.

Such a person is Dr. Holde Puchtler. Her keen mind, her knowledge
and insight, and her dedication and contributions to research and edu-
cation have brought her to a point in her career that her peers wish to
recognize her work.

Few things are so moving and personally satisfying than to be recognized
by our peers. It is the quintessence of success, for our peers are those
we most often admire and they are the ones who challenge us in our work.
It is fitting that Dr. Puchtler be so recognized. Her work in histochemistry, while unknown to most persons out of the field of medicine, ranks
high among her colleagues, worldwide. Her research has advanced,
significantly, the field of knowledge in this area. We, of the University
System of Georgia are proud of her accomplishments.

Dr. Puchtler, it must be satisfying to have contributed so much to the
field of knowledge in histological staining, but I must say that you have
contributed far more than knowledge. You have given us an example of
courage, scientific excellence, outstanding teaching, and of greatness
which "made the times." I know most surely that you would have made
your own times in the 21st or the 19th or whatever century was yours
in which to work.

Harry B. O'Rear, M.D.
Vice Chancellor for Health Affairs
University System of Georgia

Essentials of Histological Staining:
Dr. Holde Puchtler's Contribution

THEODORE H. SCHIEBLER

Dr. Puchtler, Dr. McDonald, Dr. Chandler, distinguished colleagues, ladies and gentlemen:

A wonderful day is drawing to a close -- wonderful because it has enabled us to speak about that which interests us and unites us: a day that the Medical College of Georgia has dedicated in tribute to Dr. Puchtler. It is in the spirit of this tribute that I speak to you this evening. But first please allow me, Dr. Puchtler, to extend a greeting from the Old World. Both the Histochemische Gesellschaft and the Anatomische Gesellschaft have asked me to convey their sincere affection as well as their best wishes for your personal welfare and for the continuance of your valuable scientific work. We wish you the best that people and scientists can wish one another.

When I think back upon the conversations and letters that went into the preparation for this occasion, and upon today's symposium itself, I am struck by the high esteem and respect which we feel for you, Dr. Puchtler. But more than this, we are grateful for the scientific as well as the human gifts which you have given us and continue to give. Surely there are few people who bear their own physical iniquities with such courage and optimism. I do not know which is higher -- the strength of the intellect or the strength of the soul. Certainly, both are a part of your nature and, as such, are inseparable.

Like all of us, the course of your life, both personal and professional has been shaped by your roots and by past events. If the focus of your work has been in the area of histological staining, this really is possible only because you know what the research of the past has yielded. But combined with this sense of scientific tradition is a broad understanding and appreciation of the cultural basis upon which our civilization rests, even in these unsettled times.

Both aspects of your character, the scientific as well as the cultural, were instilled and fostered by your early home life. Your father in particular, who was a great fan of Wagner's music, had a profound influence upon you. I might mention that even your first name, Holde, and that of your sister, Freia, attest to this fondness for Wagnerian opera. Of yourself you write: "My interest in history goes back to my early childhood, when I first heard my parents and their friends excitedly discussing the discovery of Tutankhamun's tomb. As soon as I was able to read, I devoured books on archeology. My interest in the history of medicine was stimulated by the lectures of Professor Elze in Wurzburg. Professor Leupold, my boss in Cologne, was interested in the history of pathology." But just as important, you were capable even as a child of listening, absorbing, and perceiving relationships.

As is so often the case, respect for the achievements of the past is combined with personal modesty. Recently you wrote me that your work is merely a continuation of the work of earlier histologists, which was interrupted by two world wars, and the events between them. You further wrote that you most admire the histologists and histochemists of the nineteenth century, who often were far ahead of the chemistry of their time. To quote you: "Much of that discovered from 1850 to 1910, from Koelliker to Heidenhain, is again becoming timely in modern cell biology, from the microfilaments of elastic membranes to the contractile structures in the protoplasm of cells." With these words you touch upon an indispensible aspect of science: an awareness of the accomplishments of the past, combined with a personal richness of ideas. But as your work so clearly demonstrates, scientific discovery is ultimately the product of individual endeavor. Studying the work of past or contemporary researchers does not

bring progress. This is achieved only by an interplay involving
one's own creativity, that of the scientific community, and the
accomplishments of our predecessors.

You first encountered histological stains during your high-
school years. Again, to quote: "I once accompanied a classmate
to the Municipal Hospital of Nuremberg, where her father was
chief of pathlolgy. We were allowed to look through a microscope, and I can still vividly recall the section that I saw -- it
was a trichrome and resorcin fuchsin-van Gieson stain of lobar
pneumonia tissue. I was fascinated and wanted to know how the
dyes reacted with the different structures. I was surprised to
learn that no one knew the chemical reactions involved, and thus
that the diagnosis of the pathologists was based not on hard
science, but on vague tradition." I personally recall the state-
ments of our anatomy instructor in Wurzburg, Professor Elze,
who said in 1942 that the anatomists of his time were only the
followers of outstanding predecessors, but that by combining
morphology with chemistry, true progress could be made. These
were certainly prophetic words. Elze did not know that the
future had already begun, for he was unaware of the published
works of Gomori and Takamatsu, who had reported independently
in 1939 on the histochemical demonstration of alkaline phospha-
tase. But Elze had a keen intellect and sensed developments
even if he did not know the details.

Your interest in histological stains blossomed during your
course in histology at the Institute of Anatomy in Wurzburg. At
that time we students were permitted to borrow histological specimens and microscopes to prepare for our exams. It was during
this time, incidentally, that you developed an aversion to hema-
lum-eosin, because it stained all structures your least favorite
color -- pink.

And then came your meeting with Emil Abderhalden, one of
the leading physiological chemists of his day. This teacher must
have been of great importance to you, for your wrote: "He
made every effort to teach us that textbooks are not repositories

of absolute truth, but only of current dogma. He analyzed laws
of physiology with obvious delight in order to show that they
were either unproved or untenable." We can probably credit
Emil Abderhalden with awakening your critical attitude as a
scientist. If I understand you correctly, he still often stands
behind you and warns you against accepting something merely
because it is printed or fashionable. Your inner independence
also makes you wary of self-proclaimed "experts." Everyone who
knows you knows that this is not arrogance, but a sign of moral
strength and thorough schooling.

Also important was your meeting with Gomori, toward whom
you felt a kinship in many regards. You wrote: "Dr. Gomori
apparently lacked all faith in authority, and we agreed in our
criticisms of various methods. On one occasion he took me to a
meeting of the Hisotchemical Society in Chicago. Most of the
lectures were new territory for me, and I was very much im-
pressed until Dr. Gomori said to me: 'It would take me ten
years to refute all the nonsense presented today.' "

Twenty-one years ago in Augusta you embarked upon your
scientific career. It is closely tied to this medical school and to
the very successful teamwork with your loyal associates Mrs.
Waldrop and Mrs. Meloan. Your idea is to establish connections
between the configuration of a dye, the nature of the solvent,
and the affinity of the dye for specific tissue structures.

A dye is a very complex substance. Knowing the chemical
formula of a dye and its charge is not sufficient to explain its
staining properties, as you have stressed time and again. A
crucial factor is the spatial constitution of the dye and the location of the charges within its structure. The problem, however,
is that commercial dyes are practically never available in pure
form, only in mixtures. As a result, the very nature of the dye
makes it difficult to find explanations for staining effects.

The other side of the problem is the tissue itself. Chemically,
it is usually even more complex than the stain. What is more,
preliminary treatment of the tissue can alter it in unpredictable

ways. Thus, the analyst of histological stains must work with
two unknowns: the dye and the tissue. Despite these difficulties, you have succeeded in elucidating the chemistry of the
binding process for a number of dyes. In so doing, you have
developed a variety of new staining methods which are summarized in the manual handed out earlier today. With your research, you are helping histologic technique to progress away
from the cookbook era toward the era of the controlled reaction,
and thus from empiricism to science.

A survey of your works reveals two main areas of interest.
The first concerns methodology, with particular emphasis upon
basic research in such areas as tissue pretreatment, dyes and
staining mechanisms. The second deals with more applied studies, particularly of intercellular substances. This afternoon you
personally reported on the histochemistry of elastin, collastin,
and other collagens. In other works you deal with amyloid.
You have done extensive studies on myoid fibrils in various cells
and tissues. And so on. But it is important to realize that
these two aspects of your work are not isolated endeavors, but
rather that they complement and enhance each other. For example, the study of staining mechanisms is essential for a critical
assessment of methods for visualizing elastic fibers. Conversely,
the traditional methods of staining elastic fibers have challenged
you to seek the underlying mechanisms.

In your critical study of stain affinities in tissues, you have
come across many absurdities in the literature. A good example
of this is the periodic acid-Schiff reaction. You simply could
not accept certain assumptions in the literature. Thus, you
showed that fuchsin can never react with two aldehyde groups in
the same chain. This means that practically none of the published structural formulas for the PAS reaction is compatible
with modern chemistry. If the accepted formulas were true, a
green reaction product should result; yet as everyone knows,
the PAS reaction actually yields a bluish-red product. You
thereupon developed your own concept, which was consistent

with theoretical constraints. In these studies you also delved
into the history of basic fuchsin and the aldehyde-Schiff reaction. If one reads these works carefully, however, one finds
not only a historical report but also an objective, well-reasoned
critique of published nonsense.

Equally absorbing are your works on the visualization of myosin with stains. These studies stem from your very early investigations, done at a time when electron microscopists could not
yet resolve any structures in the cell regions of interest. As a
result, your first reports on the light microscopic demonstration
of myoid cytoplasmic fibrils at the national meetings in 1956 and
1957 were received with skepticism. But cytoplasmic fibrils were
already well known by the second half of the nineteenth century.
The key point was that you knew that these myoid cytoplasmic
fibrils contained alpha-helix proteins, which you were able to
preserve by your fixation method. Since you also knew something about dyes and dye affinities, you were able to visualize
these structures with Levanol fast cyanin 5 RN. Today, with
improved techniques in electron microscopy, microfilaments have
been found in the nucleus and cytoplasm of many cells. Immuno-
histochemistry has also confirmed the occurrence of myosin in a
number of cells. But if we compare the labor involved in the
various methods, we find that your technique is still superior,
particularly for practical purposes. For when it is necessary to
detect the early stages of myocardial infarction, for example,
your method will surely be preferred over the more time-consum-
ing immunohistochemical and electron microscopic techniques.

This brings me, finally, to a group of your works which
have direct bearing on practical medicine, and which, if I am
correctly informed, are presently at the focus of your research.
I refer to the detection of the early stages of muscular diseases
with the aid of infrared fluorescence. You began this work
about three years ago and have succeeded in showing that muscle biopsy sections that appear practically normal under the light
microscope and display only slight changes in polarized light

show very clear and conspicuous early changes by infrared fluorescent microscopy when stained with the "correct" dye. With this technique you are opening up an entirely new field of research, for nowhere in the world literature has anyone yet explored the infrared fluorescence of stained sections. Interestingly, you were prompted in this research by your study of publications in textile chemistry, in which it was shown that the same dye shows marked differences in infrared fluorescence when applied to different fibers. Little wonder that your student-colleague, Dr. Paschal, who worked on this subject under your direction, received the national award from the American Society of Clinical Pathologists and the Bausch and Lomb medal for this research.

In conclusion, it must be said that if Dr. Puchtler's works -- of which we can only give a partial account this evening -- are viewed against the spectrum of present-day research, one finds that her field of study is being pursued in only a few quarters. This is surprising when one considers that the staining and diagnosis of histological sections is practiced world wide. But it is also true that this field of research was of widespread interest in the late nineteenth and early twentieth centuries, when dye chemistry was invented and the histologic technique was born. Once the histologists had a variety of empirically tested methods at their disposal, however, they were content to employ these methods without truly understanding them. Only a few of them appreciated the great importance of the field of research that you now pursue. Among these few was Dr. Lillie, whose memory is universally held in the highest esteem.

Today, however, I am convinced that we are close to a renaissance in your field of research. It comes from an entirely different direction -- that of computer-assisted image analysis, which is becoming an increasingly important tool in medical diagnosis. With this technique, it is possible to analyze minute color differences which the eye cannot perceive. I believe that techniques of modern image analysis, by broadening and deepening

our knowledge of the staining properites of cell and tissue structures, will one day make it possible to detect serious cell-linked
diseases early enough that help can be rendered.   Thus, it
appears to me that your field of research which may first seem
so abstract and theoretical, in fact merges with the great medical
task of bringing help to persons threatened by disease.   And
this, Dr. Puchtler, brings you back to the noble task which you
undertook when your first elected to study medicine.

Ladies and Gentlemen, I have reached the end of my remarks.
I would like to have said much more, because my heart is full,
but it is impossible to summarize a life's work in so short a time.
I have said nothing of the brilliant memory that distinguishes
Dr. Puchtler, her quickness of mind, her keen sense of humor,
her travels, her knowledge of soccer, and above all, her great
goodwill toward others.   The high admiration which you enjoy,
Dr. Puchtler, is perhaps best expressed in the words recently
written to me by Mrs. Waldrop, and which doubtlessly reflect the
opinion of many: "There are very few subjects in which she is
not well versed."

Dear Dr. Puchtler, we all wish you much continued success in
your personal and scientific life and that it may continue to
bring you much joy and satisfaction.

Index